Emergency Medicine
Examination & Board Review

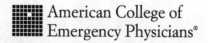
American College of
Emergency Physicians®

Accreditation Statement and Faculty Disclosure Statement

CONTINUING MEDICAL EDUCATION CREDIT

Emergency Medicine Examination and Board Review has been planned and implemented in accordance with the Essential Areas and policies of the Accreditation Council for Continuing Medical Education (ACCME).

The American College of Emergency Physicians is accredited by the Accreditation Council for Continuing Medical Education to provide continuing medical education for physicians.

The American College of Emergency Physicians designates this educational activity for a maximum of 20 Category 1 credits toward the AMA Physician's Recognition Award. Each physician should claim only those credits that he/she actually spent in the educational activity.

Emergency Medicine Examination and Board Review is approved by the American College of Emergency Physicians for 20 ACEP Category 1 credits.

CONTRIBUTOR DISCLOSURES

In accordance with the Accreditation Council for Continuing Medical Education Standards and the policy of the American College of Emergency Physicians, contributors must disclose the existence of significant financial interests in or relationships with manufacturers of commercial products that may have a direct interest in the subject matter of this publication. Contributors to this publication have characterized their relationships as follows:

The following contributors have indicated that they have no significant financial interests or relationships to disclose:

W. Clayton Bordley, MD
Kathleen J. Clem, MD
Elizabeth Magassy Dorn, MD
Worth W. Everett, MD
Karen S. Frush, MD
Ted Glynn, MD
Cherie A. Hargis, MD
H. Gene Hern, Jr., MD, MS
Loretta Jackson-Williams, MD, PhD, FACEP

Linda E. Keyes, MD, FACEP
Joel Kravitz, MD
Kenneth T. Kwon, MD, FACEP, FAAP
Luis M. Lovato, MD
Daniel C. McGillicuddy, MD
Christopher L. Moore, MD
Ronny M. Otero, MD
Robert Park, MD
Susan B. Promes, MD

Carlo L. Rosen, MD
John C. Stein, MD
Susan Stroud, MD
Suzanne H. Summer, MD, FACEP
Gary W. Tamkin, MD, FACEP
Carrie Tibbles, MD
Jason A. Tracy, MD
Corinne R. Widico, MD

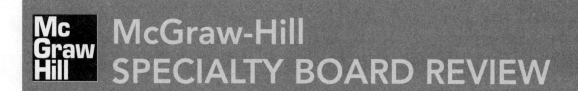

McGraw-Hill
SPECIALTY BOARD REVIEW

Emergency Medicine
Examination & Board Review

Susan B. Promes, MD, FACEP
Residency Program Director
Division of Emergency Medicine
Associate Clinical Professor of Surgery
Duke University Medical Center
Durham, North Carolina

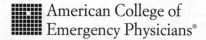
American College of
Emergency Physicians®

McGraw-Hill
Medical Publishing Division

New York   Chicago   San Francisco   Lisbon   London   Madrid   Mexico City   Milan
New Delhi   San Juan   Seoul   Singapore   Sydney   Toronto

Emergency Medicine Examination & Board Review

2 3 4 5 6 7 8 9 0   QPD/QPD   0 9 8 7 6 5

ISBN 0-07-144051-8

Notice

Medicine is an ever-changing science. As new research and clinical experience broaden our knowledge, changes in treatment and drug therapy are required. The authors and the publisher of this work have checked with sources believed to be reliable in their efforts to provide information that is complete and generally in accord with the standards accepted at the time of publication. However, in view of the possibility of human error or changes in medical sciences, neither the authors nor the publisher nor any other party who has been involved in the preparation or publication of this work warrants that the information contained herein is in every respect accurate or complete, and they disclaim all responsibility for any errors or omissions or for the results obtained from use of the information contained in this work. Readers are encouraged to confirm the information contained herein with other sources. For example and in particular, readers are advised to check the product information sheet included in the package of each drug they plan to administer to be certain that the information contained in this work is accurate and that changes have not been made in the recommended dose or in the contraindications for administration. This recommendation is of particular importance in connection with new or infrequently used drugs.

This book was set in Palatino by Rainbow Graphics.
The editor was Andrea Seils.
The production supervisor was Catherine Saggese.
Project management was provided by Roundhouse Editorial Services.
Quebecor Dubuque was printer and binder.

This book is printed on acid-free paper.

Contents

Contributors

W. Clayton Bordley, MD
Associate Professor of Pediatrics
Duke University Medical Center
Durham, North Carolina

Kathleen J. Clem, MD
Chief, Division of Emergency Medicine
Associate Professor
Department of Surgery
Duke University Medical Center
Durham, North Carolina

Elizabeth Magassy Dorn, MD
Associate Professor
Department of Emergency Medicine
University of Washington
Seattle, Washington

Worth W. Everett, MD
Assistant Professor of Emergency Medicine
Hospital of the University of Pennsylvania
Philadelphia, Pennsylvania

Karen S. Frush, MD
Chief Medical Director, Children's Services
Associate Professor of Pediatrics
Duke University Medical Center
Durham, North Carolina

Ted Glynn, MD
Assistant Director—Research
Michigan State University Emergency Medicine
    Residency
Attending Physician
Department of Emergency Medicine
Ingham Regional Medical Center
Lansing, Michigan

Cherie A. Hargis, MD
Attending Physician
Department of Emergency Medicine
Alameda County Medical Center/Highland
    Hospital
Assistant Clinical Professor
Department of Internal Medicine
University of California, San Francisco School of
    Medicine
Oakland, California

H. Gene Hern, Jr., MD, MS
Associate Residency Director
Department of Emergency Medicine
Alameda County Medical Center/Highland
    Hospital
Oakland, California
Assistant Professor of Medicine
University of California, San Francisco
San Francisco, California

Loretta Jackson-Williams, MD, PhD, FACEP
Assistant Professor of Medicine
Department of Emergency Medicine
University of Mississippi Medical Center
Jackson, Mississippi

Joel Kravitz, MD
Assistant Director
Emergency Medicine Residency Program
Department of Emergency Medicine
Albert Einstein Medical Center
Philadelphia, Pennsylvania

Linda E. Keyes, MD, FACEP
Assistant Clinical Professor of Surgery
Division of Emergency Medicine
University of Colorado Health Sciences Center
Denver, Colorado

Kenneth T. Kwon, MD, FACEP, FAAP
Director of Pediatric Emergency Medicine
Associate Clinical Professor
Department of Emergency Medicine
University of California, Irvine Medical Center
Orange, California

Luis M. Lovato, MD
Director of Emergency Critical Care
Department of Emergency Medicine
Assistant Clinical Professor
David Geffen School of Medicine at UCLA
Olive View/University of California, Los Angeles
    Medical Center
Sylmar, California

Daniel C. McGillicuddy, MD
Harvard Affiliated Emergency Medicine Residency
Beth Israel Deaconess Medical Center
Boston, Massachusetts

Christopher L. Moore, MD
Assistant Professor
Section of Emergency Medicine
Yale University School of Medicine
New Haven, Connecticut

Ronny M. Otero, MD
Senior Staff Physician
Associate Program Director
Department of Emergency Medicine
Henry Ford Hospital
Detroit, Michigan

Robert Park, MD
Assistant Clinical Professor
Director, Emergency Medicine Ultrasound
Division of Emergency Medicine
Duke University Medical Center
Durham, North Carolina

Carlo L. Rosen, MD
Program Director
Harvard Affiliated Emergency Medicine Residency
Beth Israel Deaconess Medical Center
Assistant Professor
Harvard Medical School
Boston, Massachusetts

John C. Stein, MD
Assistant Clinical Professor
Division of Emergency Medicine
University of California, San Francisco
San Francisco, California

Susan Stroud, MD
Assistant Professor of Surgery
Division of Emergency Medicine
University of Utah Health Sciences Center
Salt Lake City, Utah

Suzanne H. Summer, MD, FACEP
Attending Physician, Emergency Medicine
Kaiser Oakland Medical Center
Oakland, California

Gary W. Tamkin, MD, FACEP
Attending Physician
Alameda County Medical Center/Highland
    Hospital
Assistant Clinical Professor
University of California, San Francisco
Lafayette, California

Carrie Tibbles, MD
Associate Program Director
Harvard Affiliated Emergency Medicine Residency
Instructor in Medicine
Beth Israel Deaconess Medical Center
Boston, Massachusetts

Jason A. Tracy, MD
Assistant Program Director
Harvard Affiliated Emergency Medicine Residency
Beth Israel Deaconess Medical Center
Boston, Massachusetts

Corinne R. Widico, MD
Resident, Emergency Medicine
Alameda County Medical Center/Highland
    Hospital
Oakland, California

Preface

This book was designed as a study tool to complement the popular sixth edition of *Emergency Medicine: A Comprehensive Study Guide*, known affectionately by many emergency physicians as "Tintinalli" or "The Study Guide." This book contains over 700 questions and answers to help prepare emergency physicians for their ABEM or AOBEM written examination and residents for their annual emergency medicine in-service examination.

Dr. Kristi Koenig was the editor of the previous two editions of this book. I am indebted to her for her many years of friendship, mentorship, and most importantly the opportunity to follow in her footsteps as the current editor. Her shoes are definitely too big for me to fill—literally and figuratively! I hope to carry on her tradition of excellence with this edition of the question and answer book.

This version of the book is slightly different than previous ones. The majority of questions are referenced to the sixth edition of *Emergency Medicine: A Comprehensive Study Guide*. I am excited about the two major additions to the book. There are now sections specifically relating to the ABEM Life-Long Learning Assessment Program, and questions included in this book cover the material presented in the 2004 and 2005 ABEM articles. For those physicians who would like CME credit, 20 AMA/ACEP Category 1 CME credits are available for a small fee after completion of the POST-TEST. Please see the enclosed material for details.

I owe a special thanks to all the contributors who worked diligently on their assignments. If it weren't for these dedicated individuals, this book would not have been possible. I would be remiss if I didn't thank Marina Leusing, one of my closest friends, for her organizational skills, patience, and countless hours of work coordinating this project. Marina, you're the best! I couldn't have done it without you. Thanks to my staff assistant, Kim Brown, who always makes herself available to me no matter how overwhelmed with work she may be. I'd be lost without you, Kim. Last but definitely not least, I would have never been able to accomplish this project and so many others without the support and encouragement of my husband, Mark Haynos, and the unconditional love of my two boys, Alex and Aaron. Did I tell you that I love you?

Susan B. Promes, MD, FACEP

CHAPTER 1

Abuse and Assault Emergencies
Questions

1-1. Which of the following is the BEST evidence of failure to thrive in an infant?

(A) Prefers inanimate over animate objects.
(B) Is difficult to console.
(C) Has minimal subcutaneous fat.
(D) Gains weight in hospital.

1-2. Which of the following statements regarding psychosocial dwarfs is NOT correct?

(A) Their short statures exceed their low weights.
(B) They have bizarre, voracious appetites.
(C) They have disturbed home situations.
(D) Blunted growth hormone responses are irreversibly impaired.

1-3. A 5-year-old boy is brought in by his mother with the chief complaint of hematuria. There is no history of fever, abdominal pain, nausea, vomiting, or prior renal disease. Vital signs and physical examination are normal. The nurse happens to observe the mother covertly dripping blood from her finger into the container of urine. What is the name of this behavior?

(A) Malingering.
(B) Munchausen syndrome.
(C) Somatoform disorder.
(D) Polle's syndrome.

1-4. Which of the following statements regarding child sexual abuse is the MOST important tenet to remember for documentation?

(A) The presenting complaint may or may not be related to the genitourinary system.
(B) There is usually a time delay before the abuse is reported.
(C) The assailant is usually known to the child.
(D) The absence of physical findings does not preclude abuse.

1-5. A three-year-old boy is brought to the ED by his mother because of a bite to the left forearm, which she claims was inflicted by his 15-month-old sister 2 hours ago. Vital signs are normal. The patient has full range of motion in his left upper extremity, which is neurovascularly intact. A crescentic bite mark is on the proximal forearm. The teeth marks have caused bruising and multiple skin breaks, which have stopped bleeding. What is the NEXT most appropriate action?

(A) Irrigate the wound.
(B) Swab the site for saliva and photograph the wound.
(C) Measure the intercanine diameter.
(D) File a report of suspected child abuse.

1-6. A 30-year-old woman arrives by private vehicle with multiple contusions inflicted by her intimate partner, who struck her with the butt of a gun. She has a tender contusion and abrasions to the mid-ulnar aspect of the left forearm. There is no bony instability. The extremity is neurovascularly intact, and the remainder of the physical examination is normal. The wound is cleaned and dressed. The police have not been notified yet. A report is started by the emergency physician, and the social worker is called but is presently involved in another case. The patient says she has considered leaving the partner in the future, but for now, she plans to return home. During an argument earlier this week, the partner threatened to kill her and then commit suicide. There are no children or pets in the household. What is the next MOST appropriate action?

(A) Complete the report and discharge the patient to home.

(B) Complete the report, notify the police, and wait for arrival of law enforcement before initiating any discharge.

(C) Complete the report, discharge the patient, and have her wait in the lobby for the social worker.

(D) Complete the report and admit the patient to the hospital.

1-7. Which of the following statements regarding elder abuse is NOT correct?

(A) A victim's functional disability or acute cognitive decline may increase the risk of abuse.

(B) Situational stresses are the most likely trigger for the abuser.

(C) Incontinence, nocturnal shouting, wandering, and paranoia are common historical features in the victim.

(D) Unexplained injuries and sexually transmitted diseases suggest abuse.

1-8. A 3-year-old girl is brought to the emergency department by her mother with a chief complaint of abdominal pain for 2 hours. Fever, vomiting, and diarrhea are denied by the mother, who has been drinking alcohol. Vital signs are blood pressure 86/40 mmHg, pulse 130 beats per minute, respirations 24 per minute, temperature 37°C, and room air oxygen saturation 100%. The child's abdomen is distended and tender. A contusion is visible in the right upper quadrant, and bowel sounds are diminished. Older bruises are seen on the upper arms, anterior thighs, and buttocks. A screening ultrasound reveals fluid between the liver and the kidney. The mother denies trauma but becomes very tearful. An IV is started, and blood is sent to the laboratory. What is the next MOST appropriate sequence of events?

(A) Consult surgery, and contact social services.

(B) Ask the child what happened, consult surgery, and contact social services.

(C) Contact social services, then consult surgery.

(D) Contact surgery, and notify law enforcement directly.

Abuse and Assault Emergencies
Answers, Explanations, and References

1-1. The answer is D (Chapter 297). Children subjected to physical, nutritional, and emotional neglect in early infancy will manifest physical and behavioral traits that are signs of the failure to thrive (FTT) syndrome. Affected children are usually younger than 3 years; older children exposed to continued neglect will reflect the same traits. Physically, an infant with FTT will have minimal subcutaneous fat and a body mass index below the fifth percentile (weight is lower than height). The child's hygiene may be poor. Behaviorally, the child is wary, does not engage socially, and is difficult to console. Infants with FTT prefer inanimate over animate objects. The physician should admit the infant with suspected FTT. Information obtained about birth weight, prenatal exposure to drug or alcohol use, previous hospitalizations, and parental stature will be vital. Order a skeletal long bone study to rule out physical abuse. A medical social services consult should also be initiated. Weight gain within 1–2 weeks of hospitalization is considered proof of FTT within the original environment.

1-2. The answer is D (Chapter 297). Children older than 2–3 years who experience profound environmental neglect are at risk for becoming psychosocial dwarfs. These children have short statures which exceed their low weights, bizarre appetites (foraging from garbage cans), and disturbed home situations. Speech is often delayed or unintelligible. Their growth hormone levels are low to normal but do not increase in response to insulin or arginine stimulation. These children require admission and a formal social intervention. The blunted growth hormone responses normalize briskly after the child is removed from the original environment, either through hospitalization or foster care placement.

1-3. The answer is D (Chapter 297). Polle's syndrome is another term for Munchausen syndrome by proxy, a form of child abuse in which the parent causes or simulates an illness in a child. The apparent intent is not to harm the child but rather to gain attention for themselves from health care providers. The child may present to the ED with symptoms such as altered mental status, seizures, bleeding, vomiting, or diarrhea because insulin, warfarin, ipecac, or laxatives have been given. The child then undergoes extensive diagnostic testing, which prolongs the desired contact with health care providers. Unlike the outcome in this scenario, Munchausen syndrome by proxy is often difficult to diagnose. In some hospitals, parents have been detected by covert video. Suspected or proven cases require notification of child protective services. The child should be admitted to the hospital to provide any necessary therapy and to protect them from further parental harm. Malingering, somatoform disorder, and hypochondriasis are all behaviors or conditions directly manifested by a single patient, not through the actions of another person.

1-4. The answer is D (Chapter 297). Physical findings may be absent despite past or ongoing sexual abuse. Certain activities, such as oral-genital contact, may not cause physical trauma. In other cases, sustained injuries have healed without scarring by the time of presentation. There is usually a delay between the occurrence or initiation of sexual abuse and the disclosure; this delay may span years. If the assault is acute, e.g., less than 72 hours ago, a forensic examination is mandatory to evaluate injuries and to obtain DNA evidence. In more than 90% of cases, the child knows the assailant. Children may present to the ED with a direct disclosure of sexual abuse, or they may report symptoms referrable to the genitourinary system or unrelated symptoms. Behavioral changes may also be the reason the child is brought to the ED.

1-5.   The answer is C (Chapter 297). First, measure the wound. A bite mark with an intercanine diameter greater than 3 cm was inflicted by an adult and would indicate child abuse. In that case, forensic evidence should be gathered by swabbing the site for saliva and photographing the wound. Next, the wound should be irrigated, and the patient should receive human bite prophylaxis with amoxicillin-clavulanate. Finally, a report of suspected child abuse must be initiated.

1-6.   The answer is B (Chapter 299). Intimate partner violence and abuse (IPVA) is a more accurate and inclusive term for domestic violence, involving any intimate relationship. IPVA is a socially unacceptable behavior that occurs in members of every race, ethnicity, sexual orientation, religion, region, and socioeconomic status. Although the gun was not fired in this case, its presence during an episode of already unacceptable IPVA and the partner's threat of murder-suicide are ominous indicators for a potentially lethal future outcome. Firearms are the lethal weapons used in about 60% of IPVA homicides. Although IPVA is a crime in all 50 states, and 23 states have mandatory reporting for injuries resulting from crimes, only 7 states

specifically require a report of injuries incurred by IPVA. In this case, the key action requires direct contact of law enforcement because a police report has not yet occurred. Since the situation is high-risk and the social worker has not yet arrived, the EP should initiate or place the call to law enforcement officers, who should arrive while the patient is still in the ED. Do not discharge the patient until the officers have discussed the case with the EP, the social worker, or both. The patient must be advised of the high risk for lethal escalation, especially if she returns home. Every alternative resource should be explored first to ensure her safety, including a safe haven, and a list of community resources should be provided. Admission can be considered if no other options exist to ensure safety. Caution must be taken if the perpetrator is informed of the report but is not taken into custody, or if the patient is not given safe haven. In summary, the high-risk indicators for lethal outcome of IPVA include escalating violence; use or threat of firearms or other weapons; hostage taking; substance abuse, especially cocaine and amphetamines; homicide or suicide threats or attempts; and violent behavior outside the home.

1-7.   The answer is B (Chapter 300). An abuser's personality problems are more associated with elder abuse than are situational stressors. Abusers tend to have very dependent personalities. Alcohol or drug dependence, mental illness, or cognitive impairment will increase the likelihood of abusive or neglectful behavior in a caretaker. Elders with cognitive impairment are more likely to be abused. Incontinence, nocturnal shouting, wandering, and paranoia are common historical features in abused elders. The physician must maintain a high index of suspicion for elder abuse when eliciting the history and performing the physical examination. Unexplained traumatic injuries or sexually transmitted diseases are highly suggestive of abuse. Suspected or proven cases must be reported to adult protective services. Patients should be admitted to the hospital if medically indicated or if it is the only way to ensure their safety.

1-8. **The answer is B** (Chapter 297). In cases of suspected child abuse it is important and useful to ask the child what happened and to record the response verbatim. Regardless of the child's answer, her intra-abdominal injury takes immediate priority, so consult surgery, then social services. The EP is obligated to report all cases of suspected child abuse. Most EDs have social services workers to facilitate notification of child protec-

tive services, which would coordinate any immediate need for law enforcement. Along with head injuries, intra-abdominal injuries are the two most common causes of death from child abuse. Abdominal symptoms include pain, tenderness, vomiting, decreased bowel sounds, and distension. Obvious trauma may be absent or denied historically. Potential injuries include duodenal hematoma, hepatic or splenic rupture, intestinal perforation, traumatic pancreatitis, renal trauma, and ruptured intra-abdominal blood vessels.

CHAPTER 2

Analgesia, Anesthesia, and Sedation
Questions

2-1. A 26-year-old male has just had a successful reduction of a nondisplaced distal radial fracture. He also sustained rib fractures and a shoulder contusion in a construction accident. The patient still has significant pain, rated as 8 out of 10 after 800 mg of ibuprofen. Which of the following medication regimens is a reasonable choice for treating this patient's pain?

(A) Codeine 30 mg orally every 4 hours.
(B) Acetaminophen 325 mg/codeine 5 mg orally every 6 hours.
(C) Ibuprofen 600 mg every 6 hours and oxycodone 5 mg orally every 6 hours.
(D) Rofecoxib 25 mg orally once a day.

2-2. An opioid agonist-antagonist is associated with which of the following effects?

(A) Dose-related respiratory depression.
(B) Possible induction of withdrawal in opioid-dependent patients.
(C) Higher dosage requirements in opioid-naive patients.
(D) Lower dosage requirements than similar opioid agonists.

2-3. In which of the following situations should ketamine be used with caution?

(A) Children without intravenous access.
(B) Patients with history of asthma.
(C) Patients in whom other analgesics were not fully effective in controlling pain.
(D) Patients with suspected increased intracranial pressure.

2-4. What is the maximum dose of lidocaine with epinephrine that can be administered peripherally?

(A) 300 mg.
(B) 4.5 mg/kg.
(C) 7 mg/kg.
(D) 1.5 mg/kg.

2-5. A 35-year-old female patient drove herself to the emergency department because she sustained a small laceration to her finger. She reports the last time she received a subcutaneous injection of lidocaine she "broke out in hives" and her "throat became swollen." What is a reasonable alternative for local anesthesia in this patient?

(A) Subcutaneous administration of prilocaine.
(B) Administration of diphenhydramine 30 minutes prior to lidocaine injection.
(C) Oral diphenhydramine.
(D) Subcutaneous administration of procaine.

2-6. A 35-year-old male presents with a 4-cm laceration to his left cheek 2 cm below his lower eyelid. You explain to him that you would like to perform regional anesthesia to numb his face. Which of the following describes the appropriate procedure?

(A) A mental block can be performed by injecting 2 cc of lidocaine with epinephrine near the mental foramen.

(B) An infraorbital block can be performed by injecting 8 cc of lidocaine with epinephrine near the infraorbital foramen.

(C) A mental block can be performed by injecting 6 cc of lidocaine with epinephrine near the mental foramen.

(D) An infraorbital block can be performed by injecting 3 cc of lidocaine near the infraorbital foramen.

2-7. A 21-year-old unrestrained driver with a past medical history significant for asthma was involved in a single-vehicle automobile accident and has severe pain from an open fracture of his left tibia and fractured ribs. He is hypotensive with an initial blood pressure of 80/50 mmHg. The patient is currently receiving a liter bolus of lactated Ringer's solution. Which of the following analgesic agents is a reasonable choice in this setting of hypotension?

(A) Meperidine 50 mg intravenously.

(B) Morphine 10 mg intravenously.

(C) Fentanyl 100 mcg intravenously.

(D) Propofol 50 mg intravenously.

2-8. Which of the following is NOT one of the pharmacologic properties of etomidate?

(A) Devoid of analgesic properties.

(B) Amnestic properties.

(C) Dose-dependent cardiovascular depression.

(D) Reliable hypnosis in a short period of time.

2-9. After successful reduction of a shoulder dislocation using procedural sedation, a patient can be safely discharged from the ED upon satisfying which of the following sets of conditions?

(A) The patient can count backwards from 100 and walk in a straight line.

(B) The patient is awake and alert, can recite discharge instructions after tolerating a beverage, and has a reliable adult to accompany him or her home.

(C) The patient, although drowsy, can follow instructions.

(D) The patient is nauseous but awake and alert and can recite discharge instructions.

2-10. Which of the following agents is contraindicated in patients with head injury?

(A) Etomidate.

(B) Fentanyl.

(C) Nitrous oxide.

(D) Propofol.

Analgesia, Anesthesia, and Sedation
Answers, Explanations, and References

2-1. The answer is C (Chapter 36). Oxycodone is an effective opioid analgesic for treatment of pain. The combination of a non-steroidal anti-inflammatory drug (NSAID) and a short course of oxycodone should provide reasonable analgesia. Codeine is often used as an adjunct for pain management; however, it provides modest analgesia with significant side effects such as nausea and vomiting. Codeine is a potent antitussive agent and is still recommended for this indication when other agents are not effective. Acetaminophen and codeine are used as an adjunct for multiple painful processes. Acetaminophen is not an anti-inflammatory. Rofecoxib is a cyclooxygenase-2 inhibitor that is purported to cause less gastrointestinal distress than other NSAIDs. The once-daily dosing with acute pain may not be sufficient for this patient.

2-2. The answer is B (Chapter 36). Opioid agonist-antagonists are an infrequently used class of drugs. Due to their opioid antagonism they can precipitate withdrawal in patients on long-term opioid treatment. Opioid agonist-antagonists, because of their mixed properties on different opioid receptors, cause decreased respiratory depression. The exact dosage required to provide adequate analgesia is multifactorial. It is presumed, however, that an opioid naive patient would not require increased dosage of an opioid or opioid agonist-antagonist. It is not known whether opioid agonist-antagonists require higher dosages than similar opioid medications.

2-3. The answer is D (Chapter 38). There are concerns that ketamine may cause an increase in intracranial pressure and thus it would be contraindicated in someone who already has documented elevated intracranial pressure. One of the benefits of ketamine is that it can be given in an intramuscular dose. It is often given in combination with antisialagogues such as atropine or glycopyrrolate in the same syringe. Ketamine is associated with some bronchodilatatory properties, which may make it a good agent to use in patients with preexisting asthma. Unsuccessful complete analgesia is not a contraindication of ketamine.

2-4. The answer is C (Chapter 37). The upper-limit dose of lidocaine with epinephrine is 7 mg/kg up to a total dose of 500 mg. Due to different absorption, the dose for intercostal regional anesthesia should be a fraction (1/10) of the dose for peripheral administration. The maximum total dosage for lidocaine without epinephrine is 300 mg (4.5 mg/kg).

2-5. The answer is D (Chapter 37). Procaine is a local anesthetic with the chemical structure of an ester. There should be no cross-reaction between lidocaine, an amide, and procaine. Diphenhydramine is often given as pretreatment to "ward off" possible allergic or febrile responses to medications and blood products. The benefits of this practice are unknown. The patient arrived by a private vehicle, and if she is oversedated by oral diphenhydramine, her discharge may be delayed significantly. Subcutaneous diphenhydramine has been used as a local anesthetic, although it is associated with a burning sensation upon infiltration.

2-6. **The answer is D** (Chapter 37). An infraorbital block may be performed by either an intraoral or extraoral route. The duration of anesthesia appears to be longer by an intraoral route. The region of anesthesia includes the ipsilateral cheek, lower eyelid, upper lip, and lateral aspect of the nose. Infraorbital nerve block should be performed without epinephrine because of the proximity of the facial artery. It is recommended to limit infiltration to 2–3 cc of local anesthetic. A mental nerve block supplies anesthesia to the lower lip and chin and will not provide anesthesia to the area of concern. The mental nerve can be anesthetized by an intraoral or extraoral route. Lidocaine with epinephrine is acceptable; however, the recommended volume should be limited to 1–2 cc.

2-7. **The answer is C** (Chapter 38). Fentanyl is a potent opioid with approximately 100 times the potency of morphine but with a shorter half-life and lack of histamine release. It is uncommonly associated with hypotension. This patient's injury demands attention to the airway, breathing, circulation, and pain. Meperidine is a synthetic opioid with multiple side effects including histamine release. Histamine release has been associated with hypotension as it does cause vasodilation. The assessment of this patient can be confounded by the hyperexcitability associated with meperidine administration. Morphine is a well-known drug, and many clinicians feel comfortable with administering it in various situations. Morphine is associated with histamine release. This patient's history of asthma and current hypotension coupled with the high dose could potentially be harmful in this individual. Propofol is an anesthetic agent that is currently being evaluated in the ED setting. Its role in procedural sedation is still being defined. However, propofol has significant cardiovascular depressive ef-

fects, which should be avoided in this patient.

2-8. **The answer is C** (Chapter 38). Etomidate does not have dose-dependent cardiovascular depressant effects. The positive cardiovascular profile makes it an attractive drug for procedural sedation. Etomidate is devoid of analgesic effects, so an analgesic must be given carefully to address a patient's level of pain. Etomidate does induce amnesia, which is one of the attractive features for its use in procedural sedation. Etomidate does provide reliable hypnosis.

2-9. **The answer is B** (Chapter 38). It is important to continuously reassess a patient who has received procedural sedation. Monitoring equipment should be applied throughout the procedure. Documentation of a return to preprocedural mental status by assessing the patient's ability to understand discharge instructions is a reasonable criterion. Institutions should establish specific guidelines regarding the safe discharge of a patient who has received procedural sedation. A drowsy patient may still be under the influence of anesthesia and should be given a longer period of time to recover. A nauseous patient, particularly if actively vomiting, may not be safe to return home. This patient should be observed for a longer period of time.

2-10. **The answer is C** (Chapter 36). Nitrous oxide requires patient cooperation to be successful. Head injury is considered among the contraindications and precautions listed for administration of this agent. Etomidate and fentanyl are not contraindicated in patients with head injury. Some algorithms for intubation include fentanyl as pretreatment in patients with head injury. Propofol is relatively new to the ED setting. Although its ED applications are limited, head injury is not considered a contraindication to its use.

Cardiovascular Emergencies
Questions

3-1. Which of the following statements concerning the initial evaluation of patients presenting with acute chest pain is TRUE?

(A) The response to a "gastrointestinal cocktail" is useful in discriminating symptoms of acute myocardial ischemia from other etiologies.

(B) The pain of myocardial ischemia is always retrosternal in location and described as a sensation of heaviness or pressure.

(C) A normal electrocardiogram excludes the possibility of acute myocardial infarction in patients with acute chest pain.

(D) Resolution of chest discomfort with nitroglycerin may not be diagnostic of acute myocardial ischemia.

3-2. Which of the following statements concerning the clinical application of myocardial marker measurements is TRUE?

(A) Single-sample myocardial marker measurements are useful in excluding the diagnosis of acute myocardial infarction.

(B) Cardiac troponins remain elevated after an acute myocardial infarction for approximately 48 hours.

(C) Numerous conditions in addition to acute myocardial infarction are associated with elevated troponin levels.

(D) Abnormal cardiac troponin levels are useful in predicting patients at higher risk for adverse events regardless of CK-MB and electrocardiogram results.

3-3. Which of the following electrocardiogram patterns is most consistent with occlusion of the right coronary artery?

(A) ST-segment elevation in V_1, V_2, and V_3.

(B) R waves in V_1 and V_2 >0.04 s and R/S ratio ≥1.

(C) ST-segment elevation in I and aVL.

(D) ST-segment elevation in II, III, and aVF.

3-4. An 82-year-old female presents with 1 hour of substernal chest pressure, dyspnea, and diaphoresis. Her initial electrocardiogram is shown in Figure 3-1. No old electrocardiograms are available for comparison. Her first set of cardiac markers is negative. Which of the following is the most appropriate treatment?

(A) Admit the patient to a floor bed.

(B) Observe the patient and order serial cardiac markers.

(C) Administer thrombolytics.

(D) Cardiovert her with 50 joules.

3-5. Which of the following tachydysrhythmias, occurring shortly after the onset of acute myocardial infarction, is associated with an increased mortality?

(A) Ventricular tachycardia.

(B) Accelerated idioventricular rhythm.

(C) Atrial fibrillation.

(D) Ventricular premature beats.

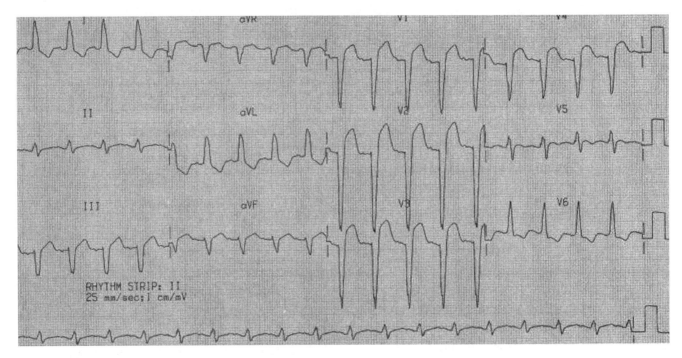

Figure 3-1.

3-6. An 85-year-old female presents with acute onset of dyspnea, inspiratory rales, and holosystolic murmur. Her electrocardiogram reveals Q waves in II, III, and aVF. Approximately five days earlier, she relates, she had a "severe bout of heartburn." Cardiac enzymes are significant for a normal CK-MB but elevated troponin. What is the most likely cause of this patient's symptoms?

(A) Left ventricular free wall rupture.

(B) Pulmonary embolism.

(C) Dressler syndrome.

(D) Papillary muscle rupture.

3-7. A 50-year-old female presents with sharp, precordial chest pain of 10 minutes duration, which has now resolved. She has a history of hypertension but no other medical problems including coronary artery disease. Her electrocardiogram reveals T-wave inversion <1 mm in the inferolateral leads. Which of the following best classifies this patient's likelihood of significant coronary artery disease?

(A) Nonexistent.

(B) Low likelihood.

(C) Intermediate likelihood.

(D) High likelihood.

3-8. Which of the following therapeutic agents has been shown to unequivocally decrease mortality in the setting of acute myocardial infarction?

(A) Aspirin.

(B) Calcium channel antagonists.

(C) Magnesium.

(D) Glycoprotein IIb/IIIa inhibitors.

3-9. A 50-year-old male presents with an acute inferior wall myocardial infarction. Following the administration of aspirin and nitroglycerin, he suddenly becomes confused and diaphoretic with a blood pressure of 70/30 mmHg. Physical examination reveals jugular venous distention, clear lung fields, and no evidence of a murmur. What combination of therapeutic agents is most likely to immediately stabilize this patient?

(A) Heparin and glycoprotein IIb/IIIa inhibitors.

(B) Angiotensin converting enzyme inhibitor and clopidogrel.

(C) Streptokinase and magnesium.

(D) Normal saline bolus and dobutamine.

3-10. A 70-year-old male presents with an acute anterior wall myocardial infarction. His electrocardiogram reveals new-onset left bundle branch block and first-degree atrioventricular block. What therapeutic intervention is indicated?

(A) Dobutamine.

(B) Prophylactic temporary pacemaker.

(C) Isoproterenol.

(D) Swan-Ganz catheter.

3-11. A 69-year-old male presents following a syncopal episode. He relates that he was mowing the lawn "for the first time this year" when he experienced precordial chest discomfort. The next thing he recalls is his wife frantically arousing him. He is currently symptom-free. His physical examination is remarkable for a holosystolic murmur best heard at the right second intercostal space. His electrocardiogram reveals a left ventricular strain pattern. What is the most likely cause of this patient's symptoms?

(A) Pulmonary embolism.

(B) Brugada syndrome.

(C) Subclavian steal syndrome.

(D) Aortic stenosis.

3-12. Which of the following is a significant predictor of sudden cardiac death or significant dysrhythmia within one year of an unexplained syncopal event?

(A) Nonspecific ST-T changes on electrocardiogram.

(B) History of neurocardiogenic syncope confirmed via tilt-table testing.

(C) History of congestive heart failure.

(D) History of atrial fibrillation.

3-13. Which of the following therapeutic agents has not been conclusively shown to decrease mortality in patients with congestive heart failure?

(A) Angiotensin converting enzyme inhibitors.

(B) Beta adrenergic blockers.

(C) Furosemide.

(D) Spironolactone.

3-14. A 70-year-old male with a history of congestive heart failure presents with a first episode of pulmonary edema. He is treated acutely and stabilized. Considering this patient's history and presentation, which of the following statements best describes the patient's condition?

(A) His 1-year mortality is approximately 50%.

(B) B-type natriuretic peptide levels are not useful.

(C) Chronic calcium channel blocker therapy would be beneficial.

(D) Prophylactic antiarrhythmic therapy would be beneficial.

3-15. What is the most common cause of systolic dysfunction leading to congestive heart failure?

(A) Hyperthyroidism.

(B) Ischemic heart disease.

(C) Chronic hypertension.

(D) Myocarditis.

3-16. Which of the following is a common electrocardiogram finding in a patient with mitral valve stenosis?

(A) Left ventricular hypertrophy.

(B) Left bundle branch block.

(C) Sinus bradycardia.

(D) Notched or biphasic P waves.

3-17. Which of the following is NOT part of the classic triad seen with aortic stenosis?

(A) Syncope.
(B) Widened pulse pressure.
(C) Dyspnea.
(D) Angina.

3-18. A 50-year-old male presents to the ED in pulmonary edema. The patient has no history of hypertension. He does complain of shortness of breath and chest pain. He has a new holosystolic murmur on exam. The murmur is loudest at the apex and radiates to the left axilla. The patient has a normal-sized heart on chest x-ray. His electrocardiogram is diagnostic for an acute myocardial infarction. What is the most likely cause of the murmur?

(A) Congestive heart failure.
(B) Aortic stenosis.
(C) Cardiac tamponade.
(D) Papillary muscle necrosis.

3-19. What is the most common cause of acute aortic insufficiency?

(A) Infective endocarditis.
(B) Trauma.
(C) Aortic dissection.
(D) Marfan's syndrome.

3-20. Which of the following electrocardiogram characteristics are rarely found in patients with dilated cardiomyopathy?

(A) Atrial fibrillation.
(B) Left ventricular hypertrophy.
(C) Normal electrocardiogram.
(D) Ventricular ectopy.

3-21. Which of the following findings is frequently found on the chest radiograph in patients with hypertrophic cardiomyopathy?

(A) Kerley's A lines.
(B) Pulmonary edema.
(C) Cardiomegaly.
(D) Normal.

3-22. Which of the following is NOT a characteristic of pericarditis?

(A) PR-segment depression.
(B) Fever.
(C) Exertional dyspnea.
(D) Sharp retrosternal pain worse when supine.

3-23. Which of the following is a late electrocardiogram finding in patients with pericarditis?

(A) "Knuckle sign" in aVR.
(B) PR depression.
(C) T-wave inversions.
(D) ST elevation.

3-24. Which of the following is NOT associated with cardiac tamponade?

(A) Pulsus paradoxus.
(B) Narrow pulse pressure.
(C) Electrical alternans.
(D) Left ventricular hypertrophy.

3-25. What is the most common cause of non-traumatic cardiac tamponade?

(A) Infection.
(B) Uremia.
(C) Malignancy.
(D) Idiopathy.

3-26. What is the most common symptom in patients presenting with a pulmonary embolism?

(A) Syncope.
(B) Angina.
(C) Shortness of breath.
(D) Pleuritic chest pain.

3-27. Which of the following tests is most helpful in ruling out a low-risk patient for a pulmonary embolism?

(A) Chest x-ray.
(B) D-dimer.
(C) Electrocardiogram.
(D) Pulse oximetry.

3-28. Which of the following is NOT associated with an adverse short-term outcome in normotensive patients with pulmonary embolism?

(A) Left ventricular hypertrophy.
(B) New T wave inversions in V_1–V_4.
(C) New right bundle branch block.
(D) Heart rate greater than systolic pressure.

3-29. Which of the following is NOT approved for the treatment of pulmonary embolism by the U.S. Food and Drug Administration?

(A) Aspirin.
(B) Unfractionated heparin.
(C) Low-molecular-weight heparin.
(D) Thrombolytic therapy.

3-30. Which of the following statements is TRUE concerning pulse oximetry readings in the diagnosis of pulmonary embolism?

(A) A normal oxygen saturation rules out pulmonary embolism.
(B) Pulse oximetry readings play no role in the diagnosis of pulmonary embolism.
(C) Pulse oximetry readings are moderately helpful in identifying patients with a pulmonary embolism.
(D) All patients with a pulmonary embolism will have abnormal pulse oximetry readings.

3-31. What systolic blood pressure identifies a patient with a hypertensive emergency?

(A) 160 mmHg.
(B) 180 mmHg.
(C) 200 mmHg.
(D) No absolute number exists.

3-32. Which is NOT associated with transient hypertension?

(A) Anxiety.
(B) Pregnancy.
(C) Alcohol withdrawal syndromes.
(D) Cocaine.

3-33. Which of the following is NOT a finding of hypertensive retinopathy?

(A) Copper and silver wiring.
(B) Cherry red spot in macula.
(C) Cotton wool spots.
(D) Papillary disc edema.

3-34. Which of the following is the drug of choice for hypertensive encephalopathy?

(A) Sodium nitroprusside.
(B) Nifedipine.
(C) Hydralazine.
(D) Methyldopa.

3-35. Which of the following is NOT a risk factor for abdominal aortic aneurysm?

(A) Syphilis.
(B) Family history of aneurysm.
(C) Smoking.
(D) Hypertension.

3-36. What is the most common symptom of a ruptured abdominal aortic aneurysm?

(A) Hematuria.
(B) Syncope.
(C) Change in level of consciousness.
(D) Pain.

3-37. Which is NOT a clinical sign of a ruptured aortic aneurysm?

(A) Cullen's sign.
(B) Scrotal hematoma.
(C) Grey Turner's sign.
(D) Femoral pulse difference.

3-38. Which of the following is NOT typical of the pain associated with an aortic dissection?

(A) Shifting locations.
(B) Slow and gradual in onset.
(C) Tearing or ripping.
(D) Abrupt and severe.

3-39. Which of the following is the best test for an unstable patient with a possible aortic dissection?

(A) Computed tomography.
(B) Aortic angiogram.
(C) Transesophageal echocardiography.
(D) Magnetic resonance imaging.

3-40. Which of the following is NOT part of Virchow's triad of risk factors for venous thromboembolism?

(A) Venous stasis.
(B) Malignancy.
(C) Vessel wall injury.
(D) Hypercoagulable state.

3-41. Which of the following is the best test for diagnosing deep vein thrombosis (DVT)?

(A) Impedance plethysmography.
(B) Physical exam.
(C) Doppler ultrasound.
(D) Latex agglutination D-dimer.

3-42. Which of the following is NOT useful in the diagnosis of DVT?

(A) Positive ultrasound.
(B) Elevated D-dimer.
(C) High score using Well's criteria.
(D) Venography.

3-43. Which drug should be avoided in pregnancy when anticoagulation is desired?

(A) Heparin.
(B) Enoxaparin.
(C) Lepirudin.
(D) Warfarin.

3-44. What is the first of sign of an arterial occlusion?

(A) Pallor.
(B) Pulselessness.
(C) Paresthesias.
(D) Pain.

3-45. What is a common electrocardiogram finding in the post–cardiac transplant patient?

(A) Left ventricular hypertrophy.
(B) Left bundle branch block.
(C) Complete heart block.
(D) Two distinct P waves.

3-46. In the resuscitation of the cardiac transplant patient, which drug has no effect?

(A) Epinephrine.
(B) Atropine.
(C) Amiodarone.
(D) Diltiazem.

3-47. What is the main role of nuclear medicine evaluation (technetium or thallium) of the heart?

(A) To predict 1-year cardiac mortality.
(B) To determine anatomic dimensions of the heart.
(C) To evaluate myocardial perfusion.
(D) To identify coronary artery anatomy.

Cardiovascular Emergencies
Answers, Explanations, and References

3-1. **The answer is D** (Chapter 49). Nitroglycerin, in addition to its utility in treating coronary ischemia, can also provide relief of symptoms caused by gastrointestinal ailments via smooth muscle relaxation. Patients with myocardial ischemia may have complete relief of their symptoms with a gastrointestinal cocktail. Unfortunately, a significant portion of patients with myocardial ischemia may not present with chest pain as their predominant symptom. A normal electrocardiogram does not rule out acute myocardial infarction. Up to 5% of patients with acute myocardial infarctions may present with this finding.

3-2. **The answer is D** (Chapter 49). Elevated troponin levels predict those patients at risk for adverse cardiovascular events and are useful in triaging patients to the appropriate level of inpatient care. In patients presenting with acute chest pain and a nondiagnostic electrocardiogram, acute myocardial infarction cannot be definitively excluded upon presentation, and serial sampling of myocardial markers is required. Cardiac troponins are highly specific for myocardial injury. In contrast, there are numerous conditions associated with elevated CK-MB levels. Following acute myocardial infarction, troponin levels begin to elevate around 6 hours, peak at 12 hours, and remain abnormal for 7 to 10 days.

3-3. **The answer is D** (Chapter 50). The electrocardiogram can be used to predict the coronary vessel causing an infarct. ST-segment elevation in lead III greater than lead II is consistent with an inferior wall injury pattern secondary to right coronary artery occlusion. A true posterior wall infarction is manifested by significant R waves in V_1 and V_2. Occlusion of the left circumflex artery is heralded by ST-segment elevation in at least one lateral lead (V_5, V_6, or aVL) with an isoelectric or elevated ST-segment in lead I.

3-4. **The answer is C** (Chapter 50). New-onset left bundle branch block (LBBB) in the setting of symptoms suggestive of acute myocardial infarction is an indication for mechanical or pharmacologic reperfusion therapy. However, ST-segment patterns may be present that indicate acute myocardial infarction in the setting of preexisting LBBB:

- ST-segment elevation of 1 mm or greater concordant with the QRS.
- ST-segment depression of 1 mm or greater in leads V_1, V_2, or V_3.
- ST-segment elevation >5 mm and discordant with the QRS.

3-5. **The answer is C** (Chapter 50). Supraventricular tachycardias are associated with an increased mortality in the setting of acute myocardial infarction. These arrhythmias result in an increased myocardial oxygen demand and are associated with increased adrenergic stimulation due to depressed systolic function. An accelerated idioventricular rhythm often reflects successful reperfusion in patients receiving thrombolytic therapy. Ventricular premature beats are the most common arrhythmia associated with acute myocardial infarction and normally do not require specific treatment. Early, transient ventricular tachycardia is not associated with an increase in mortality.

3-6. **The answer is D** (Chapter 50). Papillary muscle rupture, although rare, is most commonly seen following inferior myocardial infarction as the posteromedial papillary muscle receives its blood supply from a solitary source. Patients usually present with sudden onset of dyspnea, pulmonary congestion, and a new holosystolic murmur secondary to mitral valve regurgitation. Left ventricular free wall rupture is a catastrophic event with a greater than 90% mortality rate. If patients survive to presentation, their symptoms are consistent with cardiac tamponade, and bedside ultrasound can be diagnostic. Pulmonary embolism is certainly a diagnostic consideration in this patient but less likely based on the presenting signs and symptoms. Dressler syndrome usually presents 2 to 10 weeks following acute myocardial infarction. It may reflect an autoimmune-mediated phenomenon and is most commonly manifested by fever and chest pain.

3-7. **The answer is B** (Chapter 50). This patient has a low likelihood of significant coronary artery disease (see Table 3-1). Patients presenting to the ED with symptoms suggestive of myocardial ischemia without evidence of acute myocardial infarction require stratification based on their likelihood of significant coronary artery disease. Such individual risk stratification can help guide subsequent management and disposition.

3-8. **The answer is A** (Chapter 51). Aspirin is a simple yet powerful therapeutic weapon in the setting of acute myocardial infarction, resulting in a 23% reduction in mortality. Patients who have a significant allergy to aspirin should be given clopidogrel to ensure inhibition of platelet aggregation. The glycoprotein IIb/IIIa inhibitors are powerful antiplatelet agents. Unfortunately, the only clear mortality benefit from IIb/IIIa inhibitors is in those patients undergoing percutaneous coronary intervention. Calcium channel antagonists have not been shown to reduce mortality and in fact are more likely to cause harm in the setting of acute myocardial infarction. There is considerable conflicting evidence relating to the efficacy of magnesium in the setting of

TABLE 3-1. LIKELIHOOD OF SIGNIFICANT CORONARY ARTERY DISEASE IN PATIENTS WITH SYMPTOMS SUGGESTIVE OF UNSTABLE ANGINA

High Likelihood (85–99%)	Intermediate Likelihood (15–84%)	Low Likelihood (1–14%)
Any of the following features	*Absence of high-likelihood features and any of the following*	*Absence of high- or intermediate-likelihood features but may have*
History of prior AMI, sudden death, or other known history of CAD	Definite angina; males <60 or females <70 y of age	Chest pain classified as probably not angina
Definite angina: males ≥60 or females ≥70 y of age	Probable angina: males ≥60 or females ≥70 y of age	One risk factor other than diabetes
Transient hemodynamic or ECG changes during pain	Chest pain probably not angina in patients with diabetes	T-wave flattening or inversion <1 mm in leads with dominant R waves
Variant angina (pain with reversible ST-segment elevation)	Chest pain probably not angina and 2 or 3 risk factors other than diabetes	Normal ECG
ST-segment elevation or depression ≥1 mm	Extracardiac vascular disease	
Marked symmetric T-wave inversion in multiple precordial leads	ST depression 0.05–1 mm	
	T-wave inversion ≥1 mm in leads with dominant R waves	

Abbreviations: AMI = acute myocardial infarction; CAD = coronary artery disease; ECG = electrocardiogram.
Source: Braunwald E, Mark DB, Jones RH, et al: *Unstable Angina: Diagnosis and Management.* Clinical Practice Guideline No. 10 (amended). AHCPR Publication No. 94-0602. Rockville, MD, Agency for Health Care Policy and Research and the National Health, Lung and Blood Institute, Public Health Service, U.S. Department of Health and Human Services, 1994.

acute myocardial infarction and thus it should not be considered a routine agent in the treatment of such patients.

3-9. The answer is D (Chapter 51). This patient is suffering from a right ventricular infarction that complicates approximately one-third of all inferior wall myocardial infarcts. The mainstay of treatment is preload augmentation and inotropic support using aggressive normal saline boluses followed by initiation of dobutamine. Another key aspect of managing these patients is the preservation of atrioventricular synchrony. Atrial-augmented filling of the ventricle is vital in maintaining adequate cardiac output in the setting of ventricular systolic dysfunction as it may contribute up to 35% of the stroke volume. Synchronized cardioversion may be required to preserve this "atrial kick" in the setting of atrial tachy-dysrhythmias. Heparin, glycoprotein IIb/IIIa inhibitors, and clopidogrel may play a role in this patient's reperfusion strategy but are not as useful in the immediate stabilization phase. Streptokinase is less desirable to percutaneous coronary intervention in the setting of cardiogenic shock. Magnesium's only clear indication is in the setting of polymorphic ventricular tachycardia secondary to prolongation of the QT interval. Angiotensin converting enzyme inhibitors play a role in reducing left ventricular dysfunction and dilatation but are not necessarily initiated in the ED.

3-10. The answer is B (Chapter 51). The increased mortality in acute myocardial infarction patients with atrioventricular block is not directly caused by the conduction disturbance itself. Instead, the mortality in these patients is due to the extensive myocardial damage required to affect the intrinsic conduction system. Prophylactic temporary pacing is still indicated to prevent sudden hypotension and worsening ischemia in the setting of certain conduction disturbances, high-grade atrioventricular blocks, and symptomatic sinus bradycardia unresponsive to atropine.

Dobutamine and isoproterenol may increase myocardial work load and oxygen demand and thus are less attractive options. Atropine is indicated for symptomatic sinus bradycardia, Mobitz I second-degree atrioventricular block, and third-degree heart block.

3-11. The answer is D (Chapter 52). The classic presentation of aortic stenosis is one of chest pain, dyspnea, and exertional syncope. This diagnosis should be entertained in all elderly patients presenting with syncope. Subclavian steal syndrome, certainly a consideration in this patient, occurs as a result of proximal subclavian stenosis and resultant "shunting" of blood away from the ipsilateral vertebral artery. Such patients are unlikely to experience chest discomfort or dyspnea. Although less common, patients with pulmonary embolism may present with syncope as a part of their symptom complex due to profound (but transient) right ventricular outflow obstruction. Brugada syndrome is a syndrome manifested by syncope due to polymorphic ventricular tachycardia. Such patients have a unique electrocardiogram that reveals ST-segment elevation in leads V_1–V_3 associated with a right bundle branch block pattern (see Figure 3-2). Patients with this disorder are at high risk for sudden cardiac death and require treatment with an automatic implantable cardioverter defibrillator (AICD).

3-12. The answer is C (Chapter 52). The patient with unexplained syncope despite an initial ED evaluation (up to 50% of such patients) requires risk stratification based on clinical and electrocardiographic characteristics. Depending on the risk of near-term events, patients may either be admitted for evaluation and further cardiac monitoring or discharged with the intent of further outpatient evaluation. Significant predictors of sudden cardiac death or significant dysrhythmia within one year of a syncopal event are abnormal electrocardiogram (excluding nonspecific ST-T changes), age >45

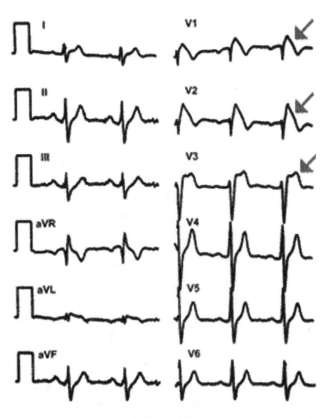

Figure 3-2.

years, history of ventricular dysrhythmia, and history of congestive heart failure. Patients with confirmed reflex-mediated syncope do not have increased risk of cardiovascular morbidity or mortality. Patients with atrial fibrillation are at increased risk for cerebrovascular complications but not sudden cardiac death.

3-13. **The answer is C** (Chapter 53). Although loop diuretics are indicated for acute pulmonary edema and decompensated heart failure, these agents are not used alone in the chronic management of congestive heart failure due to a lack of mortality benefit. Beta adrenergic blockers and angiotensin converting enzyme inhibitors decrease mortality in patients with symptomatic left ventricular dysfunction. Spironolactone is useful in New York Heart Association Class III and IV heart failure patients with continued symptoms despite the use of other agents.

3-14. **The answer is A** (Chapter 53). Heart failure has a substantial impact in both human and economic terms. It is the leading cause of hospitalization in patients over 65 years of age. Heart failure patients who present with a first episode of pulmonary edema have 1-year mortality rates of 50%. B-type natriuretic peptide levels have significant utility in the acute and chronic management of patients with congestive heart failure. The use of calcium channel blockers should be avoided in the heart failure patient due to their negative effects on inotropic function. Despite their increased risk for malignant dysrhythmias, prophylactic antiarrhythmic therapy is contraindicated in heart failure patients as it appears to increase mortality.

3-15. **The answer is B** (Chapter 53). Ischemic heart disease is the most common cause of systolic dysfunction in patients in developed nations. Chronic hypertension is more often associated with heart failure due to diastolic dysfunction. Less common in occurrence, acute congestive heart failure resulting from myocarditis and thyrotoxicosis is usually reversible with treatment of the underlying disease process.

3-16. **The answer is D** (Chapter 54). Mitral valve stenosis leads to progressive dilatation of the left atrium. This finding on the electrocardiogram classically is the notched or biphasic P wave as the distended atrium conducts the P wave. Another finding in mitral stenosis may be right axis deviation. Left ventricular hypertrophy usually does not occur as the left ventricle characteristically does not have the increased pressures from mitral stenosis. Sinus bradycardia is not typically seen in mitral valvular disease. In fact, quite often the patient develops a tachycardic rhythm, namely, atrial fibrillation.

3-17. **The answer is B** (Chapter 54). Clinically, aortic stenosis has a narrow pulse pressure. Aortic insufficiency, on the other hand, causes a widened pulse pressure. This is sometimes manifested by a "water hammer pulse" or head bobbing. As aortic stenosis progresses, dyspnea is the first symptom, followed by paroxysmal nocturnal dyspnea, exertional syncope, and angina.

3-18. **The answer is D** (Chapter 54). Mitral regurgitation from papillary necrosis would produce a holosystolic murmur loudest at the apex. Aortic stenosis produces a loud systolic murmur but is loudest at the second right intercostals space and radiating to the carotids. Congestive heart failure does not cause a murmur but rather an extra heart sound from fluid overload. Cardiac tamponade can cause muffled heart tones and could cause shortness of breath and chest pain but does not cause a murmur.

3-19. **The answer is A** (Chapter 54). Infective endocarditis causes most cases of acute aortic insufficiency. Other common acute causes are trauma and aortic dissection. Marfan's syndrome, syphilis, calcific degeneration, congenital bicuspid valves, and rheumatic heart disease are examples of chronic causes of aortic insufficiency.

3-20. **The answer is C** (Chapter 55). Patients with dilated cardiomyopathy almost always have a very abnormal electrocardiogram. As the cardiac function declines and the chambers enlarge, atrial fibrillation and ventricular ectopy are quite common. The most common finding, however, is left ventricular hypertrophy and left atrial enlargement. Q waves and poor R-wave progression across the precordium are also common findings.

3-21. **The answer is D** (Chapter 55). Patients with hypertrophic cardiomyopathy frequently have no abnormality seen on chest x-ray. Evidence of pulmonary vascular congestion or edema is highly unusual, as is cardiomegaly. The asymmetrical hypertrophy of the septum classically produces symptoms of dyspnea with exertion, but it has more to do with an abrupt elevation in the left ventricular filling pressures in the hypertrophic heart.

3-22. **The answer is C** (Chapter 55). Patients with pericarditis tend to not have exertional dyspnea. If they have any dyspnea, it is due to increased pericardial irritation with inspiration. Low-grade fevers and pain when supine are classic findings. Dysphagia is caused by local irritation of the esophagus by the inflamed posterior pericardium.

3-23. **The answer is C** (Chapter 55). Initially (Stage 1), patients have the classic findings of diffuse ST elevation, PR depression, and a "knuckle sign" in the PR segment of aVR. In Stage 2, the ST segment returns to baseline and the T-wave amplitude decreases. T-wave inversions are classically a late finding (Stage 3) in the electrocardiograms of patients with pericarditis. Stage 4 is the resolution of the repolarization abnormalities.

3-24. **The answer is D** (Chapter 55). Patients with cardiac tamponade usually do not have underlying heart disease. The most common causes are malignancy and pericarditis. In fact, the electrocardiogram classically has very low voltage. Electrical alternans (beat-to-beat amplitude variation) is seen in about 20% of cases. Pulsus paradoxus and a narrow pulse pressure are commonly seen in tamponade.

3-25. **The answer is C** (Chapter 55). Metastatic malignancy accounts for 40% of nontraumatic tamponade. Acute idiopathy accounts for 15%; bacterial and tubercular infections account for 10%. Uremia also accounts for 10% of nontraumatic pericardial tamponade.

3-26. **The answer is C** (Chapter 56). Shortness of breath is the most common symptom of a pulmonary embolism, occurring in approximately 90% of patients with the diagnosis. Chest pain is the second most common presenting symptom. Syncope is an uncommon finding but one that perhaps carries a more serious prognostic value as syncope is a sign that the cardiopulmonary system is severely compromised.

3-27.   **The answer is B** (Chapter 56). A normal D-dimer suggests that the patient does not have an active thrombosis. In a low-risk patient, a negative D-dimer can effectively rule out a pulmonary embolism. A normal chest radiograph and normal electrocardiogram occur quite frequently and are not reassuring.

3-28.   **The answer is C** (Chapter 56). Factors associated with an adverse short-term outcome in normotensive patients include syncope or seizure with respiratory distress at presentation, age >70, presence of congestive heart failure, chronic obstructive pulmonary disease, prior pulmonary embolism, >50% pulmonary vascular occlusion, T-wave inversions in V_1–V_4 or new incomplete right bundle branch block, heart rate/systolic pressure ratio >1.0, room air pulse oximetry <94%, and increased troponin levels.

3-29.   **The answer is A** (Chapter 56). Aspirin has not been approved by the FDA for treatment of pulmonary embolism. However, other drugs that inhibit thrombin or accelerate fibrinolysis have been approved. While thrombolytic therapy of pulmonary embolism has been approved, there is little data supporting a survival benefit.

3-30.   **The answer is C** (Chapter 56). A normal pulse oximetry reading and even a normal PaO_2 is not helpful in excluding the diagnosis of pulmonary embolism. Up to 25% of patients without underlying lung disease will have a PaO_2 >80 mmHg. Many diseases in the differential diagnosis of pulmonary embolism can produce hypoxia. A normal pulse oximetry reading does not eliminate the possibility of pulmonary embolism.

3-31.   **The answer is D** (Chapter 57). A hypertensive emergency is not defined by any absolute blood pressure measurement but rather by a relative increase from the patient's baseline pressure and the evidence of end organ damage (encephalopathy, LV failure with pulmonary edema, renal compromise, etc.).

3-32.   **The answer is B** (Chapter 57). Pregnancy tends to lower blood pressure. The other choices (cocaine, anxiety, alcohol withdrawal) all elevate blood pressure transiently. The blood pressure will eventually return to baseline once the underlying condition is reversed or treated.

3-33.   **The answer is B** (Chapter 57). The finding known as the cherry red spot is found in central retinal vein occlusion, not in hypertensive retinopathy. The central macula has a separate blood supply and so appears to be a focal area of redness in the middle of a pale macula (from the central artery occlusion). Copper and silver wiring are early (Stage II) retinopathy findings. Cotton wool spots represent focal ischemia of Stage III retinopathy. Papillary disc edema is found in malignant hypertension and is Stage IV of hypertensive retinopathy.

3-34.   **The answer is A** (Chapter 57). Sodium nitroprusside is the drug of choice for hypertensive encephalopathy. Patients require immediate and titratable lowering of the blood pressure. Sodium nitroprusside has a rapid onset with a relatively short half-life. Intravenous nitroglycerin and labetalol have been used, but nitroprusside is still the best agent. The other choices are not well suited for the emergency setting because they are difficult to adjust quickly if the patient becomes too hypotensive. The patient's mean arterial pressure should not be lowered by more than 20–25% within the first hour.

3-35.   **The answer is A** (Chapter 58). Syphilis is not a risk factor for abdominal aortic aneurysm. Classic risk factors include factors associated with atherosclerosis, such as hypertension and smoking. These factors contribute to weakness within the aortic wall and the development of aneurysms.

3-36. **The answer is D** (Chapter 58). Pain is the most common presenting symptom, though the others listed can be part of the clinical picture. Syncope and an altered sensorium are due to blood loss and hypotension. Hematuria is often mistakenly attributed to a renal calculus.

3-37. **The answer is D** (Chapter 58). Femoral pulse difference is not seen in aortic aneurysms. It is a widely held misconception that the femoral pulses are incongruent, but the aneurysm typically does not alter the pulse. The other options are all signs of a retroperitoneal hematoma. Cullen's sign is peri-umbilical ecchymosis. Grey Turner's sign is flank ecchymosis.

3-38. **The answer is B** (Chapter 58). Pain associated with an aortic dissection is typically described as abrupt in onset and as a tearing or ripping sensation. In addition, the pain tends to migrate down the back as it travels distally down the thoracic aorta.

3-39. **The answer is C** (Chapter 59). While all of the answers have excellent sensitivity for aortic dissection, the transesophageal echocardiograph (TEE) is the test of choice for the unstable patient or the patient who requires close clinical monitoring. TEE can be performed in the ED at the patient bedside and has a sensitivity between 97% and 100%.

3-40. **The answer is B** (Chapter 59). Virchow's classic triad includes vessel wall injury, venous stasis, and hypercoagulable state. While malignancy is certainly a risk factor, it is not one of the classic factors described by Virchow.

3-41. **The answer is C** (Chapter 59). Doppler ultrasound (Duplex) has a sensitivity that approaches 97%. Physical exam is a poor predictor of DVT. Impedance plethysmography has poor sensitivity of only 80%. Not only is

latex agglutination D-dimer the worst D-dimer test, but D-dimers should be used only to rule out disease, not to rule in disease. In other words, a negative D-dimer tells the clinician that DVT is unlikely.

3-42. **The answer is B** (Chapter 59). A high D-dimer is NOT helpful in diagnosing DVT. All the other tests mentioned have excellent specificity and sensitivity and can aid the diagnosis. An elevated D-dimer does not help to rule in or out the diagnosis of DVT. Only a low or normal D-dimer will help to rule out the diagnosis. A high D-dimer must be followed up with further testing.

3-43. **The answer is D** (Chapter 59). Warfarin is contraindicated in pregnancy. It is teratogenic and causes fetal bleeding. All forms of heparin are compatible with pregnancy. Since pregnant patients are at higher risk of thromboembolism, they must be placed only on heparin and not on coumadin. No form of heparin crosses the placenta, so it is safe in pregnancy. Lepirudin is a class B drug in pregnancy and can be used for anticoagulation when heparin-induced thrombocytopenia occurs.

3-44. **The answer is D** (Chapter 59). Pain is the first presenting symptom of an arterial occlusion. It may occur alone and be the only indication of a serious threat to the limb. The other P's include pallor, paresthesias, pulselessness, polar (cold), and paralysis. High clinical suspicion is required to salvage the limb at risk. As the ischemic time increases, anesthesia and paralysis portend severe injury and likely loss of the limb.

3-45. **The answer is D** (Chapter 60). The technique of cardiac transplantation preserves both the donor and recipient sinus nodes. This produces the classic finding of two electrically distinct P waves on the electrocardiogram. The atrial suture line keeps the nodes electrically isolated from one another. The donor heart should not have any other abnormalities on the electrocardiogram.

3-46. **The answer is B** (Chapter 60). Posttransplant patients have no sympathetic innervation. Therefore, vagally induced bradycardias do not exist in these patients, and atropine will have no clinical effect. Other drugs that act directly on the cardiac tissue will have more clinical effects.

3-47. **The answer is C** (Chapter 61). Nuclear medicine scanning techniques use potassium analogues to identify areas of cardiac perfusion defects. The heart is pharmacologically stressed and the potassium analogues are taken up by the cardiac muscle. Areas with less uptake of the radioactive analogue have decreased perfusion to that area. This type of test is a functional and physiologic test rather than an anatomic one.

CHAPTER 4

Disorders of the Skin Emergencies
Questions

4-1. Which of the following topical agents is NOT associated with cutaneous atrophy?

(A) Triamcinolone acetonide.

(B) Betamethasone.

(C) Mometasone furoate.

(D) Fluocinonide.

4-2. A previously healthy 20-year-old man presents with a 3-day history of rash, fever, malaise, red eyes, and mouth sores. He has been unable to eat due to mouth pain. He denies arthralgias, penile discharge, new medications, drug allergies, or prior similar episodes. Vital signs are blood pressure 100/60 mmHg, pulse 110 beats per minutes, 20 respirations per minute, and temperature 38°C. The patient appears alert but uncomfortable. He has multiple vesiculobullous lesions on his conjunctivae and mouth. Visual acuity is 20/20. Target lesions are found on his palms and soles. What is the next MOST appropriate action?

(A) Discharge with analgesics, antihistamines, and mouth rinses.

(B) Discharge after 1–2 L normal saline IV; prescribe analgesics, antihistamines, oral prednisone, and mouth rinses.

(C) Admit and administer 1–2 L normal saline IV; analgesics, antihistamines, and mouth rinses.

(D) Admit and administer 1–2 L normal saline IV; oral prednisone, analgesics, antihistamines, and mouth rinses.

4-3. Which of the following statements regarding toxic epidermal necrolysis (TEN) and staphylococcal scalded skin syndrome (SSSS) is TRUE?

(A) Nikolsky's sign is positive, and the entire epidermis is involved in both conditions.

(B) Mucous membranes are affected in both conditions.

(C) Ocular morbidity occurs in both conditions.

(D) Tender erythroderma precedes bullous lesions.

4-4. Which of the following statements regarding the rash of meningococcemia and Rocky Mountain spotted fever (RMSF) is TRUE?

(A) The rash coincides with the onset of fever, headache, and myalgias.

(B) The rash is petechial and spreads from the extremities to the trunk.

(C) The rash involves the palms, soles, and mucous membranes.

(D) Purpura fulminans can be a serious complication.

4-5. A 30-year-old man with Hodgkin's disease presents with 36 hours of fever, malaise, dyspnea, and multiple vesicular lesions widely distributed across the head, trunk, and extremities (see Figure 4-1). Intact vesicles are clustered and have an erythematous base. Some lesions are pustular, and others are crusted. His vital signs are blood pressure 120/80 mmHg, pulse 100 beats per minute, respiratory rate 28 breaths per minute, temperature 38°C, and room air oxygen saturation 93%. The patient is alert but appears ill. There is no corneal uptake of fluorescein nor dendritic lesions. His neck is supple, and the neurologic examination is normal. Auscultation of the lungs reveals diffuse, bilateral rales. An IV is started, and blood is sent for lab work and culture. A urinalysis is normal. What is the next MOST appropriate action?

(A) Contact the local health authority and the Centers for Disease Control and Prevention.

(B) Perform computed tomography of the head and chest.

(C) Perform computed tomography of the chest and abdomen.

(D) Administer oxygen, perform a chest radiograph, give intravenous acyclovir, and admit.

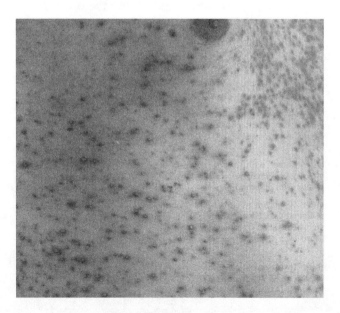

Figure 4-1.

4-6. A 50-year-old woman presents with a 2-day history of blisters on her gums, inner cheeks, and lips. The intraoral blisters have broken and are tender, but she is eating. She denies prior similar episodes, medications, or drug allergies. Vital signs are normal. The patient has excellent dental hygiene. Small, 1-cm, flaccid bullae are visible on the vermillion border of the lips. Nikolsky's sign is positive. Tender superficial erosions are on the gingiva and buccal surface. The gingiva is not inflamed or bloody. The tongue is not ulcerated. Blisters are absent from the remainder of the face and body. There is no corneal fluorescein uptake. The remainder of the physical examination is normal. What is the next MOST appropriate action?

(A) Analgesics, chlorhexidine oral rinses, discharge.

(B) Analgesics, reassurance, discharge.

(C) Analgesics, dermatologic consult (or referral), discharge.

(D) Analgesics, routine dental referral, discharge.

4-7. A 6-month-old girl presents with a papular and vesiculopapular rash involving the scalp, face, palms, and soles. She has scratched the lesions. The mother is concerned because her 5-year-old son just finished a treatment for scabies, following an outbreak at his preschool. What is the MOST appropriate action?

(A) Reassure the mother because scabies does not involve the face or scalp.

(B) Perform a scabies preparation; if positive, prescribe lindane (Kwell).

(C) Perform a scabies preparation; if positive, prescribe crotamiton (Eurax).

(D) Prescribe permethrin 5% cream (Elimite).

4-8. Which of the following statements regarding tinea capitis is TRUE?

(A) It is transmitted only by direct person-to-person contact.

(B) Microsporum species are the main cause of infection.

(C) A kerion is a complication due to bacterial infection.

(D) Treat with ultramicrosized griseofulvin and a selenium sulfide or ketoconazole shampoo.

4-9. Which of the following skin lesions has an "almost pathognomonic" association with Hodgkin's disease?

(A) Acanthosis nigricans.

(B) Dermatomyositis.

(C) Generalized erythroderma.

(D) Ichthyosis.

4-10. A 17-year-old boy presents with a 2-day history of an erythematous, pruritic rash involving both cheeks, lips, and chin. The rash is not oozing and the lower eyelids are spared. After he shaved himself two days ago he applied an aftershave product that belonged to his older brother. In addition to advising him to avoid the product in the future, what is the MOST appropriate treatment?

(A) Topical hydrocortisone and oral antihistamines for 10 days.

(B) Topical hydrocortisone and oral antihistamines for 3–5 days.

(C) Topical triamcinolone and oral antihistamines for 3–5 days.

(D) Topical triamcinolone and oral antihistamines for 10 days.

CHAPTER 4

Disorders of the Skin Emergencies
Answers, Explanations, and References

4-1. **The answer is C** (Chapter 245). Mometasone furoate (Elocon) is not fluorinated. Triamcinolone, betamethasone, and fluocinonide are all fluorinated steroids. Cutaneous atrophy is associated with the use of fluorinated steroids. High-potency preparations should not be used on the face. Fluorinated steroids should not be prescribed to pregnant women due to risk of fetal adrenal suppression.

4-2. **The answer is D** (Chapter 246). The patient has signs suggestive of Stevens-Johnson syndrome, the severe, multisystemic, potentially fatal variant of erythema multiforme. Vesiculobullous lesions commonly affect mucous membranes. Death is usually due to infection and dehydration. Mortality rates range from 10% to 15%. As in this case, patients with severe disease should be admitted. Therapy consists of intravenous fluids, oral prednisone, analgesics, antihistamines, mouth rinses, and skin care. No causative factor can be found in 50% of cases. Known triggers include anticonvulsants, antibiotics, herpes, and mycoplasma infection.

4-3. **The answer is D** (Chapter 246). Both TEN and SSSS involve tender erythroderma followed by skin shedding. Nikolsky's sign is positive when skin is loosened with minimal rubbing or with lateral pressure and is seen in both conditions. However, in TEN, the cleavage plane is between the epidermis and the dermis; shedded skin exposes the dermis. In SSSS, the cleavage plane is intraepidermal; shed skin exposes the deep

epidermal layer. TEN commonly involves the mucous membranes, which are usually spared in SSSS. Secure the airway early in TEN as the airway epithelium may slough. A severe, purulent conjunctivitis occurs with TEN, which may cause permanent injury. SSSS may be initiated by a conjunctivitis, but the subsequent process does not involve the eyes. Tender erythroderma preceeds bullous lesions in both conditions. TEN is associated with drugs, vaccinations, and lymphoma. SSSS follows a staphylococcal infection and involves an exotoxin. Both conditions require fluid replacement and admission. Ideally, patients with TEN should be admitted to a burn unit or a critical care unit.

4-4. **The answer is D** (Chapter 246). Fever, headache, and myalgias occur with the onset of meningococcemia and RMSF. Usually, the rash in RMSF occurs within 2 to 4 days (range 1–15 days) but may be absent for the entire course of the disease in 15% of patients. The rash is evident upon presentation in many patients with meningococcemia. In RMSF, red macules, which blanch with pressure, appear on the wrists and ankles. The RMSF rash rapidly spreads from the distal extremities to the trunk and face and transforms into hemorrhagic macules or petechiae especially evident on the palms and soles. The RMSF rash does not characteristically involve mucous membranes. In meningococcemia, the rash is more protean. Petechiae macules, maculopapules, urticaria, or hemorrhagic vesicles may be evident. Classically the lesions of meningococcemia involve the trunk and extremities, but they may also occur on the head, mucous membranes, palms, and soles. Purpural fulminans is a serious complication in RMSF and meningococcemia. Purpura fulminans occurs when the patient has vascular shock or develops disseminated intravascular coagulation. The classic triad of skin findings includes widespread ecchymoses, hemorrhagic bullae, and epidermal necrosis. Dermal vascular thrombosis causes gangrene of the extremities, nose, ears, and genitalia.

4-5. The answer is D (Chapters 135, 246). The patient has disseminated herpes zoster and signs of pulmonary involvement. He needs oxygen and a chest radiograph. Disseminated herpes zoster occurs in immunocompromised patients such as those with Hodgkin's lymphoma, leukemia, and AIDS. These patients are at risk for ocular, lung, and CNS involvement and require admission and antiviral therapy. The emergency physician should include smallpox in the differential diagnosis of fever and vesicular rash. The local health authority and the Centers for Disease Control and Prevention should be contacted in cases of suspected smallpox. The lesions of classic smallpox are deeper, most prominent on the face and extremities, and are all in the same stage. Varicella lesions are more superficial, most prominent on the trunk, and are in different stages (vesicles, pustules, crusts, and scabs). The emergency physician should always evaluate the corneas for dendritic lesions when vesicles are located in the distribution of the first division of the trigeminal nerve. Since CNS involvement is highly likely, many practitioners would give IV ceftriaxone, get a head computed tomography (CT) scan to rule out mass lesions, and perform a lumbar puncture. Emergent CT of the chest and abdomen are not indicated in this case.

4-6. The answer is C (Chapter 246). The patient has a bullous disease mainly involving the mouth. The differential diagnosis includes

pemphigus vulgaris, bullous pemphigoid, and toxic epidermal necrolysis. An HSV-1 infection would be vesicular and is more common in children than adults. The patient does not have gingivitis and does not need chlorhexadine rinses or a dental referral. Follow up is required with a dermatologist for a skin biopsy with immunofluorescence. Pemphigus vulgaris is a rare but serious autoimmune, mucocutaneous blistering disease. Men are affected more than women. Age of onset is 40–60 years. Over 50% of patients have oral lesions that precede cutaneous blisters. Nikolsky's sign is positive—the flaccid blister spreads with light lateral pressure. Skin biopsy with direct immunofluorescence is diagnostic. Serum autoantibodies to a skin glycoprotein may be detected by indirect immunofluorescence. Patients are treated with high-dose systemic corticosteroids after dermatologic consultation. The average age of onset of bullous pemphigoid is 70 years. The blisters are tense. Oral and cutaneous lesions tend to occur simultaneously. Skin biopsy with immunofluorescence is diagnostic. Serum anti–basement membrane autoantibodies may be detected by indirect immunofluorescence. Treatment involves systemic corticosteroids. Patients with either condition can present with dehydration due to decreased oral intake and significant fluid and electrolyte loss due to the bullae formation. Dermatologic consultation is advised.

4-7. The answer is D (Chapter 250). Infants and young children with scabies develop papular or vesiculopapular lesions involving the scalp, face, palms, and soles. In general, a positive scabies preparation is preferable to empiric treatment. In this case, however, another family member is already affected, which raises the likelihood of infection. Lindane is neurotoxic and contraindicated for use in infants, children, and pregnant women. Permethrin 5% cream is the recommended treatment for scabies in infants and children. Permethrin is more scabicidal than crotamiton and more effectively reduces pruritus and secondary bacterial infection. Apply permethrin 5% cream over the entire body for **8 hours** according to a pediatric dermatology reference. Repeat the treatment in 1 week.

4-8. **The answer is D** (Chapter 247). Tinea capitis is a scalp infection caused by the dermatophyte *Trichophyton tonsurans,* currently epidemic in the United States. Infections during the 1940s and 1950s were caused by *Microsporum audouinii.* Preschool children are most commonly infected, but tinea capitis also affects neonates, infants, and adults. Tinea can spread by direct close contact or by combs, brushes, hats, towels, and pillowcases. *Trichophyton tonsurans* causes seborrheic-like scaling and less alopecia and is not fluorescent on Wood light examination. A kerion is a severe inflammatory reaction from the dermatophyte, causing a tender, boggy, pustular, and indurated plaque, which is not due to a secondary bacterial infection. To mitigate scarring due to a kerion, give prednisone 1 mg/kg/day for 1–2 weeks, in addition to the antifungal medication. Ultramicrosized griseofulvin starting at 15 mg/kg/day with a meal is the treatment of choice, which in conjunction with selenium sulfide 2.5% or ketoconazole 2% shampoo will decrease the shedding of the contagious spores. Topical agents alone are not effective treatment for tinea capitis.

4-9. **The answer is C** (Chapter 164). Generalized erythroderma, which is intensely pruritic, is considered "almost pathognomonic" for Hodgkin's disease. Erythroderma is also common in lymphocytic leukemia. Acanthosis nigricans is strongly associated with adenocarcinoma of the stomach and is also found in cases of breast and lung cancer. Dermatomyositis is associated with carcinomas of the breast, ovary, gastrointestinal tract, and female genital tract. Ichthyosis may be familial or acquired. Hodgkin's disease is the most common malignant disease associated with acquired (nonfamilial) ichthyosis.

4-10. **The answer is B** (Chapter 247). The patient has a mild contact dermatitis of the face due to direct application of an irritant. A brief, 3-to-5-day course of low- to medium-potency topical hydrocortisone is indicated, along with an oral antihistamine to treat pruritus. Care must be taken to avoid getting topical corticosteroids in the eyes due to the potential risk of glaucoma and cataracts. Triamcinolone is a fluorinated corticosteroid that should not be used on the face because it causes cutaneous atrophy. A 10-to-14-day course of systemic steroids is required for severe cases and those with periocular involvement. This patient's case was mild.

Emergency Wound Management
Questions

5-1. Which of the following statements is TRUE with regard to the management of mammalian bites?

(A) Puncture wounds, wounds >24 hours old, and most wounds on the hand and foot should be left open.

(B) Cephalexin, dicloxacillin, erythromycin, or clindamycin are all adequate prophylactic single-agent coverage choices for cat bites.

(C) Although a minority of dog bites become infected, those occurring in postsplenectomy or other immunocompromised patients should have prophylactic antimicrobial coverage initiated.

(D) Cat-scratch disease typically develops 1 to 2 days following a cat bite or scratch.

5-2. Which statement is MOST correct in regard to wound preparation for primary closure?

(A) Local anesthesia should be performed following irrigation to avoid introduction of bacteria deeper into the wound.

(B) Irrigation with normal saline at 5–8 psi is the most effective means of decreasing wound bacterial counts.

(C) Hair that interferes with wound closure should be removed by shaving to prevent entrapment within the wound.

(D) Wounds should be lightly scrubbed to remove particulate matter, followed by irrigation with a povidone-iodine solution.

5-3. What are some benefits of cyanoacrylate tissue adhesives compared to standard suture material for wound closure?

(A) Rapid and painless application.

(B) Decreased rate of wound dehiscence.

(C) Increased wound tensile strength.

(D) Improved cosmetic outcome.

5-4. Which of the following eyelid wounds is not a clear indication for ophthalmologic referral for further management?

(A) Laceration of the inner surface of the lid.

(B) Lid margin lacerations.

(C) Medial lacerations involving the lacrimal system.

(D) Lateral wounds running parallel to the lid margin.

5-5. A 21-year-old male presents with a lower extremity laceration that occurred after falling out of his canoe in a nearby river approximately 4 hours prior to arrival. What statement is most correct regarding this patient's injury?

(A) Irrigation of the wound is not required as the wound was immediately cleansed while submerged in the water.

(B) Infectious complications in this type of wound usually occur in a delayed fashion at 7–10 days postinjury.

(C) Antimicrobial prophylaxis is not indicated.

(D) *Aeromonas hydrophila* exposure should be considered.

5-6. A 22-year-old night club bouncer presents with a dorsal hand laceration following an altercation the night prior to arrival. The wound is approximately 0.5 cm in length, overlying the third metacarpophalangeal joint. What statement is correct in considering this patient's management?

(A) Radiography is rarely indicated unless bone or joint tenderness is present.

(B) Evidence of infection necessitates immediate hand surgeon consultation.

(C) Meticulous wound inspection through range of motion is required.

(D) *Eikenella corrodens* is the most common bacterial species implicated in human bite infections.

5-7. A 40-year-old carpenter presents with a digital fingertip amputation. There is a soft tissue defect (approximately 1 cm × 1 cm) of the volar pad without bony exposure. Which of the following statements best describes the optimal management of this injury?

(A) Primary closure is indicated, via undermining of the wound edges, even if significant wound tension exists.

(B) Immediate hand specialist consultation is required.

(C) Use of the amputated portion for full thickness grafting clearly results in the best functional and cosmetic outcome.

(D) Conservative management with serial dressing changes is indicated.

Emergency Wound Management
Answers, Explanations, and References

5-1. **The answer is C** (Chapter 49). A rare but serious complication of dog bites, due to the bacterium *Capnocytophaga canimorsus,* is associated with overwhelming sepsis and most commonly occurs in immunocompromised patients. Approximately 60–80% of cat bites will become infected, with a significant portion of these due to *Pasteurella multocida. Pasteurella,* although sensitive to penicillin, is inadequately covered by cephalexin, dicloxacillin, erythromycin, or clindamycin. Primary closure of mammalian bite wounds >6 hours old is contraindicated in most situations. *Bartonella henselae* is the causative agent in cat-scratch disease resulting in regional lymphadenopathy approximately 7–12 days following innoculation.

5-2. **The answer is B** (Chapter 41). Proper wound preparation is the cornerstone of wound management by allowing for an optimal cosmetic result while restoring function and minimizing the risk of infection. Irrigation at 5–8 psi can be accomplished using a 19-gauge plastic catheter attached to a 35–65-mL syringe. Sterile normal saline is the least tissue-toxic irrigant. Irrigants that contain providone-iodine, chlorhexidine, and hydrogen peroxide actually increase a wound's susceptibility to infection. Local anesthesia should be performed before irrigation or debridement and is not associated with an increased risk of wound infection. If hair removal is required to facilitate suturing, clipping is recommended as shaving will significantly increase the rate of wound infection.

5-3. **The answer is A** (Chapter 42). Octyl-cyanoacrylate tissue ahesives allow for rapid and painless wound closure. This can often be accomplished without the use of needles, even if wound anesthesia is required, by using topical anesthetics. The tissue adhesives have equivalent cosmetic outcomes and a small increase in absolute wound dehiscence rates. Tissue adhesives are equivalent in strength to standard 5-0 suture material and thus should not be used for wound edges requiring more than gentle hand or forcep approximation.

5-4. **The answer is D** (Chapter 43). Eyelid injuries require a meticulous evaluation due to the delicate yet complex anatomical structures. Errors in wound management can result in significant cosmetic as well as functional morbidity. Management of laterally located eyelid lacerations running parallel to the wound margin is within the emergency medicine physician's scope of practice. Injuries involving the lid margins can result in a notched appearance if not perfectly aligned. Lacrimal system injuries may be difficult to diagnose initially and if not properly repaired can result in chronic tearing. Palpebral conjuctival lacerations as well as injuries resulting in ptosis clearly require specialist referral for definitive management.

5-5. **The answer is D** (Chapter 45). *Aeromonas hydrophila* is associated with lacerations sustained in freshwater lakes and streams. Such infections occur within 8–48 hours, are rapidly progressive, and are associated

6-7. Which one of the following classes of medications is know to adversely affect glycemic control?

(A) Anticonvulsants.

(B) Antihistamines.

(C) Antidepressants.

(D) Calcium channel blockers.

6-8. Which one of the following types of infections is proven to be more frequent in patients with diabetes?

(A) Pneumonia.

(B) Urinary tract infections.

(C) Sinusitis.

(D) Otitis media.

6-9. A well-known alcoholic patient presents to your ED with anorexia, vomiting, and abdominal pain. He does not have a "surgical abdomen" on exam. He is found to have blood glucose of 250 mg/dL and a wide anion gap metabolic acidosis without a history of toxic ingestion. Which of the following is TRUE regarding the therapy of this patient?

(A) A negative urinary ketone test effectively rules out alcoholic or diabetic ketoacidosis.

(B) The patient should be aggressively hydrated with normal saline.

(C) The patient should be aggressively hydrated with D_5NS.

(D) The patient should immediately receive a loading dose of insulin.

6-10. Which of the following is a possible mechanism for the lack of ketoacidosis seen in patients with hyperosmolar hyperglycemic nonketotic syndrome compared to patients with diabetic ketoacidosis?

(A) Higher levels of counterregulatory hormones.

(B) Higher levels of endogenous insulin.

(C) Lower levels of glucagon.

(D) Higher levels of lipolysis.

6-11. Which of the following is a diagnostic criterion for hyperosmolar hyperglycemic nonketotic syndrome?

(A) Plasma glucose >250 mg/dL.

(B) Arterial pH >7.25.

(C) Serum bicarbonate >15 mEq/L.

(D) Anion gap >12.

6-12. A 70-year-old female is brought to the ED because of altered level of consciousness. The building manager found the patient in her apartment after she had not been seen for several days. There is no past medical history available. The patient is delirious and presents with a fever of 103°F, systolic blood pressure of 90 mmHg, and a heart rate of 160 beats per minute that appear to be sinus tachycardia on the monitor. The patient is unable to provide you with any past medical history, but you find an Atrovent inhaler and bottle of propylthiouracil in her purse. The patient becomes combative and requires paralysis and intubation to manage her medical condition. Following her intubation she is placed on a monitor, and two large-bore IVs are established and aggressive fluid hydration begun. What is the next medication you should administer?

(A) Propanolol.

(B) Esmolol.

(C) Propylthiouracil.

(D) Iodine.

6-13. Which of the following is the most common etiology of hyperthyroidism?

(A) Thyroiditis.

(B) Excessive thyroid hormone ingestion (thyrotoxicosis facticia).

(C) Toxic multinodular goiter.

(D) Graves' disease.

6-14. Which one of the following is an electrocardiogram change consistent with myxedema coma?

(A) Prolongation of the QT interval.

(B) Premature ventricular contractions.

(C) Premature atrial contractions.

(D) Left ventricular hypertrophy.

6-15. Which of the following is the most common infectious cause worldwide of primary adrenal insufficiency?

(A) Human immunodeficiency virus.

(B) Cytomegalovirus.

(C) Tuberculosis.

(D) *Pseudomonas* organisms.

CHAPTER 6

Endocrinologic Emergencies
Answers, Explanations, and References

6-1. **The answer is C** (Chapter 210). Metformin, a biguanide, improves the end organ sensitivity to insulin and acts by a number of mechanism in diabetic patients, including a reduction in hepatic glucose output and enhanced peripheral glucose uptake. Metformin is considered an antihyperglycemic drug rather than a hypoglycemic agent such as the sulfonylureas and insulin. While less likely than the sulfonylureas, the nonsulfonylureas are also associated with a hypoglycemic response.

6-2. **The answer is A** (Chapter 210). The condition of alcoholics, the elderly, and others with depleted glycogen stores will generally not improve with glucagons. Octreotide is only recommended after initial glucose therapy has been initiated in the sulfonylurea ingestion. It should be considered when oral hypoglycemic agent (OHA) induced hypoglycemia is not responding to dextrose therapy. Steroid administration should be considered for hypoglycemia that is either resistant to aggressive glucose replacement therapy or associated with signs of adrenal insufficiency. Untreated hypoglycemia is deleterious to the medically or traumatically injured brain.

6-3. **The answer is D** (Chapter 211). Insulin's main action occurs at the three principal tissues of energy storage and metabolism (i.e., liver, adipose tissue, and skeletal muscle). Insulin acts on the liver to facilitate the uptake of glucose and its conversion to glycogen while inhibiting glycogen breakdown (glycogenolysis) and suppressing gluconeogenesis. Insulin's effect on lipid metabolism is to increase lipogenesis in the liver and adipose cells by the production of triglycerides from free fatty acids and glycerol while inhibiting the breakdown of triglycerides. Insulin stimulates the uptake of amino acids into muscle cells while preventing the release of amino acids from muscles and hepatic sources.

6-4. **The answer is C** (Chapter 211). Only 2% of total-body potassium is intravascular. The initial serum concentration is usually normal or high because of the intracellular exchange of potassium for hydrogen ions during acidosis, the total-body fluid deficit, and diminished renal function. Initial hypokalemia indicates severe total-body depletion. During initial therapy for DKA, the serum potassium concentration may fall rapidly, primarily due to the action of insulin. As a general guideline, an initial serum potassium level >3.3 mEq/L and <5.0 mEq/L coupled with urine output calls for 10 mEq potassium chloride per hour replacement in intravenous fluid for at least 4 hours.

6-5. **The answer is D** (Chapter 211). Young age and new-onset diabetes are risk factors for the development of cerebral edema secondary to the treatment of DKA. Any change in neurologic function early in the therapy of DKA should prompt the clinician to immediately administer mannitol (1–2 g/kg), which should be at the bedside of high-risk patients. Mannitol should be given prior to obtaining confirmatory computed tomography scans because serious morbidity and mortality may be prevented. Other aggressive measures such as intubation, hyperventilation, and fluid restrictions may be necessary following your initial treatment with mannitol.

6-6. **The answer is B** (Chapter 211). The older terminology for type 2 diabetes includes non-insulin-dependent diabetes mellitus or adult-onset-diabetes mellitus. Unlike type 1 diabetes, type 2 diabetes can be prevented or delayed with lifestyle interventions. Patients with type 2 diabetes often require insulin at some point in their course of therapy. Therapy of type 2 diabetes typically is initiated stepwise from diet/exercise to oral agents to insulin or combination oral agent–insulin therapies. It is estimated that 100 million people worldwide have diabetes, with 85 to 90 percent of cases being type 2.

6-7. **The answer is A** (Chapter 211). The most common glucose-altering medications include corticosteroids, sympathomimetics, diuretics, anticonvulsants, salicylates, and β-adrenergic receptor antagonists.

6-8. **The answer is B** (Chapter 211). While there are possible epidemiologic associations between diabetes and many infectious diseases, only urinary tract infections, other urogenital infections, and skin infections have been shown to be more frequent in diabetic patients than control groups in retrospective or prospective studies.

6-9. **The answer is C** (Chapter 213). This patient's diagnosis is alcoholic ketoacidosis (AKA). The standard test for ketone detection is serum or urine nitroprusside test. While β-hydroxybuterate is the predominant ketone present in AKA, acetoacetate is the only ketone normally detected by the nitroprusside test. Since patients with AKA may have only mildly elevated acetoacetate levels, it is important to not exclude the diagnosis of AKA with a negative test. Therapy is aimed at both glucose adminis-

tration and volume replacement. The fluid of choice is D_5NS. Insulin is of no proven benefit and may be dangerous because patients often have depleted glycogen stores and normal or low glucose levels.

6-10. **The answer is B** (Chapter 214). The reason for the absence of ketoacidosis in hyperosmolar hyperglycemic nonketotic syndrome is not clearly understood. The relative lack of ketoacidosis has been attributed to three possible mechanisms: (1) lower levels of counterregulatory hormones, (2) higher levels of endogenous insulin, which strongly inhibits lipolysis, and (3) inhibition of lipolysis by the hyperosmolar state. There is controversy about the role of counterregulatory hormones such as glucagon.

6-11. **The answer is C** (Chapter 214). The diagnostic criteria for hyperosmolar hyperglycemic nonketotic syndrome includes a plasma glucose >600 mg/dL, arterial pH >7.30, serum bicarbonate >15 mEq/L, small amount of urine and serum ketones, effective serum osmolarity >320 mOsm/L, anion gap <12, and the presence of stupor or coma.

6-12. **The answer is B** (Chapter 215). This patient's fever and tachycardia out of proportion to the fever along with her altered level of consciousness, and the fact that propylthiouracil was found in her purse, all point to a presumptive diagnosis of thyroid storm. Initial therapy is stabilization, airway protection, oxygenation, intravenous fluids, and monitoring. β-blockers are first-line therapy to treat the severe adrenergic symptoms that are resulting in her hemodynamic instability. While propanolol is the treatment of choice in most patients, it is contraindicated in patients with a history of asthma, congestive heart failure, or chronic obstructive pulmonary disease (COPD). A selective β-1 medication such as esmolol should be used in this patient given the likelihood of her having a COPD history based upon the Atrovent found in her purse. Decreasing synthesis of additional hormone is a second-line therapy and can be accomplished with the administration of propylthiouracil. Iodine decreases the release of preformed thyroid hormone but must not be administered until the synthetic pathway has been blocked.

6-13.   **The answer is D** (Chapter 215). Graves' disease is the most common etiology of hyperthyroidism, accounting for more than 80% of cases in the United States. Toxic multinodular and toxic nodular goiters are the next most frequent etiologies. Graves' disease is common in the third and fourth decades of life and is caused by an autoimmune thyroid-stimulating antibody that activates the thyrotropin receptor on thyroid cells.

6-14.   **The answer is A** (Chapter 216). Electrocardiogram changes seen in myxedema coma include sinus bradycardia, prolongation of the QT interval, and low voltage with flattening or inversion of T waves.

6-15.   **The answer is C** (Chapter 217). Worldwide, tuberculosis is the most common infectious cause of primary adrenal insufficiency. In the United States, however, infection with the human immunodeficiency virus (HIV) is the most common cause. HIV may cause adrenal insufficiency via opportunistic infections (principally cytomegalovirus), the use of medications such as ketokonazole, or inhibition of the hypothalamic–pituitary–adrenal (HPA) axis by cytokines released by macrophages.

Environmental and Unique Environments Emergencies
Questions

7-1. Which of the following statements is TRUE regarding cold-related injuries?

(A) Chilbain (pernio) is more common in men than women.

(B) Dry heat is the best method for rewarming frostbite.

(C) Early surgical intervention is required for severe frostbite.

(D) Trench foot may result in irreversible damage.

7-2. Which of the following is NOT a predisposing factor for hypothermia?

(A) Extremes of age.

(B) Hyperglycemia.

(C) Severe burns.

(D) Alcoholism.

7-3. Which of the following types of heat injury is correctly paired with the appropriate treatment?

(A) Heat exhaustion and rapid evaporative cooling.

(B) Heat stroke and oral rehydration.

(C) Heat cramps and fluid and electrolyte replacement.

(D) Prickly heat and talc or baby powder.

7-4. What is the MOST common finding in a patient with a brown recluse spider bite?

(A) Severe itching.

(B) Local tissue necrosis.

(C) Severe muscle cramps.

(D) Anaphylaxis.

7-5. A 25-year-old man complains of pain and swelling in his hand and forearm, perioral numbness, and vomiting after trying to catch a rattlesnake. His blood pressure is 90/60 mmHg. Which of the following therapies is NOT indicated?

(A) Fluid resuscitation.

(B) Immediate fasciotomy of the arm.

(C) Administration of 10 vials of antivenin.

(D) Measurement of coagulation factors and platelets.

7-6. Which of the following is TRUE regarding marine envenomations?

(A) Jellyfish nematocysts are inactivated by fresh water rinsing.

(B) Sponge dermatitis is treated with antibiotics against gram-negative organisms.

(C) Hot water immersion is an effective pain reliever for venomous fish and stingray injuries.

(D) Tetrodotoxin poisoning from an octopus bite may be reversed with antivenin.

7-7. A 55-year-old male diver begins complaining of back pain and urinary retention 1 hour after a dive. What is the MOST likely diagnosis?

(A) Barotrauma to the bladder.

(B) Neurotoxin from a marine envenomation.

(C) Nitrogen narcosis.

(D) Decompression sickness.

7-8. An unconscious teenage near-drowning victim is brought to the ED by ambulance after diving into the shallow end of his friend's pool at a party. A brief period of ventilation was required poolside. Which of the following tests is LEAST likely to impact patient management?

(A) Core temperature.
(B) Electrolytes.
(C) Chest radiograph.
(D) C-spine radiographs.

7-9. Which of the following patients does NOT require referral to a specialized burn care facility?

(A) A 60-year-old diabetic with a full-thickness burn of his entire forearm.
(B) A 25-year-old woman with full-thickness burns of both hands and lower arms.
(C) A 35-year-old man with a few small areas of partial-thickness burns on his back and small full-thickness burns on his upper arm.
(D) A 40-year-old house fire victim with a few small partial-thickness burns on her arms, soot in her nasal pharynx, and wheezing.

7-10. Which of the following statements about chemical burns is TRUE?

(A) Acids cause deeper tissue injury than alkalis.
(B) Finding and treating with chemical-specific antidotes is usually more critical than irrigation with water or saline.
(C) Calcium gluconate is a specific antidote for sulfuric acid burns.
(D) Time of exposure is the most important factor in determining the extent of tissue damage.

7-11. Which of the following is TRUE regarding electrical injuries?

(A) Household voltage (110 V) may cause ventricular fibrillation without evidence of electrical burns.

(B) Low-voltage AC is more likely to produce transient ventricular asystole, and high-voltage AC is more likely to cause ventricular fibrillation.
(C) Labial artery bleeding commonly occurs immediately after oral electrical burns.
(D) Delayed cardiac arrhythmias are common after household voltage electrical injuries.

7-12. A 35-year-old man presents complaining of a headache, weakness, nausea, and vomiting after working on his car in a closed garage. Which of the following statements regarding management of this patient's problem is TRUE?

(A) Pulse oximetry can aid in assessing the severity of illness.
(B) Hyperbaric oxygen therapy is indicated.
(C) The patient may be discharged if his symptoms resolve after treatment with 100% oxygen.
(D) Severe metabolic acidosis may be present.

7-13. Which of the following best describes a patient with *Amanita phalloides* mushroom intoxication?

(A) Visual hallucinations and ataxia within 30 minutes after ingestion.
(B) Flushing, tachycardia, and palpitations several hours after mushroom ingestion and shortly after drinking a martini.
(C) Symptoms of the SLUDGE syndrome within 30 minutes after ingestion.
(D) Nausea, vomiting, and diarrhea within 24 hours of ingestion followed by hepatic failure in 3 days.

7-14. Which of the following plants is correctly matched with its toxic effects?

(A) Foxglove and neuromuscular blockage.
(B) Hemlock and mucous membrane pain and burning.

(C) Jimson weed and hallucinations.

(D) Castor bean and cardiac arrhythmias.

7-15. A patient presents with fever and malaise but without rash, pulmonary, or gastrointestinal symptoms. She returned to the United States 1 week ago after traveling in West Africa for 2 weeks. What is the most likely diagnosis?

(A) Malaria.

(B) Hepatitis A.

(C) Tuberculosis.

(D) Rickettsial infection.

7-16. Which of the following travel exposures is correctly matched to its specific associated infection?

(A) Undercooked meat and schistosomiasis.

(B) Untreated water products and amebiasis.

(C) Rodent contact and African sleeping sickness.

(D) Tsetse flies and viral hemorrhagic fevers.

7-17. Which of the following statements regarding typhoid fever is TRUE?

(A) The vaccine is highly effective.

(B) The disease is transmitted by insect bites.

(C) Patients usually present with constipation rather than diarrhea.

(D) It is an uncommon cause of prolonged fever in returning travelers.

7-18. Which of the following statements about traveler's diarrhea is TRUE?

(A) Viral causes account for about 50–70% of all acute cases of traveler's diarrhea.

(B) *Giardia lamblia* is the most commonly identified cause of chronic diarrhea.

(C) Amebiasis typically causes nonbloody diarrhea without fever.

(D) Antibiotic treatment does not improve outcomes in patients with cholera.

7-19. Which of the following statements regarding acclimatization to high altitude is TRUE?

(A) Increased ventilation is the primary initial adaptation to high altitude.

(B) Erythropoetin levels rise only after several weeks at high altitude.

(C) Water retention facilitates adaptation to high altitude.

(D) Given enough time, the body will eventually adapt to any altitude.

7-20. Which of the following is NOT a common high-altitude syndrome?

(A) Allergic asthma.

(B) Peripheral edema.

(C) Bronchitis and pharyngitis.

(D) Retinopathy.

7-21. Which of the following statements regarding Antarctic medicine is TRUE?

(A) Telemedicine has not proved to be helpful to medical practitioners in Antarctica due to polar cap absorption (PCA) radio blackouts.

(B) Practicing medicine at the South Pole does not require specialized knowledge of Antarctica-specific diseases and ailments.

(C) Cold-related injuries are common in Antarctica.

(D) During summer months medical evacuations can easily be obtained when a serious emergency occurs.

7-22. Which of the following is TRUE about medical problems in space?

(A) Adverse psychological reactions are common due to the enclosed living conditions.

(B) Hemostasis is more difficult in microgravity than on Earth.

(C) Space motion sickness is rare.

(D) Ocular foreign bodies are common problems in microgravity.

Environmental and Unique Environments Emergencies
Answers, Explanations, and References

7-1. **The answer is D** (Chapter 191). Trench foot develops from exposure to wet, cold but nonfreezing conditions over hours to days. Early on, tissue damage is reversible but can become permanent if the foot is not removed from the cold environment. Rapid rewarming in warm water (40–42°C) is the primary therapy for frostbite. Dry heat from fires or car exhaust should be avoided as it may cause thermal damage on top of the cold injury. Early surgical intervention is not indicated as the extent of injury is difficult to assess initially and areas of eschar may be protective to underlying healing tissue. Chilbain is more common in women than men.

7-2. **The answer is B** (Chapter 192). Hypoglycemia, not hyperglycemia, may lead to hypothermia secondary to hypothalmic dysfunction. Other endocrine disorders such as hypothyroidism and hypoadrenalism predispose to hypothermia because of decreased metabolic rate. Severe burns and other dermal diseases may impair the skin's ability to thermoregulate or prevent vasoconstriction. Patients at the extremes of age are more vulnerable to hypothermia. The use of any drug, including alcohol, that causes altered sensorium places a patient at higher risk for hypothermia.

7-3. **The answer is C** (Chapter 193). Heat stroke is defined as a body temperature of greater than 40°C (104°F) accompanied by altered mental status and anhidrosis. Patients with heat stroke should be aggressively cooled to a temperature of 40°C (104°F), at which

point cooling measures should stop to avoid overshoot hypothermia. Heat exhaustion is a heat-related illness with severe volume depletion where sweating and mental status are preserved and temperature does not get above 40°C. It is treated with volume and electrolyte replacement, and oral rehydration may be sufficient. Heat cramps occur after vigorous exercise in individuals who have been sweating profusely and replacing fluid losses with water alone. Treatment consists of oral or IV fluid and salt replacement. Prickly heat is a pruritic, maculopapular rash due to inflammation of blocked sweat ducts. Antihistimines and chlorhexidine cream are the treatment of choice for the acute phase.

7-4. **The answer is B** (Chapter 194). Brown recluse species *(Loxosceles reclusa)* are among the most common spiders in the United States. A necrotic wound that may take weeks or months to heal often follows a bite. Wounds may be resistant to treatment and result in long-term disability. Severe muscle cramping, particularly of the abdominal musculature, is the hallmark of black widow spider envenomation. Anaphylaxis may result from insect stings, the most common being yellow jacket stings.

7-5. **The answer is B** (Chapter 195). The mainstay of treatment following rattlesnake bites is neutralization of the venom with antivenin. Large amounts of antivenin may be required. Coagulation factors and platelets should be checked in all snakebite victims to help determine the severity of envenomation. Supportive care, including fluid resuscitation, is important for all patients with pit viper envenomation. If compartment syndrome is suspected, pressures should be measured. Fasciotomy should be performed only when compartment pressures remain >30 mmHg after medical treatment.

7-6. **The answer is C** (Chapter 196). Hot water immersion can relieve pain in patients who have been stung by a stingray or venomous fish. Fresh water rinsing may stimulate nematocyst discharge and make jellyfish stings worse. Vinegar is the treatment of choice. Sponge dermatitis is a painful, itchy, inflammatory reaction, not an infection, and is treated with antihistamines and steroids in severe cases. Marine-associated infections are most commonly caused by normal skin flora, but gram-negative rods, especially *Vibrio* species, are the most common marine bacteria. There is no antivenin available for tetrodotoxin, but with supportive care, including mechanical ventilation if needed, full recovery is usual.

7-7. **The answer is D** (Chapter 197). Decompression sickness (DCS) is caused by formation of gas bubbles in tissues after ascent from a dive and results in vascular occlusion, usually in the venous circulation. DCS may have cutaneous manifestations including rash and pruritis. It classically causes joint and back pain and may be associated with neurologic symptoms secondary to spinal cord involvement. Patients with neurologic or other severe forms of DCS should be referred for hyperbaric oxygen therapy. Barotrauma is the most common affliction of divers and usually affects the ears, sinuses, lungs, and rarely the gastrointestinal tract. The bladder is not involved. Nitrogen narcosis is due to the anesthetic effects of breathing nitrogen at high partial pressures and causes divers to become altered on deep dives.

7-8. **The answer is B** (Chapter 198). Electrolytes are rarely abnormal in near-drowning vic-

tims unless a large amount of salt water has been aspirated. Near-drowning victims require aggressive resuscitation and evaluation. A core temperature must be obtained as near-drowning patients are frequently hypothermic and require rewarming. Chest radiographs (CXR) may demonstrate pulmonary edema but may be initially normal. Patients with a normal CXR may still be hypoxic, and oxygenation should be measured by arterial blood gases or pulse oximetry. Because many near-drownings occur secondary to trauma, all victims need their C spines evaluated for injury.

7-9. **The answer is C** (Chapter 199). Criteria for major burns requiring specialized burn center admission include: (1) patients ages 10–50 with partial-thickness burns greater than 25% of total body surface area (TBSA); (2) full-thickness burns to greater than 10% TBSA in anyone; (3) patients younger than 10 or older than 50 years with partial-thickness burns greater than 20% TBSA; (4) burns involving the face, hands, feet, or perineum; (5) burns crossing major joints; (6) circumferential limb burns; (7) patient with burns and inhalation injury; (8) electrical burns; (9) any patient with burns and underlying medical problems; (10) burns in infants and elderly patients; and (11) burns complicated by fractures or other trauma.

7-10. **The answer is D** (Chapter 200). Acids generally cause protein denaturation and coagulation necrosis that creates a tough eschar, limiting the spread of the toxic compound. Alkalis cause liquifaction necrosis, allowing the agent to penetrate more deeply into the tissue and cause more extensive damage. The mainstay of therapy for all chemical burns is reducing the length of time of exposure to the compound by immediate, copious irrigation with water. In addition, hydrofluoric acid (not sulfuric acid) burns should be treated with calcium gluconate gel or injection.

7-11. **The answer is A** (Chapter 201). Cutaneous burns tend to be minimal with household voltages (110 V). Electrical burns are absent in more than 40% of cases of low-voltage electrocution deaths because 110 V AC is capable of producing ventricular fibrillation but deposits relatively little heat energy into the skin. High-voltage injuries generally cause severe skin burns and are more likely to cause transient ventricular asystole than ventricular fibrillation. There is little risk of delayed cardiac arrhythmias after household voltage electrical injury. Labial artery bleeding is a common delayed complication from oral electrical burns.

7-12. **The answer is C** (Chapter 203). Carbon monoxide (CO) exposure occurs from many sources, including fires, engines, home furnaces, and heaters. CO binds hemoglobin with a 250 times greater affinity than oxygen. Pulse oximetry cannot be used to determine arterial oxygenation in the setting of CO intoxication because the device confuses carboxyhemoglobin (COHb) for oxyhemoglobin, thus giving a spuriously high reading for oxygen saturation. Hyperbaric oxygen treatment is indicated in patients with severe manifestations including altered mental status, seizures, myocardial ischemia, or pregnancy with COHb >15%. Patients with mild symptoms that resolve after treatment with 100% oxygen may safely be discharged. The presence of a high COHb level and a severe metabolic acidosis should suggest concomitant intoxication with cyanide, as can commonly occur in house or industrial fires. CO alone does not cause a severe metabolic acidosis.

7-13. **The answer is D** (Chapter 204). Nearly all deaths in the United States from mushroom poisoning are due to the *Amanita* species. *Amanita phalloides*, as well as other *Amanita* species and *Gyromitra esculenta*, cause delayed gastrointestinal symptoms that appear 6–24 hours after ingestion and then progress to cause hepatic failure and death. *Psilocybe* mushrooms cause hallucinations. *Coprinus* mushrooms can cause a disulfi-

ram reaction, and *Inocybe* and *Clitocybe* mushrooms cause a muscarinic (SLUDGE) syndrome.

7-14. **The answer is C** (Chapter 205). Jimson weed causes hallucinations due to its anticholinergic properties. Foxglove contains cardiac glycosides similar to digitalis and can cause hyperkalemia and cardiac arrhythmias. Poison hemlock contains coniine alkaloids similar to nicotine that can induce neuromuscular blockade. Castor bean contains the potent ricin toxin that has severe cytotoxic effects on multiple organ systems. Capsicum, as frequently encountered in police pepper spray, causes mucous membrane irritation with burning and pain.

7-15. **The answer is A** (Chapter 206). Malaria is a common infection in most tropical and subtropical areas, including West Africa, and is one of the most common causes of fever in returning travelers. Hepatitis A generally presents with gastrointestinal symptoms and jaundice and has a longer incubation period. Tuberculosis has an incubation period of months and would be unusual for a tourist to acquire. Rickettsial infections are also common sources of fever in returning travelers but are classically associated with a rash and history of a tick bite.

7-16. **The answer is B** (Chapter 206). Undercooked meat is a common source for trichinosis and salmonella. Schistosomiasis is associated with exposure to freshwater. Ingestion of untreated water is associated with amebiasis as well as salmonella, shigella, and hepatitis. Rodent contact is a risk factor for viral hemorrhagic fevers, and tsetse flies are the vector for trypanosomiasis, African sleeping sickness.

7-17. **The answer is C** (Chapter 206). Typhoid fever is a common cause of fever in returning travelers. Also called enteric fever, it is caused by *Salmonella typhi* and *S. paratyphi* and is transmitted by fecal-oral contamination. Vaccine is recommended but is only

75% effective. Patients usually present with fever and headache. Gastrointestinal symptoms commonly include abdominal distention and constipation rather than diarrhea.

7-18. **The answer is B** (Chapter 206). Giardiasis is the most commonly identified cause of chronic diarrhea. Most cases of acute traveler's diarrhea are bacterial, and viral causes account for only 5–10% of cases. Amebiasis is another cause of chronic diarrhea that is associated with bloody diarrhea and fever. Antibiotics for cholera can shorten the illness course, diminish vomiting, lessen volume resuscitation needs, and ensure that bacteria are eradicated from stool.

7-19. **The answer is A** (Chapter 207). Increased ventilation is the primary initial adaptation to high altitude as a result of the hypoxic ventilatory response (HVR). Erythropoetin levels rise within 2 hours of ascent to altitude; however, red cell mass takes weeks to increase. Water loss, as a result of bicarbonate diuresis from respiratory alkalosis and suppression of antidiuretic hormone and aldosterone, results in decreased plasma volume and hemoconcentration. Diuresis is considered a healthy response to high altitude, and antidiuresis is a hallmark of acute mountain sickness. The body cannot acclimatize to all altitudes. At extreme altitudes over 5,490 m (18,000 ft) the body will not adjust but will gradually deteriorate.

7-20. **The answer is A** (Chapter 207). High altitudes do not exacerbate asthma, and patients with allergic asthma do better at high altitudes because of the reduced allergens. Swelling of the hands and face is common at high altitudes and may be associated with acute mountain sickness. Bronchitis and pharyngitis are often seen in persons exercising at altitudes over 2,500 m due to cold, dry air and increased ventilation. Several types of retinal abnormalities have been described at high altitudes. Retinal hemorrhages are common.

7-21. **The answer is B** (Chapter 208). Although the South Pole is unique because of the remoteness and isolation, there are no known Antarctica-specific diseases. Persons practicing in Antarctica must have a broad range of knowledge and skills, because even in summer medical evacuation cannot be guaranteed. Telemedicine has been important for medical practice and research in Antarctica, providing remote access to educational materials, specialist consultation, and clinical support. Transmission of medical and biomedical data from Antarctica to home countries occurs regularly and is not impeded by PCA radio blackouts. Trauma and accidents are the most common conditions in Antarctica, and cold-related injuries are uncommon.

7-22. **The answer is D** (Chapter 209). In the absence of gravity, small airborne particles can injure the eye, and ocular foreign bodies have been a common problem. Hemostasis does not present any different challenges in space than it does on Earth. Bleeding responds to direct pressure, cauterization, and wound repair. Space motion sickness is the most common medical problem in space. No adverse psychological reactions have been reported from any of the numerous space missions.

8-3. A 66-year-old woman with a history of hypertension and allergy to "sulfa" complains of acute onset of left eye pain, headache, and vomiting. On physical exam she has a steamy cornea, fixed mid-dilated pupils, photophobia, and an intraocular pressure of 60 mmHg. What is the most appropriate course of action?

(A) Administer intravenous analgesics, antiemetics, mannitol, and acetazolamide. Give topical β-blockers and mydriatics. Call for emergent ophthalmologic consultation.

(B) Administer intravenous analgesics, antiemetics, and mannitol. Give topical β-blockers, steroids, and miotics. Call for emergent ophthalmologic consultation.

(C) Administer intravenous analgesics, antiemetics, mannitol, and acetazolamide. Give topical β-blockers, steroids, and miotics. Call for emergent ophthalmologic consultation.

(D) Administer intravenous analgesics, antiemetics, and mannitol. Give topical β-blockers, steroids, and mydriatics. Call for emergent ophthalmologic consultation.

8-4. A woman comes in complaining of 12 hours of diplopia in all directions except right lateral gaze. She has a dilated right pupil that can look only to the right. What is the most likely diagnosis?

(A) Wernicke's encephalopathy.
(B) Carotid dissection.
(C) Aneurysm.
(D) Diabetes mellitus.

8-5. A 16-year-old with sickle cell disease was hit in the eye with a fist. His visual acuity is normal. On physical exam, he has mild periorbital edema, mild enophthalmos, and upward gaze diplopia; fundus is normal. Slit lamp exam is normal except for a small dependent hyphema, and his intraocular pressure measures 30 mmHg. Which of the following is the MOST appropriate treatment?

(A) He should be treated with topical β-blockers, steroids, cycloplegics, and intravenous acetazolamide to reduce intraocular pressure (IOP), get an orbital computed tomography (CT) scan, and have immediate ophthalmologic consultation.

(B) He should be treated with topical β-blockers, steroids, cycloplegics, and intravenous acetazolamide to reduce IOP, get an orbital CT scan, and have ophthalmology follow-up within 24 hours.

(C) He should be treated with topical β-blockers, steroids, and cycloplegics to reduce IOP, and get an orbital CT scan and immediate ophthalmologic consultation.

(D) He should be treated with topical β-blockers, steroids, and cycloplegics to reduce IOP, get an orbital CT scan, and follow-up with ophthalmology in 24 hours.

8-6. A 7-year-old girl scraped her eye with an apple stem. Her visual acuity is 20/20. She has moderate photophobia and is rubbing her eye, crying. On slit lamp exam, she has a 6-mm superficial linear abrasion of her cornea in the temporal inferior quadrant. Seidel's test is negative. The anterior chamber is quiet. What is the MOST appropriate treatment?

(A) Erythromycin ointment, an eye patch, pain medication, and ophthalmologic follow-up in 24 hours.

(B) One drop of homatropine, plus tobramycin eyedrops, an eye patch, pain medication, and ophthalmologic follow-up in 24 hours.

(C) One drop of homatropine, plus erythromycin ointment, pain medication, and ophthalmologic follow-up in 24 hours.

(D) Tobramycin eyedrops, topical steroids, pain medication, and ophthalmologic follow-up in 24 hours.

8-7. Which of the following statements about acute hearing impairment is MOST accurate?

   (A) Sudden hearing loss (SHL) is defined as hearing loss occurring within 10 days.

   (B) Pharmacological side effects are the cause of tinnitus in 40% of cases.

   (C) Antidepressants are the most commonly implicated drugs in tinnitus.

   (D) Tinnitus may be heard by the examiner.

8-8. Which of the following statements is MOST accurate about outer ear infections?

   (A) The most common organisms implicated in otitis externa are *Streptococcus pyogenes* and *Pseudomonas aeruginosa*.

   (B) *Candida* is the most common cause of otomycosis.

   (C) Patients presenting with otitis media who have a history of diabetes or HIV or are elderly should get a CT scan of the head.

   (D) Corticosporin solution eardrops are safe with perforated tympanic membranes.

8-9. A 22-year-old man is brought in after being caught in an avalanche while snowshoeing. Among his injuries he has a white non-tender right auricle with vesicles on it and a swollen, tender, ecchymotic left auricle and perforated left tympanic membrane without hemotympanum. What is the MOST appropriate treatment?

   (A) Place warm gauze soaks on the right auricle. Do not violate the skin of the left auricle. Begin IV antibiotics.

   (B) Place warm gauze soaks on the right auricle while you aspirate the subcutaneous blood from the left auricle. Begin IV antibiotics.

   (C) Place lukewarm soaks on the right auricle and debride the vesicles that have formed. Incise and remove the subcutaneous blood from the left auricle and place a sutured bolster dressing on that ear.

   (D) Place warm soaks on the right auricle, but do not debride the vesicles. Incise and remove the subcutaneous blood and place a sutured bolster dressing on the left auricle.

8-10. A 67-year-old man with a history of hypertension and diabetes comes in complaining of left jaw pain for 2 weeks that began when he was singing in the gospel choir and is now occurring with increasing frequency and severity. He notices it now even without singing; it makes him nauseous and is accompanied by a feeling of fullness in his throat. His temperature is 100°F, blood pressure 160/70 mmHg, pulse 105 beats per minute, respiratory rate 22 breaths per minute. On physical examination, there is no facial swelling or trismus. His temporomandibular joint, mandible, teeth, and oropharynx are without swelling, erythema, or tenderness. What is the most appropriate management plan for this patient?

   (A) Order a complete blood count (CBC), blood cultures, and CT of the head and neck, and administer antibiotics.

   (B) Order a CBC, blood cultures, and soft tissue radiograph of the neck, and give antibiotics.

   (C) Order a CBC, blood cultures, CT of the head and neck, and electrocardiogram.

   (D) Order a CBC, soft tissue radiograph of the neck, electrocardiogram, and cardiac enzymes.

8-11. A 27-year-old woman presents to the ED complaining of inability to close her jaw after yawning widely this morning. On physical exam, she has a gaping jaw with the mandibular teeth protruding anterior to the alveolar teeth. What is the MOST appropriate management plan?

(A) Take a panoramic radiograph, administer intravenous narcotics and muscle relaxants, grab the posterior mandibular molars with padded thumbs, and exert steady pressure downward and posteriorly.

(B) Administer 2 cc of 2% lidocaine to the preauricular space bilaterally, grab the posterior mandibular molars with padded thumbs, and exert steady pressure downward and posteriorly.

(C) Take a panoramic radiograph, administer intravenous narcotics and muscle relaxants, and exert steady pressure on the mentum posteriorly.

(D) Take a panoramic radiograph, administer intravenous antibiotics, and call for an oral surgery consultation.

8-12. A 19-year-old man presents to the ED with pain in his right temporomandibular joint after being hit in the partially open mouth with a fist. His physical exam shows malocclusion of his teeth with posterior dislocation of the mandibular teeth occlusive surface. CT of the mandible shows superior dislocation of bilateral condyles without fracture. What is the MOST appropriate plan of action?

(A) Give intravenous narcotics and muscle relaxants and exert steady downward pressure on the posterior mandibular molar.

(B) Give intravenous narcotics, muscle relaxants, and antibiotics and call for a head and neck surgical consultation.

(C) Give intravenous narcotics and order CT of the brain. Check for cranial nerve defects and hearing loss, and call for a head and neck surgical consultation.

(D) Give intravenous narcotics and muscle relaxants. Then exert steady pressure on the posterior mandibular molar, first anteriorly, then downward and posteriorly.

8-13. A 28-year-old woman complains of 2½ weeks of nasal congestion and nocturnal coughing and now has had 7 days of a "pressure-like" anterior headache and pain behind her eyes, worse when she beds down. Her physical exam shows normal vital signs, tenderness to percussion over the forehead, and purulent rhinorrhea. What is the MOST appropriate treatment?

(A) Perform CT of the head to rule out complications, discharge with nasal vasoconstrictors, and recommend follow-up with her doctor in 5 days.

(B) Perform Waters' view radiograph to confirm diagnosis, discharge with nasal vasoconstrictors, and recommend follow-up with her doctor in 5 days.

(C) Discharge with trimethoprim-sulfamethoxazole, nasal vasoconstrictors, and nasal steroids, and recommend follow-up with her doctor in 5 days.

(D) Discharge with amoxicillin-clavulanate, nasal vasoconstrictors, and antihistamines, and recommend follow-up with her doctor in 5 days.

8-14. A 45-year-old man presents with swelling over his right temple, fever, trismus, and difficulty swallowing 3 days after having extraction of his third upper molar. The pharynx cannot be well visualized secondary to trismus, but there is no sublingual edema. What is the MOST appropriate course of action?

(A) Give intravenous narcotics and cephalexin, and order facial CT.

(B) Emergently intubate the patient using a nasal approach, give intravenous narcotics and cephalexin, and order facial CT.

(C) Give intravenous narcotics and clindamycin, and order facial CT.

(D) Emergently intubate the patient with a cricothyroidotomy kit and ENT at the bedside, give intravenous narcotics, and order facial CT.

8-15. An otherwise healthy man presents with severe pain at the site of his third mandibular molar extraction 2 days ago. He is afebrile and has no trismus or facial or gingival swelling. The space at the site of his third molar is without bleeding or exudate but is exquisitely tender. Which of the following is TRUE?

(A) This man presents with postextraction alveolar osteitis and should have a panoramic radiograph to rule out retained root tip or foreign body and then be given an inferior alveolar nerve block, irrigation, and packing with oil-of-clove-soaked gauze. He should be seen by his dentist in 24 hours.

(B) This man presents with postextraction alveolar osteitis due to fibrin clot loss at the site of extraction and is at risk for bleeding. He should be given an inferior alveolar nerve block, irrigation, and packing with thrombin-impregnated gauze. He should be seen by his dentist in 24 hours.

(C) This man presents with early postextraction infectious complication and should have CT to rule out masticator space infection and then be given intravenous antibiotics and analgesics. He should be seen by his dentist in 24 hours.

(D) This man presents with common postextraction pain and should be given an inferior alveolar nerve block and analgesics. He should be seen by his dentist in 24 hours.

8-16. A 27-year-old man with a history of HIV and a CD4 count of 450 presents with pain and a foul metallic taste in his mouth. On exam he is afebrile with normal vital signs and has fetid breath, normal tongue and pharynx, edematous ulcerated gingival edema with "punched out" interdental papilla, and a grey pseudomembrane that bleeds easily on removal. Which of the following is TRUE?

(A) The patient had herpes gingivomastitis and is best treated with intravenous antivirals and referral to an oral surgeon within 24 hours.

(B) This patient has hand-foot-and-mouth disease and is best treated with pain medication, hydration, and follow-up in 2–4 days with an oral surgeon.

(C) This patient has acute necrotizing ulcerative gingivitis and should be given intravenous penicillin and admitted to the hospital.

(D) This patient has acute necrotizing ulcerative gingivitis and should be prescribed chlorhexidine washes, oral analgesics, oral antibiotics that cover anaerobes, and follow-up with an oral surgeon within 24 hours.

8-17. Which of the following statements is MOST accurate in evaluating an oral ulcer?

(A) Aphthous ulcers involve the nonkeratinized surfaces of the mouth, especially the buccal mucosa and soft palate, and are best treated with topical steroids.

(B) Herpes simplex ulcers involve primarily nonkeratinized surfaces of the mouth, especially the buccal mucosa and soft palate, and are best treated with oral antivirals.

(C) Herpangina caused by coxsackievirus leads to painful ulcers on both keratinized (tongue, gingival, hard palate) and nonkeratinized (buccal and pharyngeal mucosa) surfaces of the mouth and is best treated with pain medication.

(D) Hand-foot-and-mouth disease is commonly associated with coxsackie type A16 virus and is characterized by vesicles and ulcers of the nonkeratinized mouth surfaces (buccal and pharyngeal mucosa). It is best treated with pain medication.

8-24. A 36-year-old man comes in complaining of neck pain, swelling, and hoarse voice since being punched in the neck at a poker game approximately 20 minutes prior. On physical exam he is speaking with a hoarse voice and has edema and crepitus over his anterior midline neck. What is the MOST appropriate course of action?

(A) Place the patient in a cervical collar, order emergent CT of the neck, and then have an anesthesiologist perform a fiberoptic endotracheal tube placement.

(B) Administer intravenous dexamethasone and racemic epinephrine by nebulizer. Order CT of the neck, then have an anesthesiologist perform a fiberoptic endotracheal tube placement.

(C) Perform an immediate cricothyroidotomy, then obtain an anesthesia consultation for definitive airway placement.

(D) Perform an immediate fiberoptic endotracheal intubation, then place the patient in a cervical collar and order CT.

8-25. A 62-year-old woman, recently started on lisinopril, presents with 2 hours of swelling of her lips and tongue. She has no stridor or wheezing, and her sublingual space is normal. What is the next BEST course of action?

(A) Give 50 mg diphenhydramine and 125 mg of methylprednisone intravenously. Perform nasopharyngoscopy; if there is no laryngeal edema, the patient can be discharged after several hours of observation if clinically improved.

(B) Give racemic epinephrine nebulizer. Give 50 mg diphenhydramine and 125 mg of methylprednisone intravenously. Admit to the intensive care unit.

(C) Give 50 mg diphenhydramine and 125 mg of methylprednisone intravenously. Admit to the intensive care unit.

(D) Give epinephrine 0.3 mg subcutaneously. Give 50 mg diphenhydramine and 125 mg of methylprednisone intravenously. Avoid nasopharyngoscopy. The patient can be discharged after several hours of observation if clinically improved.

8-26. A 4-year-old girl is brought in after placing a yellow bead up her nose. Physical exam is normal except for a round yellow bead visualized just proximal to the inferior meatus of her right naris. What is the BEST procedure for removing the foreign body?

(A) Administer a nasal pharyngeal nebulizer of 1 mL of phenylephrine and 3 mL of 4% lidocaine, then grasp the bead with alligator forceps and remove.

(B) Administer a nasal pharyngeal nebulizer of 1 mL of phenylephrine and 3 mL of 4% lidocaine. Pass a Fogarty vascular catheter past the object, inflate the catheter, and remove both the object and the catheter.

(C) Administer a nasal pharyngeal nebulizer of racemic epinephrine, then have the caregiver give a puff of air over the child's mouth while the left naris is occluded.

(D) Administer a nasal pharyngeal nebulizer of racemic epinephrine, then grasp the bead with alligator forceps and remove.

8-27. A 45-year-old woman with a history of hypertension comes in complaining of spontaneous copious bleeding from her nose over the past 2 hours despite pressure and elevation. On physical exam her blood pressure is 190/100 mmHg. Other vital signs are normal. She has bright red blood oozing from the septum in her right naris. What is the MOST appropriate next step?

(A) Administer an oral antihypertensive medication.

(B) Administer an intravenous antihypertensive medication.

(C) Use silver nitrate liberally on the septum.

(D) Spray the nares with vasoconstrictor.

8-28. A 59-year-old homeless man complains of 1 week of lower posterior molar pain and for the past 24 hours has had a sore throat, difficulty swallowing, and night sweats. On physical exam he is anxious, he has significant trismus and edema of the upper midline neck, his tongue is elevated, and he is unable to protrude it beyond his teeth. The sublingual space is indurated and elevated. What is the next BEST course of action?

(A) Perform rapid sequence endotracheal intubation, administer intravenous ampicillin-sublactam, and order CT and emergent head and neck surgery consultation.

(B) Perform awake fiberoptic endotracheal intubation, administer intravenous ampicillin-sublactam, and order CT and emergent head and neck surgery consultation.

(C) Perform cricothyroidotomy, administer intravenous ampicillin-sublactam, and order CT and emergent head and neck surgery consultation.

(D) Perform rapid sequence endotracheal intubation, administer intravenous broad-spectrum fluoroquinolone, and order CT and emergent head and neck surgery consultation.

CHAPTER 8

Eye, Ear, Nose, Throat, and Oral Emergencies
Answers, Explanations, and References

8-1. **The answer is A** (Chapter 238). Seidel's test involves brushing a moistened fluorescein strip across the anesthetized cornea under blue light to check for streaming indicative of corneal violation with a projectile foreign object. Black tissue imbedded in the sclera is suggestive of uveal tissue herniation through a rent in the sclera caused by a foreign body. Any suspicion of foreign body violation of the eye should be worked up by CT or ultrasound and treated with intravenous antibiotics, a tetanus booster, and ophthalmic consultation. A negative Seidel's test with a superficial corneal abrasion does not require CT or intravenous antibiotics. Rust rings or deeply embedded foreign bodies in the visual axis should not be removed by an emergency physician but be deferred to the ophthalmologist.

8-2. **The answer is C** (Chapter 238). Central retinal artery occlusion is most common secondary to an embolus from a thrombus in the heart as occurs in atrial fibrillation or a cholesterol plaque from an arterial source. The treatments for all the listed causes of acute visual loss are correct, but the physical findings for each disorder is incorrect. Central vein thrombosis presents with a "blood and thunder" retina. A vitreal hemorrhage would usually obscure visualization of the retina or appear as a preretinal bleed. Optic neuritis presents with decreased red perception before visual loss and a normal fundus with normal or edematous optic disk.

8-3. **The answer is B** (Chapter 238). The proper management of acute angle glaucoma is intravenous analgesics, antiemetics, mannitol, and acetazolamide, plus topical β-blockers and steroids to lower intraocular pressure, followed by a miotic. However, in this patient, acetazolamide is contraindicated with allergy to sulfonamides. Miotics (pupillary constrictors) not mydriatics (pupillary dilators) are effective when the intraocular pressure has been brought under control by the other measures and pull the iris away from the cornea to avoid recurrence. Emergent ophthalmologic consultation is needed for definitive treatment.

8-4. **The answer is C** (Chapter 238). This patient is presenting with a third nerve palsy and pupil dilation. Acute CN III palsy with ipsilateral pupillary dilatation is a posterior circulation aneurysm until proven otherwise. The expanding aneurysm causes compression on the pupillomotor fibers that ride on the outside of the third nerve. Emergent blood pressure management, neuroimaging, and neurosurgical consultation are indicated. Although diabetes and hypertension are the most frequent causes of third nerve palsy, they usually spare the pupil as the mechanism is secondary to insufficiency of the vaso vasorum (penetrating feeding vessels into the nerve), and thus ischemic to the central fibers first. Carotid dissection would cause Horner's syndrome, which presents as papillary miosis, not dilatation, along with ptosis and anhydrosis and does not affect the third nerve. Wernicke's encephalopathy affects the abductors (CN VI) rather than CN III and is associated with altered mental status.

8-5. The answer is D (Chapter 238). This patient presents with two complications from blunt injury to the eye, namely, a traumatic hyphema and a blowout fracture of the orbit with entrapment. Traumatic hyphemas occur because of bleeding from a ruptured iris vessel. Treatment involves keeping the head elevated, paralyzing the iris with cycloplegics and topical prednisone, and lowering the IOP with topical β-blockers. If IOP is elevated, carbonic anhydrase inhibitors (CAI) are indicated *except* in sickle cell anemia, in which the CAI can lower the pH of the aqueous humor and cause sickling of the cells, thereby clogging the outflow tract of the trabecular matrix. Intravenous mannitol may be used as an alternative. Hyphemas occupying greater than one-third of the anterior chamber should be seen by an ophthalmologist immediately. Rebleeding occurs in 3–5 days in up to 30% of cases. Ophthalmologic consultation should be sought as some ophthalmologists like to admit patients with hyphemas to the hospital for observation. Blowout fractures should be evaluated with CT to rule out sinus fracture, and oral antibiotics are often recommended. All blowout fractures should be referred to an ophthalmologist for a comprehensive eye exam to rule out retinal tears or detachment (CT or ultrasound may help). Immediate bedside consultation is not necessarily indicated unless the consulting ophthalmologist prefers to admit patients with hyphemas.

8-6. The answer is C (Chapter 238). Cycloplegics help considerably decrease the pain from corneal abrasion, though adjunct oral pain medications are often needed. Both tobramycin and erythromycin are adequate topical antimicrobial agents, but abrasions from organic sources have potential for fungal infections and should not be patched. There is no role for steroids in the treatment of corneal abrasion.

8-7. The answer is D (Chapter 239). Tinnitus can be divided into objective, heard by the examiner (i.e., secondary to AV malformations, arterial bruits, mechanical abnormalities), and subjective (i.e., secondary to cochlear/neurosensory insult from toxins or vascular insufficiency). Pharmacological side effects are the cause of tinnitus in 10% of cases. Aspirin, nonsteroidal anti-inflammatory drugs, and antibiotics such as aminoglycosides are the most commonly implicated pharmacological causes of tinnitus. Antidepressants, however, are the only class of drug found to be useful in alleviating idiopathic tinnitus. SHL is defined as hearing loss occurring within 3 days or fewer. Idiopathy is the most common cause of SHL, though infectious causes such as mumps, genetic degenerative diseases, vascular insufficiency from a variety of causes, and toxic effects of drugs need to be considered in the differential diagnosis.

8-8. The answer is C (Chapter 239). For elderly patients, diabetic or HIV patients, patients with persistent otitis media (OM) despite two weeks of treatment, or any patient with associated cranial nerve palsy or fever, order a CT scan to rule out malignant OM, which requires parenteral antibiotics, admission, and ENT consultation. *Staphylococcus aureus* and *Pseudomonas aeruginosa* are the most common organisms implicated in otitis externa (OE). Otomycosis, or fungal OE, accounts for 10% of OM, with increased incidence in tropical climates and in HIV and diabetic patients. *Aspergillus*, not *Candida*, accounts for 80–90% of the cases. Corticosporin otic preparations have not been approved by the FDA for OE with perforations due to the theoretical concern of the neomycin (aminoglycoside) toxicity on the inner ear. However, the ENT literature recommends the *suspension* but not the *solution*, which is more easily absorbed across the round window. Ofloxacin is the only antibiotic drop approved by the FDA for OE with perforated tympanic membranes.

8-9.   **The answer is D** (Chapter 239). This patient has both frostbite of his right ear and a traumatic injury of his left ear. Frostbite injuries should be quickly rewarmed with asceptic warm (38–40°C) saline-soaked gauze. Vesicles that form should not be debrided but be allowed to reabsorb. The left ear, which presents with a traumatic hematoma, needs to be debrided and the blood evacuated to prevent necrosis of the cartilage and formation of cauliflower ear. Incision and drainage with a sutured bolster dressing has the best outcome. Antibiotics should be reserved for immunocompromised patients.

8-10. **The answer is D** (Chapter 240). Patients who complain of jaw pain that has occurred with exertion and now with rest and who have normal physical exams must be considered for coronary ischemia. This patient's electrocardiogram and cardiac enzymes were positive for acute myocardial infarction. In the differential is deep tissue infection such as the pterygoid space or prevertebral pharyngeal abscess, which can be normal on physical exam, though these usually present with trismus and dysphagia. A history of dental surgery or mandible fracture should be sought. A CT would be indicated to rule these out.

8-11. **The answer is B** (Chapter 240). This patient presents with a nontraumatic jaw dislocation. A radiograph is not required unless the reduction is unsuccessful or difficult. This procedure does not require consultation services unless there are other issues or time constraints. The proper method would be to anesthetize either locally or with intravenous narcotics and muscle relaxants, grab the posterior mandibular molars with padded thumbs, and exert steady pressure downward and posteriorly.

8-12. **The answer is C** (Chapter 240). Superior dislocation forces the condylar head up-

ward and may protrude into the auditory canal. It is associated with cerebral contusions and cranial nerve palsies, thus CT imaging of the brain and head and neck surgery consultation are indicated. Reduction in the ED should not be attempted. Antibiotics are not indicated unless there are associated fractures.

8-13. **The answer is C** (Chapter 241). This patient presents with simple acute sinusitis of her frontal and ethmoid sinuses. Acute sinusitis is usually preceded by a viral cold and presents with 7 days or greater of sinus pressure symptoms. Retro-orbital pain is associated with ethmoid sinusitis. Retro-orbital pain without visual symptoms, proptosis, diplopia, fever, or symptoms of meningitis does not mandate CT. Acute sinusitis is a clinical diagnosis, and plain films are not indicated. Broad-spectrum antibiotics are not indicated for initial treatment, and antihistamines, which may make secretions dry and impair drainage, are indicated only for allergic sinusitis. Nasal steroids improve symptoms compared to antibiotics alone.

8-14. **The answer is C** (Chapter 240). This patient presents with history and symptoms suspicious of masticator space infections, which occur most commonly after third molar surgery or mandible fracture. Swelling over the temple indicates the temporal space, which is associated with significant trismus. Airway compromise is rare but should be considered if the trismus does not abate with pain medication, vomiting is present, phlegmon is identified on CT, or other signs of impending airway compromise occur. Clindamycin or ampicillin-sublactam would be the antibiotics of choice as the offending organism is usually anaerobic.

8-15. **The answer is A** (Chapter 242). Although third molar extraction can be complicated by deep masticator space infection, this is unlikely in the afebrile patient without trismus or gingival edema and thus CT and intravenous antibiotics are not indicated. This patient does have postoperative pain and could probably be managed with local anesthesia and oral analgesics, but this patient's presentation is most consistent with postextraction alveolar osteitis or "dry socket" and is most properly managed with a panoramic radiograph to rule out retained root tip or foreign body, an inferior alveolar nerve block, irrigation, packing with oil-of-clove-soaked gauze, and follow-up with his dentist in 24 hours. Thrombin-impregnated gauze is not indicated.

8-16.   **The answer is D** (Chapter 242). This patient has acute necrotizing ulcerative gingivitis, also known as Vincent's disease or trench mouth, and should be treated with chlorhexidine washes, analgesics, oral antibiotics that cover anaerobes, and follow-up with an oral surgeon within 24 hours. Although this disease is most difficult to differentiate from herpes gingivomastitis (HG), HG usually has more systemic symptoms and a lack of interdental papilla involvement. Hand-foot-and-mouth disease involves other surfaces of the mouth as well, not just the gingival.

8-17.   **The answer is A** (Chapter 242). The location of mouth ulcerations can help differentiate the pathological entities. Aphthous ulcers involve the nonkeratinized surfaces of the mouth (buccal mucosa and soft palate) and are best treated with topical steroids. Herpes simplex ulcers involve primarily keratinized surfaces of the mouth (gingival hard palate, outer lip) and are treated with oral antivirals. Herpangina caused commonly by coxsackievirus leads to shallow, painful ulcerations primarily on nonkeratinized mucosa (soft plate, tonsilar pillars, sparing the buccal mucosa and keratinized surfaces) and is best treated with pain medication. Hand-foot-and-mouth disease, commonly associated with coxsackie type A16 virus, is characterized by vesicles and ulcers of all surfaces in the oral cavity and is best treated with pain medication.

8-18.   **The answer is B** (Chapter 242). This patient presents with an Ellis class II fracture, which accounts for 70% of tooth fractures. The treatment of Ellis class II (dentin exposed) and Ellis class III (pulp exposed) fractures is the same. The dried tooth should be sealed with glass ionomer dental cement or calcium hydroxide base to decrease dental contamination by oral bacteria and given 24 hours until dental follow-up. Oral analgesics are indicated. Topical analgesics should be avoided. No antibiotic treatment is necessary.

8-19.   **The answer is B** (Chapter 242). Total avulsion of the tooth requires reimplantation as soon as possible and can be successful if done within 3 hours of avulsion. Teeth should be kept moist with the mouth or suspended in Hank's balanced salt solution, sterile normal saline, or milk in transport. If the teeth have been dry for 20–60 minutes, they should be soaked in Hank's balanced salt solution for 30 minutes. Radiography is not necessary if physical exam does not suggest alveolar fracture. The teeth should be placed in the sockets with gentle, firm pressure and secured to the surrounding teeth with periodontal dressing. The patient should follow-up with a dentist within 24 hours.

8-20.   **The answer is A** (Chapter 243). This patient presents with classic viral pharyngitis and thus should be asked about risk factors for the 3 viral causal organisms that require diagnostic testing: mononucleosis, influenza, and HIV. More than 70% of primary infections with HIV are associated with acute pharyngitis developing 2–4 weeks after exposure. She does not meet 3 of the 4 CDC criteria for GABHS, which are tonsilar exudates, tender anterior cervical adenopathy, absence of cough, and history of fever. Fungal pharyngitis, suggested in choice B, presents with hyperemia and exudates and usually has buccal mucosal involvement.

9-6. Which of the following is the BEST statement about the etiology and treatment of Ogilvie's syndrome?

(A) Immediate laparotomy is needed for reduction of the obstruction.

(B) Use of neostigmine has been shown to be an effective treatment.

(C) Barium enemas have been shown to relieve the colonic obstruction.

(D) The condition can be misdiagnosed as renal colic.

9-7. Which of the following is the MOST common cause of abdominal pain requiring surgical treatment in the elderly?

(A) Appendicitis.

(B) Biliary tract disease.

(C) Abdominal aortic aneurysm.

(D) Bowel obstruction.

9-8. Which of the following would NOT be considered appropriate in the initial management of a hypotensive patient with a history of known esophageal varices presenting with hematemesis?

(A) Sengstaken-Blakemore tube placement.

(B) Large-bore intravenous lines.

(C) Nasogastric lavage.

(D) Volume repletion with normal saline.

9-9. Which of the following is the MOST common source of upper gastrointestinal bleeding?

(A) Esophageal varices.

(B) Mallory-Weiss tears.

(C) Epistaxis.

(D) Peptic ulcer disease.

9-10. Which of the following diagnostic studies yields the LEAST information among patients presenting with acute lower gastrointestinal bleeding?

(A) Colonoscopy.

(B) Plain abdominal radiographs.

(C) Tagged erythrocyte bleeding scans.

(D) Angiography.

9-11. Which of the following is the MOST common obstructive cause of dysphagia?

(A) Zenker's diverticulum.

(B) Esophageal stricture secondary to gastroesophageal reflux disease.

(C) Neoplasm.

(D) Schatzki's ring.

9-12. Which of the following statements is NOT considered routine practice in a patient presenting with symptoms suggestive of an esophageal perforation?

(A) The patient should be observed for 4 hours and, if pain improves, discharged home.

(B) The diagnostic studies of choice are computed tomography and emergency endoscopy.

(C) Appropriate resuscitation includes hemodynamic stabilization, airway protection, and broad-spectrum antibiotic coverage.

(D) Emergent gastroenterology and/or surgical consultation should be obtained in every patient with a suspected esophageal perforation.

9-13. When considering the disposition of a 50-year-old patient with symptoms that are felt to be esophageal in origin, which of the following strategies is MOST appropriate?

(A) In the absence of risk factors for heart disease, cancer, or systemic diseases, diagnostic studies are not necessary.

(B) A minimum of an electrocardiogram and chest radiographs should be obtained in atypical cases of chest pain.

(C) Emergency physicians should use caution when prescribing medications for gastroesophageal reflux disease.

(D) A patient with dysphagia can be safely discharged home with a nasogastric tube in place for fluid administration.

9-14. Which of the following is NOT considered a contributing factor to the development of gastroesophageal reflux disease?

(A) Cholesterol-lowering medications.

(B) Nicotine.

(C) Pregnancy.

(D) Diabetes mellitus.

9-15. All of the following maneuvers, procedures, and medications have been proposed as methods to remove impacted food boluses, ingested coins, and batteries. Which choice matches the MOST appropriate treatment with the patient presentation?

(A) A 3-year-old child swallowed a coin over 24 hours ago, which is now located at the region of C6. Remove the coin using a Foley catheter.

(B) A 48-year-old man presents with a 1-hour history of food bolus impaction. Administer a proteolytic enzyme.

(C) A 75-year-old female presents after choking on a piece of steak. Administer sublingual nifedipine.

(D) A 2-year-old ingested a button battery, and x-rays indicate the battery is in the proximal small bowel. Observe the patient and carefully examine the child's stool for the battery.

9-16. A 16-year-old male presents after ingesting a battery. Figure 9-1 shows the upright abdominal radiograph of this patient. What is the recommended treatment?

(A) Prepare for emergent endoscopy.

(B) Induce vomiting with syrup of ipecac.

(C) No emergency intervention is required other than repeat abdominal x-rays.

(D) Insert a Foley catheter and remove the battery.

9-17. A 30-year-old male presents to the ED complaining of intermittent epigastric burning for the past 2 months. He reports no associated back pain, vomiting, or melena. The symptoms improve after meals. He has not tried any medications. His physical exam is normal except for mild epigastric tenderness. Laboratory studies including a complete blood count, lipase, and fecal occult blood testing are all normal. Which of the

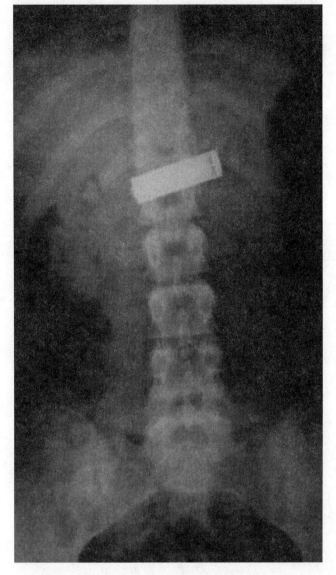

Figure 9-1. Photograph courtesy of Edward Dickinson, MD.

following is the MOST appropriate management for this patient?

(A) Consult gastroenterology and admit for endoscopy.

(B) Order serologic testing, start symptomatic treatment for *Helicobacter pylori* infection, and refer to a gastroenterologist.

(C) Begin antibiotics for *H. pylori.*

(D) Order a urea breath test, and recommend that the patient begin using histamine receptor antagonists.

9-18. Which of the following is NOT a complication arising from peptic ulcer disease?

(A) Gastrointestinal perforation.

(B) Gastric outlet obstruction.

(C) Pernicious anemia.

(D) Gastrointestinal hemorrhage.

9-19. Which one of the following unique patient populations DOES NOT commonly present with atypical features of appendicitis?

(A) Elderly.

(B) Intravenous drug users.

(C) Pregnant patients.

(D) Immunocompromised patients.

9-20. Which one of the following is NOT suggestive of acute appendicitis on computed tomography or ultrasound?

(A) Appendicolith with surrounding phlegmon.

(B) Fat stranding in the right lower quadrant.

(C) Pericecal inflammation.

(D) Compressible tubular structure in the right lower quadrant.

9-21. Which of the following statements is TRUE regarding bowel obstructions?

(A) The most common causes of large bowel obstruction are surgical adhesions and hernias.

(B) The most common causes of small bowel obstructions are carcinomas and strictures.

(C) Patients with small bowel obstructions have a stepladder appearance on plain films.

(D) Intestinal pseudo-obstruction typically involves the small bowel.

9-22. Which one of the following abnormalities DOES NOT typically occur with bowel obstructions?

(A) Vomiting and decreased oral intake.

(B) Volume depletion with hemoconcentration.

(C) Gastrointestinal bleeding.

(D) Abnormal bowel sounds.

9-23. Which one of the following statements is TRUE regarding bowel obstructions?

(A) Pelvic exams should be performed in female patients presenting with symptoms suggestive of bowel obstruction.

(B) Treatment for closed-loop obstruction is bowel rest, rehydration, and antibiotics.

(C) Surgery is the definitive treatment for Ogilvie's syndrome.

(D) Feculent vomitus is associated only with large bowel obstruction.

9-24. Which of the following treatments is recommended for a painful inguinal hernia?

(A) Mechanical compression with a pessary in women should be attempted to reduce the need for operative management.

(B) Failed manual reduction is an indication for emergent surgical repair.

(C) Only nonoperative management is recommended for elderly patients.

(D) Operative management is the standard for indirect hernias, whereas direct inguinal hernias are best treated with antibiotics and pain medications.

9-25. A 45-year-old male presents with a painless lump in the region of his groin that is diagnosed as a reducible inguinal hernia. Which of the following is NOT a component of the management for this patient?

(A) Inform the patient the condition is not life threatening but consultation with a general surgeon is advisable to consider elective repair.

(B) Tell the patient to avoid heavy lifting and excessive straining with bowel movements.

(C) Recommend minimizing sexual intercourse as it may aggravate the hernia and necessitate emergency surgery.

(D) Give the patient instructions on manual reduction of the hernia and tell him to return if it becomes painful or if reduction is not successful.

9-26. Antibiotics are NOT indicated for which one of the following situations?

(A) A 19-year-old male with an upper gastrointestinal imaging series showing small intestine segmental narrowing and mucosal destruction who presents to the ED with crampy diarrhea.

(B) A 65-year-old female admitted for severe diarrhea after finishing a 1-month course of antibiotics to treat a chronic sinus infection.

(C) A patient with ulcerative colitis presenting with severe abdominal pain, vomiting, bloody diarrhea, and a fever of 40°C.

(D) A 45-year-old nontoxic-appearing patient with sigmoid diverticulitis who is afebrile and tolerating oral fluids.

9-27. Which of the following is the MOST common etiology of painful rectal bleeding?

(A) Internal hemorrhoid.
(B) Perianal abscess.
(C) Venereal proctitis.
(D) Anal fissure.

9-28. Which of the following is NOT a common cause of anorectal infection among sexually active patients?

(A) Herpes simplex virus.
(B) *Chlamydia trachomatis.*
(C) Condylomata lata.
(D) Candidiasis.

9-29. Which type of anorectal abscess can consistently be safely and adequately treated in the ED?

(A) Isolated ischiorectal abscess.
(B) Isolated perianal abscess.
(C) Perirectal abscess.
(D) Intersphincteric abscess.

9-30. A healthy 35-year-old male presents for evaluation of nonbloody diarrhea that started 3 days after returning from a business trip to the Caribbean. Which of the following tests is the MOST appropriate diagnostic study?

(A) Stool ova and parasite.
(B) *Clostridium difficile* toxin assay.
(C) Wright's stain of the stool.
(D) No study indicated.

9-31. Regarding the treatment of diarrhea, which of the following statements BEST describes the current treatment recommendations for antimotility agents?

(A) Avoid their use in the elderly.
(B) In combination with antibiotic therapy, they can reduce duration of symptoms.
(C) They should not be used with oral hydration therapy.
(D) Anticholinergic effects of diphenoxylate can be problematic in patients with cardiac conditions.

9-32. Which of the following is an important cause of unconjugated hyperbilirubinemia?

(A) Viral hepatitis.
(B) Acetaminophen toxicity.
(C) *Amanita* toxin.
(D) Hemolytic anemia.

9-33. A 65-year-old diabetic woman complains of right upper quadrant pain for 1 day. Physical examination reveals an uncomfortable woman who is febrile without jaundice but with significant right upper quadrant tenderness and a positive Murphy's sign. Diagnostic tests reveal a normal white blood count and normal liver function tests and lipase level. Bedside ultrasound by the emergency physician shows no obvious gallstones but tenderness on examination. What is the MOST likely diagnosis?

(A) Acalculous cholecystitis.
(B) Gallstone pancreatitis.
(C) Ascending cholangitis.
(D) Malignancy.

9-48. A 70-year-old nursing home patient complains that his chronic jejunostomy tube fell out a few hours ago. No replacement jejunostomy tubes are available in the ED, and interventional radiology will not be able to replace the tube for a few days. What is the MOST appropriate temporary catheter to use in this patient?

(A) 16 F Foley with the balloon inflated.

(B) 16 F Foley with the balloon deflated.

(C) 12 F Foley with the balloon inflated.

(D) 12 F Foley with the balloon deflated.

9-49. Where is the first place jaundice is MOST likely to be detected?

(A) Sclera.

(B) Mucous membrane.

(C) Skin.

(D) Subungual area.

9-50. A 40-year-old male presents 3 weeks after liver transplantation with fevers, abdominal pain, and elevated liver enzymes. What is the MOST likely etiology of this patient's problems?

(A) Infection.

(B) Rejection.

(C) Biliary leak.

(D) Hepatic artery thrombosis.

9-51. What is the MOST common organism seen in spontaneous bacterial peritonitis?

(A) *Streptococcus pneumoniae.*

(B) *Enterobacteriaceae.*

(C) Anaerobes.

(D) *Pseudomonas aeruginosa.*

9-52. A 35-year-old male comes to the ED complaining of right upper quadrant pain for 2 days. Laboratory tests are as follows: total serum bilirubin 0.9 mg/dL, AST 1500 IU/L, ALT 600 IU/L, alkaline phosphatase 80 IU/L, and lipase 5 IU/L. What is the MOST likely diagnosis?

(A) Alcoholic hepatitis.

(B) Viral hepatitis.

(C) Choledocholithiasis.

(D) Acute cholecystitis.

9-53. Biliary leak after liver transplantation is associated with which of the following vascular complications?

(A) Portal vein thrombosis.

(B) Hepatic vein thrombosis.

(C) Hepatic artery thrombosis.

(D) Mesenteric ischemia.

9-54. A patient presents with minimal drainage from the stomal site of a gastrostomy tube placed endoscopically a few days ago. No fevers, vomiting, or abdominal pain are noted, and physical examination reveals minimal seropurulent drainage from the stomal site with no cellulitis. What is the MOST appropriate management of this patient?

(A) Culture the drainage and start empiric antibiotics.

(B) Provide local skin care with hydrogen peroxide.

(C) Call a gastroenterologist to replace the tube with a larger one.

(D) Obtain radiographs to check tube placement and evaluate possible gastric rupture.

9-55. Intussusception is suspected in a 2-year-old toddler. What is the preferred procedure?

(A) Barium enema.

(B) Gastrograffin enema.

(C) Water enema.

(D) Air enema.

CHAPTER 9

Gastroenterologic Emergencies
Answers, Explanations, and References

9-1. **The answer is C** (Chapter 72). Appendicitis and nonspecific abdominal pain are common diagnoses among all age groups presenting to the ED complaining of abdominal pain. Pelvic inflammatory disease accounts for a small proportion of causes of abdominal pain but is almost entirely a disease process of young women. Among older patients (>50 years) bowel obstruction, biliary tract disease, and pancreatitis are much more common and can have subtle presentations compared to younger cohorts.

9-2. **The answer is D** (Chapter 72). The diagnostic study of choice for abdominal aortic aneurysm is computed tomography (CT). While bedside sonography may be useful and more timely, it does not provide critical information about dissection or leakage. Angiography and magnetic resonance imaging are also not widely available and not considered part of the emergency evaluation of abdominal aortic aneurysms. The intravenous pyelogram, a dye-contrast imaging study used to diagnose renal colic and to identify ureteral stones, is time consuming and not useful in patients with renal disorders or dye allergies. It is an informative study, when available, and can appropriately inform clinical decision making in many cases. However, noncontrast CT has the added benefit of assessing the surrounding structures, most notably the aorta in the case of a leaking aortic aneurysm, which can masquerade as renal colic. Therefore, CT is the study of choice in renal colic. Sonography is the initial diagnostic study of choice for biliary tract disease including cholelithiasis, acute cholecystitis, and common duct obstructions. Plain films have limited utility in this setting, and CT, while useful in considering alternative diagnoses, is not recommended as the initial study for localized right upper quadrant pain. In distinct contrast, small bowel obstructions should be evaluated using CT as the study of choice, with the utility of plain films riddled with unacceptably low sensitivities and specificities.

9-3. **The answer is C** (Chapter 72). In young females the diagnosis of pregnancy and in particular ectopic pregnancy must always be considered for any complaints of abdominal pain with or without vaginal bleeding. Pregnancy tests are now highly accurate, and determination of pregnancy should not depend on the date of the last menstrual period or a verbal report of last sexual activity. Verification of a pregnancy by either serum or urine β-HCG testing should not deter a complete pelvic examination, during which appropriate cervical and vaginal samples can be obtained for culture. Palpation of the adnexa may reveal a mass, which in the absence of a pregnancy may be indicative of an ovarian cyst, a large tubo-ovarian abscess, or other pelvic pathology. However, determination of the presence or absence of a pregnancy should be the first diagnostic decision. The use of progesterone in assisting with pregnancy determination is not recommended. Culdocentesis is a procedure with little discriminatory power to help guide management in the setting of pregnancy. Transvaginal sonography is the cornerstone of establishing whether a pregnancy is intrauterine or not and can rapidly guide management of abnormal gestations, especially in the setting of ectopic pregnancy. While pelvic sonography may also play a role in the diagnostic evaluation of nonpregnant patients, its use is most appropriate after the initial diagnosis of pregnancy is established.

9-4.   **The answer is D** (Chapter 72). The use of opioid analgesics is recommended in the management of acute abdominal pain. Studies have shown no detrimental effects associated with opioid medication use. Its judicious use may permit a better history of the illness to be uncovered as well as possibly enhancing the abdominal exam. Concomitant medications for control of associated symptoms, like antiemetics for nausea and vomiting, or acetaminophen for fevers, are also recommended. In the setting of hypotension, use of vasopressor medications may be required. Depending on the patient's comorbidities and the suspected reason for the hypotension, preferred medications include dopamine, norepinephrine, or dobutamine. Septic shock may be one cause of hypotension in patients presenting with abdominal pain, and early aggressive treatment with antibiotic therapy is required. However, not all patients with fever and abdominal pain need antibiotic therapy. Patients with peritoneal signs and cases of suspected sepsis warrant antibiotic therapy.

9-5.   **The answer is B** (Chapter 73). The complaint of abdominal pain among the elderly should prompt clinicians to lower their threshold for considering more serious intra-abdominal conditions. Patients who have low cardiac output conditions like congestive heart failure or who take medications, such as digoxin, should be considered at high risk for the elusive condition of mesenteric ischemia. A history of sudden onset of abdominal pain, with increasing

severity, but with a normal physical exam, should prompt consideration of mesenteric ischemia. The condition is associated with a high mortality rate, and initial diagnosis is often incorrect. The diagnostic study of choice is angiography. Sigmoid volvulus is two to three times more frequent than cecal volvulus among the elderly and presents with gradually increasing abdominal pain, nausea, and vomiting. Cholecystitis is the most common surgical emergency in older patients, but patients often localize pain to the right upper quadrant. There is no association of cholecystitis to the comorbid conditions listed. Perforated peptic ulcer often presents with acute onset of pain and gastrointestinal bleeding and can be a similarly challenging condition to diagnose. The diagnostic study of choice for this condition is computed tomography.

9-6.   **The answer is B** (Chapters 73, 79). Colonic distention in the immobile, chronically ill, and elderly can mimic large bowel obstruction and is characteristic of intestinal pseudo-obstruction, also commonly known as Ogilvie's syndrome. Acute abdominal radiographs show massively dilated loops of large bowel without air-fluid levels. Patients have a distended abdomen that is tympanic to percussion. Treatment modalities are conservative. Surgical intervention is not recommended due to the absence of a mechanical obstruction to reduce and is associated with very poor outcomes. Barium enemas should also be avoided because the barium may not be evacuated, further complicating the condition. Colonoscopy has been used successfully to decompress the distention. Neostigmine, a cholinesterase inhibitor, has been used successfully to relieve this condition.

9-7.   **The answer is B** (Chapter 73). The most common surgical emergency among older patients is acute cholecystitis. Acute appendicitis is less frequent among the elderly, but the presentation is commonly atypical, necessitating consideration of appendicitis in every older patient complaining of abdominal pain. Bowel obstruction occurs commonly in the elderly, but it is less frequent than biliary tract disease. The incidence of abdominal aortic aneurysms increases dramatically after age 55 in men and after age 70 in women. Surgical or medical treatment is guided by the size of the aneurysm and patient comorbidities.

9-8. **The answer is A** (Chapter 74). Upper gastrointestinal bleeding is defined as a bleeding source originating proximal to the ligament of Treitz. Patients typically present with hematemesis or melena, and possibly hematochezia in the setting of brisk proximal bleeding. Primary treatment of any gastrointestinal bleed must include placement of large-bore intravenous lines, initial volume resuscitation with crystalloid solutions such as normal saline, cardiac monitoring, and supplemental oxygen. Nasogastric lavage is recommended in all gastrointestinal bleeding patients in order to help guide identification of the bleeding source. A common myth is that nasogastric lavage is contraindicated in the setting of known esophageal varices. Whereas esophageal varices are associated with a high mortality and rebleed rate, initial treatment of gastrointestinal bleeding is the same for all types of bleeds, regardless of any history of known esophageal varices. If initial resuscitative efforts fail or a patient remains hypotensive, more aggressive measures may be required. Establishment of a definitive airway then takes precedence; next are considerations of Sengstaken-Blakemore tube placement to physically tamponade a presumed esophageal or gastric bleeding source, and/or medications such as somatostatin and octreotide to assert vasoconstricting sclerotherapeutic properties.

9-9. **The answer is D** (Chapter 74). Peptic ulcer disease is the most prevalent etiology of upper gastrointestinal bleeding. Duodenal ulcers account for approximately 29% of all ulcers, while gastric ulcers constitute about 16%. Other causes of upper gastrointestinal

bleeding include swallowed blood from nasopharyngeal sources, esophageal mucosal tears known as Mallory-Weiss bleeds, esophagitis and duodenitis, and esophageal or gastric varices. Varices are common among alcoholics and patients with portal hypertension. Less common causes include aortoenteric fistulas, arteriovenous malformations, and malignancies.

9-10. **The answer is B** (Chapter 74). The degree of active bleeding, the stability of the patient, and local availability of the various modalities along with the gastroenterology consultant's preferences guide the choice of diagnostic study ordered to evaluate a lower gastrointestinal bleed. Angiography is a useful study in the setting of brisk (0.5 to 2.0 mL per minute) lower tract bleeding sources. Relatively slower lower tract bleeding (0.1 to 0.5 mL per minute) is amenable to technetium-radiolabeled red blood cell scans. In both cases, the diagnostic study can then guide embolization or sclerotherapy. Colonoscopy has the advantage of being both diagnostic and therapeutic in localizing distal bleeding sources. Plain radiographs bear no influence on the initial management of lower gastrointestinal bleeding conditions.

9-11. **The answer is D** (Chapter 75). The common causes of obstructive dysphagia, which refers to physical hindrances to the passage of food boluses, include neoplasms (adenocarcinomas comprise approximately 95% of esophageal neoplasms), esophageal strictures from scarring induced by gastroesophageal reflux disease, Schatzki's rings, esophageal webs, and diverticula. Among these, Schatzki's rings are found in approximately 15% of the population, making it the most common cause of obstructive dysphagia.

9-12. **The answer is A** (Chapter 75). Esophageal perforations are associated with high morbidity and mortality and therefore require a high degree of vigilance among patients presenting after recent endoscopy or other invasive procedures in and around the esophagus. In typical cases, patients complain of severe, acute, diffuse pain in the neck, chest, and upper abdomen that is exacerbated by swallowing. In less acute cases, the symptoms may be less dramatic. The desired diagnostic studies are either computed tomography of the chest or emergency endoscopy, and the decision is often guided by the consultant's preference, whether a gastroenterologist or a surgical consultant. Due to concerns over sepsis and diffuse necrotizing mediastinitis, broad-spectrum antibiotics should be started in conjunction with airway and hemodynamic stabilization. Patients require aggressive monitoring, endoscopy, or CT, and all require emergent consultation with either gastroenterology or surgery.

9-13. **The answer is B** (Chapter 75). It is recommended that patients presenting with symptoms suggestive of an esophageal origin, because of the inability to distinguish esophageal symptoms from those of cardiac or pulmonary disease, should have at a minimum an electrocardiogram and chest x-rays. When the history is suggestive of gastroesophageal reflux disease as the diagnosis, empiric treatment with histamine blockers or proton pump inhibitors is recommended. Patients being evaluated for new esophageal-related symptoms, particularly dysphagia or odynophagia, should not be discharged home with newly placed nasogastric tubes. Rather, patients with worrisome presentations, such as cachexia, dehydration, or the inability to either swallow or control their secretions, should be admitted for further diagnostic testing.

9-14. **The answer is A** (Chapter 75). The three categories of factors that predispose one to gastroesophageal reflux disease are (1) elements that lower the tone of the lower esophageal sphincter (including high-fat foods, caffeine, nicotine, peppermint, spearmint, pregnancy, and medications such as calcium channel blockers, nitrates, progesterone, and estrogen), (2) conditions

that decrease esophageal motility (diabetes, scleroderma, achalasia), and (3) situations that prolong gastric emptying (high-fat foods, gastroparesis, outlet obstruction, and anticholinergic medication). Cholesterol-lowering medications are not independently associated with reflux disease.

9-15. **The answer is D** (Chapter 76). The pediatric population accounts for the majority of foreign body ingestions. Fortunately, up to 90% of ingested foreign bodies pass spontaneously. Coin removal is optimally performed by an experienced endoscopist. When endoscopy is not readily available, removal of the coin using a Foley catheter can be attempted with caution about securing an airway before attempting the removal. However, coins that have been lodged for greater than 24 hours should be removed via endoscopy because of lower success rates with the Foley catheter method. Food bolus impactions are also optimally removed using endoscopy. Alternative suggested methods to dislodge a food impaction include proteolytic enzymes, glucagon, and calcium channel blockers. Proteolytic enzymes are not recommended due to complications including esophageal perforation. Following a test dose, glucagon can be administered in an attempt to relax the esophageal smooth muscle. The calcium channel blocker medication nifedipine has also been reported to successfully dislodge impacted food boluses. However, hypotension side effects make it a second choice in the elderly when endoscopy is available. Button batteries can be problematic when they are lodged in the esophagus. However, detection of a battery that is distal to the pylorus does not require intervention and will be passed normally in the stool.

9-16. **The answer is C** (Chapter 76). Figure 9-1 shows a battery (size AA) in the region of the stomach ingested by the 16-year-old patient. The majority of ingested objects pass through the gastrointestinal tract spontaneously without the need for any intervention. Special cases that require specific intervention include ingestion of sharp objects, such as razor blades or pins, or especially long or wide objects that are not likely to pass (>5 cm long or 2 cm wide). Button battery and lithium battery ingestions also require specialized care due to concerns of esophageal erosion. Induced vomiting or attempted removal by gastric lavage is not recommended for any ingested foreign body.

9-17. **The answer is B** (Chapter 77). A definite diagnosis of peptic ulcer disease is difficult to make without visualizing regions of ulceration. The preferred diagnostic tests, therefore, are endoscopy or upper gastrointestinal barium contrast radiography. Studies for diagnosing *H. pylori* infection include serologic tests and cultures, but these are not readily available in many locations, and the results are not available for immediate interpretation. The sensitivities and specificities of the tests are variable. The urea breath test involves the use of radioactive carbon isotopes and is the study of choice for confirming cure of infection. For stable patients with normal labs presenting to the ED with physical exam findings that do not suggest another more likely alternative diagnosis, it would be appropriate to begin symptomatic treatment for *H. pylori*, order serologic tests, and then refer the patient to his primary care physician and/or gastroenterologist to arrange for initiation of antibiotic therapy. Cost-effective analysis and consensus opinion suggest that antimicrobial treatment for *H. pylori* should be ordered only in patients with persistent symptoms. Recommendations should also be given about dietary adjustments; however, there is no evidence linking alcohol use or diets with high fat content to the development of peptic ulcer disease.

9-18. **The answer is C** (Chapter 77). Due to the high prevalence of peptic ulcer disease and the high recurrence rates in the setting of incomplete or untreated disease, there is a high rate of associated morbidity. The main

complications that occur as a result of severe, untreated, or complicated peptic ulcer disease include gastrointestinal hemorrhages from gastric or duodenal ulcers, intestinal perforation, and intestinal obstructions near the gastric outlet resulting from chronic scarring or inflammation and edema. Pernicious anemia results from an autoimmune disease in which the body develops antibodies to the acid-secreting cells in the gastric mucosa, with ensuing loss of intrinsic factor, vitamin B_{12} malabsorption, and development of the anemia.

9-19. **The answer is B** (Chapter 78). Acute appendicitis can be difficult to diagnose in some special patient populations. Extremes of age present particular problems due to communication issues and the lack of "typical" signs and symptoms. Abdominal pain can be poorly localized, fevers may not be mounted, and the delay in seeking care may be misleading. Acute appendicitis is the most common nonuterine surgical emergency among pregnant patients. Functionally immunocompromised patients, including those with AIDS and those on immune suppression medications such as transplant patients, are also considered in the category of patients that may commonly have atypical presentations. Intravenous drug use is not associated with deceptive presentations and is not an independent risk factor for appendicitis.

9-20. **The answer is D** (Chapter 78). Computed tomography is considered the diagnostic study of first choice in considering appendicitis. Radiographic findings that are highly suggestive of acute appendicitis include the following: pericecal inflammation, abscess in the right lower quadrant, periappendiceal phlegmon, periappendiceal fluid collections, and fat stranding in the right lower quadrant. Ultrasonography is being used to diagnose appendicitis as well. Findings with graded compression studies include visualization of a noncompressible appendix with a diameter of at least 6 cm, evidence of an appendicolith, or

9-45. **The answer is B** (Chapter 86). Hepatic encephalopathy should be considered as a diagnosis only after other life-threatening causes are ruled out. Cirrhotic patients are at increased risk of spontaneous subdural hematomas due to coagulopathy and thrombocytopenia, and thus emergent head imaging is indicated in these patients who present with altered mental status. Precipitants of hepatic encephalopathy include infection and gastrointestinal bleeding, and diagnostic evaluation for these entities should be undertaken if clinically indicated. Lactulose is standard treatment for hepatic encephalopathy. Oral antibiotics such as neomycin and rifaximin can also be given to prevent bacterial growth and protein metabolism. Patients with known hepatic encephalopathy with mild symptoms of apathy, lethargy, drowsiness, or variable orientation (Stage I or II) may be managed as outpatients after other emergent causes are excluded.

9-46. **The answer is C** (Chapter 91). This ultrasound image is a clear-cut example of acute appendicitis. An inflamed appendix is a tubular structure, usually located off of the cecum, which is larger than 6 mm, fluid filled, noncompressible, and tender. Frequently, the appendix is difficult to visualize even by experienced ultrasonographers, with a false-negative rate of 6–14%. A negative or nondiagnostic bedside emergency ultrasound by an emergency physician should be followed up with formal radiologic ultrasonography or computed tomography, or with surgical intervention if there is high clinical suspicion for appendicitis. In this case, further imaging is not necessary and surgical consultation is indicated.

9-47. **The answer is A** (Chapter 87). Ranson's criteria on admission to predict patient outcome in acute pancreatitis include the following: age >55 years, blood glucose >200 mg/dL, white blood cell count >16,000/L, alanine aminotransferase (ALT or SGOT) >250 IU/L, and lactate dehydrogenase (LDH) >700 IU/L. Hypotension is not part

of Ranson's criteria but may indicate a complicated course. Although Ranson's criteria are thought to have poor predictive value in the acute setting, they may aid to identify patients at risk for complications and can help to determine the level of inpatient care needed.

9-48. **The answer is D** (Chapter 89). Since jejunostomy tracts are smaller than gastrostomy tracts, smaller tubes should be used when replacing a jejunostomy tube with a temporary catheter. Typically 8–14 F Foley catheters are used for jejunostomies, as opposed to 16 F Foley catheters for gastrostomies. When replacing a dislodged or dysfunctional jejunostomy tube with a Foley catheter, the balloon should not be inflated as this can lead to jejunal damage or bowel obstruction. The balloon can be inflated for gastrostomies once proper positioning is suspected. For both jejunostomy and gastrostomy tube replacements, efforts should be aborted if any resistance is met.

9-49. **The answer is A** (Chapter 84). The sclera has a high concentration of elastin, which binds bilirubin readily; thus jaundice is usually first detected in the eyes and can be seen with bilirubin levels greater than 2 mg/dL. Jaundice is harder to detect in people with darker complexions due to the innate darker color of the skin and sclera in many of these patients. Jaundice can also be falsely suspected in those with high blood carotene levels resulting from ingestion of foods high in β-carotene, which can cause a yellow-orange skin discoloration.

9-50. **The answer is A** (Chapter 90). Infection is the most common complication following liver transplantation, seen in over 60% of patients. Other common complications include rejection (usually seen at 7–14 days), biliary leaks/strictures/obstruction, and vascular complications such as hepatic artery thrombosis.

9-51. **The answer is B** (Chapter 86). Common organisms seen in spontaneous bacterial peritonitis are *Enterobacteriaceae* (63%) such as *Escherichia coli* and *Klebsiella,* followed by *Streptococcus pneumoniae*, enterococci, and anaerobes. Empiric treatment for suspected spontaneous bacterial peritonitis includes third-generation cephalosporins, ticarcillin-clavulanic acid, piperacillin-tazobactam, or ampicillin-sulbactam.

9-52. **The answer is A** (Chapters 85, 86). These liver function tests are most consistent with alcoholic hepatitis. An AST/ALT ratio >2 is more indicative of alcoholic hepatitis, whereas a ratio <1 is more commonly seen in viral hepatitis. Biliary disease such as cholecystitis and choledocholithiasis tends to raise alkaline phosphatase in addition to transaminases.

9-53. **The answer is C** (Chapter 90). Because the hepatic artery solely supplies the biliary system, hepatic artery thrombosis is associated with biliary leaks or abnormalities. Duplex ultrasonography should be performed on any patient suspected of having a biliary abnormality after a liver transplant to evaluate for hepatic artery thrombosis, which is the most common vascular complication following liver transplantation.

9-54. **The answer is B** (Chapter 89). Minimal drainage around a gastrostomy stomal site shortly after placement is typical of a foreign body reaction due to the catheter. In the absence of systemic symptoms and local cellulitis, local wound care with warm water and hydrogen peroxide should be sufficient treatment. If more voluminous drainage or gastric content leakage is suspected, replacement with a larger size tube is indicated. No signs or symptoms point to a misplaced tube, gastric perforation, or systemic infection in this patient.

9-55. **The answer is D** (Chapter 91). Air is the preferred contrast medium when performing a diagnostic and reduction enema for intussusception. Barium has an increased peritonitis risk if perforation occurs with resultant spillage into the peritoneum. However, barium does offer the advantage of better contrast visualization under fluoroscopy. Gastrograffin, a water-soluble substance, is a less preferred radiographic contrast agent in neonates and infants due to its potential for fluid shifts and resultant electrolyte abnormalities.

Gynecologic and Obstetric Emergencies
Questions

10-1. Which of the following gynecologic malignancies generally does not present with vaginal bleeding?

(A) Cervical cancer.

(B) Vaginal cancer.

(C) Ovarian cancer.

(D) Uterine cancer.

10-2. Which of the following statements regarding the diagnosis and management of vaginal bleeding is TRUE?

(A) All patients presenting to the ED with vaginal bleeding who are not pregnant can be referred to clinic without further ED evaluation.

(B) Blood clots are abnormal in vaginal bleeding.

(C) Patients with vaginal bleeding who are hemodynamically unstable are resuscitated according to standard practice.

(D) Ultrasonography has no role in the evaluation of nonpregnant patients with vaginal bleeding.

10-3. Which of the following statements regarding leiomyomas is TRUE?

(A) Leiomyomas or fibroids are uncommon pelvic tumors.

(B) Most patients with leiomyomas are symptomatic.

(C) Leiomyomas decrease in size during menopause.

(D) These tumors decrease in size during pregnancy.

10-4. A 49-year-old female presents to the ED with a complaint of right flank pain and mild nausea. She had an abdominal hysterectomy 5 days prior to presentation. She has no dysuria or hematuria. Which of the following tests would be LEAST helpful?

(A) Abdominal and pelvic CT scan without contrast.

(B) Intravenous pyelogram.

(C) Renal function tests.

(D) Urinalysis.

10-5. Which of the following is NOT consistent with hyperemesis gravidarum?

(A) Abdominal pain.

(B) Hypokalemia.

(C) Ketonuria.

(D) Weight loss.

10-6. A 25-year-old female presents to the ED with a complaint of dysuria and nausea. She is 6 weeks pregnant by dates. Her evaluation indicates that she has a simple urinary tract infection (UTI). Which of the following medications is not safe in pregnancy?

(A) Cephalexin.

(B) Ciprofloxacin.

(C) Nitrofurantoin.

(D) Metoclopramide.

10-7. A 30-year-old female with type 2 diabetes presents to the ED with a complaint of nausea, vomiting, polydipsia, and polyuria for a week. Despite being compliant with her oral hypoglycemic agents, her glucose checks at home have been in the 280–350 mg/dL range. Her screening urine test for β-hCG is positive. What is the MOST appropriate next step in management?

(A) Give an oral fluid challenge, double the oral hypoglycemic agent, and have the patient follow up with OB at the next available appointment.

(B) Give an oral fluid challenge, check electrolytes and serum glucose, and have the patient follow up with OB at the next available appointment.

(C) Give intravenous fluids, check electrolytes and serum glucose, double the oral hypoglycemic agent, and have the patient follow up with OB at the next available appointment.

(D) Give intravenous fluids, check electrolytes and serum glucose, stop the oral hypoglycemic agent, and call for an appointment with OB within the week.

10-8. Which of the following statements regarding vulvovaginitis is TRUE?

(A) Symptoms can occur in sexually active, virgin, and postmenopausal women.

(B) Microscopic evaluation of vaginal secretions is not necessary to establish a diagnosis.

(C) Polymicrobial infections are uncommon.

(D) The most common cause of vulvovaginitis is trichomoniasis.

10-9. A previously healthy 27-year-old female G_1P_0 at 16 weeks gestation presents to the ED with a complaint of continued nausea and vomiting and new vaginal bleeding. She has no abdominal pain. Her blood pressure is 160/90 mmHg with a heart rate of 110 beats per minute. What is the MOST likely diagnosis?

(A) Implantation bleeding.

(B) Ectopic pregnancy.

(C) Molar pregnancy.

(D) Preeclampsia.

10-10. A 28-year-old female presents to the ED with a complaint of left lower abdominal pain and vaginal bleeding. She has a history of irregular menses. She has 2 healthy children at home. Which of the following tests would narrow the differential and help determine disposition?

(A) Complete blood count.

(B) β-HCG.

(C) Urinalysis.

(D) Rh factor.

10-11. A 44-year-old female presents to the ED with a complaint of a white nipple discharge that has been present for a week. She thought the symptoms would resolve. She has no pain and has felt no masses. Her neurological exam is normal. The urine pregnancy test is negative. Which of the following statements is TRUE?

(A) Decreased cortisol levels can cause galactorrhea.

(B) Decreased prolactin levels can cause galactorrhea.

(C) This patient can be worked up by her primary care provider.

(D) This patient requires neurosurgery evaluation.

10-12. A 54-year-old female presents to the ED with a complaint of a breast mass. Which of the following statements is TRUE?

(A) The most common cause for breast disease in postmenopausal women is fibrocystic disease.

(B) All women with a palpable mass should be referred to a breast specialist.

(C) Fibrocystic changes of the breast include skin thickening, discoloration, and discharge.

(D) Patients over the age of 40 with a normal exam do not need a mammogram.

10-13. A 64-year-old female with a history of diabetes presents to the ED with a complaint of progressive urinary incontinence over the past 3 weeks with the sensation of never completely emptying her bladder. Which of the following studies would be MOST appropriate to order to determine which type of incontinence is present?

(A) Postvoid residual.

(B) Glucose.

(C) Urinalysis.

(D) Intravenous pyelogram.

10-14. Which of the following statements regarding gynecologic malignancies is TRUE?

(A) The diagnosis of cervical cancer in an HIV-positive patient is an AIDS-defining illness.

(B) Lymphedema is treated surgically for patient comfort.

(C) Human papillomavirus is not a risk factor for cervical and vulvar cancers.

(D) Gastrointestinal obstruction is the most common oncologic complication.

10-15. A 25-year-old female presents to the ED with a complaint of lower abdominal pain, vaginal bleeding, and fever. She underwent an induced abortion 2 weeks prior to presentation. Which of the following tests is MOST helpful in the management of this patient?

(A) Pelvic ultrasound.

(B) Complete blood count.

(C) Urinalysis.

(D) Urine β-hCG.

10-16. Which of the following is NOT a risk factor for pelvic inflammatory disease (PID)?

(A) Multiple sex partners.

(B) Frequent vaginal douching.

(C) Lack of barrier contraceptive.

(D) Pregnancy.

10-17. Which of the following is LEAST helpful in the diagnosis of PID?

(A) Leukorrhea on wet preparations of vaginal secretions.

(B) Thickened fluid-filled fallopian tubes with free pelvic fluid seen with transvaginal pelvic ultrasound.

(C) Leukocytes and bacteria from culdocentesis.

(D) Elevated C-reactive protein levels.

10-18. Treatment of bacterial vaginosis in pregnancy does NOT include which of the following regimens?

(A) Metronidazole 250 mg po bid for 7 days.

(B) Clindamycin cream 2% intravaginally qhs for 7 days.

(C) Clindamycin 300 mg po bid for 7 days.

(D) Metronidazole gel 0.75% intravaginally bid for 5 days.

10-19. Which of the following statements regarding labor in the pregnant patient is TRUE?

(A) False labor or Braxton Hicks contractions are characterized by irregular, brief contractions that lead to changes in the cervix.

(B) True labor is characterized by painful, repetitive uterine contractions that increase steadily and lead to changes in the cervix.

(C) Cervical dilatation of the cervix refers to the process of thinning that occurs during labor.

(D) Effacement describes the diameter of the internal cervical os and is used as an indicator of the progression of labor.

10-20. A 25-year-old G_1P_0 female presents to the ED frantic because her "water broke." She states that she is from out of town and does not know a physician in the area. She is 37 weeks gestation by dates and has a blood pressure of 118/65 mmHg and a heart rate of 110 beats per minute. Which of the following statements regarding spontaneous rupture of membranes (SROM) is TRUE?

(A) Rupture of membranes can be confirmed by nitrazine paper changing to red.

(B) Ferning is diagnostic of vaginal fluid.

(C) A speculum and digital exam should not be performed if SROM is suspected.

(D) SROM signals the end of active labor.

10-21. Which of the following physiologic changes does NOT take place during normal pregnancy?

(A) Delayed gastric emptying.

(B) Increased respiratory rate.

(C) Delayed gallbladder emptying.

(D) Increased renal blood flow.

10-22. Which of the following statements regarding ovarian cysts is TRUE?

(A) Typical presentation is unilateral pelvic pain.

(B) Ultrasonography should be done immediately for all patients with suspected ovarian cysts.

(C) Cysts that are >8 cm, unilocular, and unilateral are observed.

(D) Complications include rupture, hemorrhage, torsion, and infection.

10-23. Which of the following statements regarding diagnostic evaluation of the female patient of childbearing age with abdominal and pelvic pain is TRUE?

(A) Ultrasonography is the test of choice for evaluating suspected pelvic and gynecologic pathology.

(B) An elevated white blood cell count is sensitive for an acute surgical condition.

(C) Positive urinalysis findings are specific for urine pathology.

(D) Laparotomy is the gold standard for diagnosing PID.

10-24. A 36-year-old female presents to the ED with a complaint of abdominal pain and vaginal spotting. Figure 10-1a and 10-1b shows the ultrasound images that were obtained. Which of the following statements does NOT apply to this patient's diagnosis?

(A) Abdominal pain or discomfort is the most common symptom.

(B) Vital signs are usually normal.

(C) A low progesterone level aids in the diagnosis.

(D) A negative urine pregnancy test rules out the diagnosis.

10-25. Which of the following is NOT appropriate management for a patient with an ectopic pregnancy?

(A) Methotrexate.

(B) Laparoscopy in the hemodynamically unstable patient.

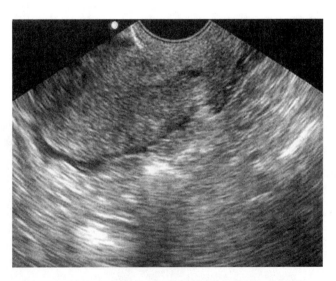

Figure 10-1a. Longitudinal view of pelvis.

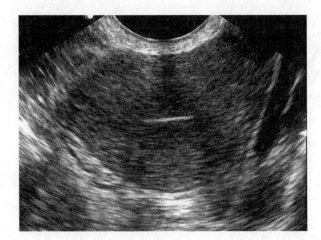

Figure 10-1b. Transverse view of pelvis.

(C) Anti-Rh$_0$ immunoglobulin in an Rh-negative patient.

(D) Expectant management with serial β-hCG levels and ultrasound.

10-26. Which of the following statements regarding the diagnosis and management of thromboembolism in pregnancy is TRUE?

(A) Perfusion lung scan with technetium 99m is harmful to the fetus.

(B) Iodine-125 fibrinogen scanning should not be used in pregnancy.

(C) Warfarin can be used safely in pregnancy.

(D) Heparin cannot be used safely in pregnancy.

10-27. A 28-year-old female presents to the ED in active labor. On visual inspection the fetal head is seen at the introitus. Which of the following should NOT be done?

(A) Support the inferior portion of the perineum with a sterile towel.

(B) Immediately suction the infant's nose and mouth after delivery of the infant's head.

(C) Maintain control of the slippery newborn so that inadvertent dropping does not occur.

(D) Transfer the patient to the labor and delivery ward.

10-28. Which of the following statements regarding complications of delivery is TRUE?

(A) Decelerations in fetal heart rate must be treated with immediate delivery of the infant.

(B) In the event of a prolapsed cord the examiner's hand should be used to elevate the presented fetal part until the patient is prepared for cesarean section.

(C) Breech presentations occur most frequently in term pregnancies.

(D) During suspected shoulder dystocia fundal pressure should be applied to assist in delivery.

10-29. A 21-year-old female presents with a complaint of severe pain on urination, subjective fever, and headache. She states that she has "bumps" on her vulva. She has no history of similar episodes. Which of the following is NOT a treatment option?

(A) Confirm the diagnosis by culture and treat with acyclovir 400 mg tid for 7–10 days.

(B) Confirm the diagnosis by culture and treat with acyclovir 400 mg bid daily.

(C) Confirm the diagnosis by polymerase chain reaction (PCR) and treat with famciclovir 250 mg tid for 7–10 days.

(D) Confirm the diagnosis by PCR and treat with valacyclovir 1 g bid for 7–10 days.

10-30. While a 35-week pregnant patient is in the ED for headache, she has a generalized seizure. She does not have a history of seizure disorder. She is now postictal and unable to give further information. Which of the following is LEAST helpful in management?

(A) Neurology consultation.

(B) Obstetrics consultation.

(C) Administration of magnesium sulfate.

(D) Repeat vital signs.

10-31. Which of the following statements regarding HELLP syndrome is TRUE?

(A) Platelet count is >100,000.

(B) Patients are hypertensive.

(C) Most patients are multigravid.

(D) The coagulation profile is normal.

Gynecologic and Obstetric Emergencies
Answers, Explanations, and References

10-1. **The answer is C** (Chapters 106, 111). One of the difficulties in the diagnosis of ovarian cancer is that the presenting symptoms are nonspecific. The symptoms include abdominal pain, bloating, early satiety, and weight loss. All of these symptoms could be caused by many other diagnoses. In contrast, cervical, uterine, and vaginal cancers present with symptoms of abnormal, postcoital, or postmenopausal vaginal bleeding.

10-2. **The answer is C** (Chapters 31, 101, 113). Standard practice for a hemodynamically unstable patient with vaginal bleeding is fluid and blood resuscitation until the underlying cause can be corrected. After it is determined that a patient is not pregnant and is hemodynamically stable in the ED, several diagnoses should be ruled out prior to outpatient referral. Those diagnoses include trauma, bleeding dyscrasias, infection, and foreign body presence. Patients are often concerned about the presence of blood clots with vaginal bleeding. Blood clots are not abnormal in women with heavy bleeding when there may be insufficient time for fibrinolysis to occur. Ultrasonography is an important imaging modality in the nonpregnant patient who may have structural changes such as leiomyomas as a cause of abnormal vaginal bleeding.

10-3. **The answer is C** (Chapters 101, 102, 113). Leiomyomas decrease in size during menopause. Growth at this time is suspicious for malignant transformation. In contrast, these tumors increase in size during pregnancy and have the potential to cause complications. Leiomyomas are the most common pelvic tumor and the most common indication for major surgery in women. They are typically asymptomatic but can undergo torsion or degenerate and cause acute pain.

10-4. **The answer is A** (Chapter 112). Operative injury to the ureter occurs more often during the performance of abdominal hysterectomy than any other pelvic surgery. In the patient who develops flank pain shortly after surgery, suspect ureteral injury. Tests for functional status should be ordered. Those tests include abdominal and pelvic CT scan with contrast, an intravenous pyelogram, renal function tests, and a urinalysis.

10-5. **The answer is A** (Chapter 106). Severe nausea and vomiting in pregnancy with weight loss, volume depletion, and laboratory changes showing hypokalemia and ketonemia is hyperemesis gravidarum. If the patient has abdominal pain, other diagnoses should be considered. Patients are treated with intravenous fluids containing 5% glucose to replete volume and reverse ketonuria and antiemetics as needed until correction of electrolyte imbalance and successful trial of oral fluids.

10-6. **The answer is B** (Chapter 104). Pharmaceutical companies have not traditionally tested drugs in pregnant women to determine potential fetal effects. Antimicrobial agents considered safe in pregnancy are cephalosporins, azithromycin, nitrofurantoin, and penicillins. Antiemetics considered safe in pregnancy are promethazine, prochlorperazine, metoclopramide, and odansetron. Fluoroquinolones have caused fetal cartilage abnormalities in animals and are contraindicated in pregnancy.

10-7.   **The answer is D** (Chapters 105, 106). Nausea and vomiting in pregnancy are generally seen in the first 12 weeks. Treatment is with intravenous fluids and antiemetics as needed. Oral fluids should be started after the nausea and vomiting are controlled but prior to discharge. Oral hypoglycemic agents are not used during pregnancy because they do not provide adequate glucose control, and some agents have been associated with an increased risk of congenital anomalies, hyperbilirubinemia, and irreversible β-cell hyperplasia in exposed infants. The oral hypoglycemic agent should be discontinued and the patient referred as a high-risk patient for urgent follow-up in OB.

10-8.   **The answer is A** (Chapter 108). Vulvovaginitis is an inflammation of the vulva and vaginal tissues and has the potential to develop in any female. The most common etiologies are infections, irritant or allergic contact, local reaction to foreign body, and atrophy. The most common cause of vulvovaginitis is bacterial vaginosis. Polymicrobial infections are not uncommon. When signs of vulva inflammation with minimal discharge and no vaginal pathogens are present, noninfectious causes of vulvovaginitis should be considered. Microscopic evaluation of secretions will provide a diagnosis in most instances and is mandatory because symptoms are nonspecific.

10-9.   **The answer is C** (Chapters 103, 106). The most likely diagnosis is molar pregnancy. This patient is still in the first half of pregnancy. She has passed the time frame for implantation bleeding. Ectopic pregnancy

has to be considered in the differential diagnosis. The patient, however, does not have abdominal pain, which is the most common symptom of ectopic pregnancy. Finally, preeclampsia always occurs after 20 weeks of gestation unless gestational trophoblastic disease (GTD) is present. Patients with GTD may present with intractable vomiting. When hypertension in pregnancy is seen prior to 24 weeks gestation, the possibility of a molar pregnancy should be considered.

10-10.   **The answer is B** (Chapters 101, 103). The differential for this patient's symptoms is broad. The differential narrows considerably once pregnancy is established. Urine tests can be performed rapidly at the bedside and are therefore the best first test for pregnancy. Ectopic pregnancy must be considered with a positive test and remains in the differential until it is excluded with conviction. If the patient is not pregnant, the differential remains broad, but most diagnoses would allow the patient to be discharged with an outpatient workup.

10-11.   **The answer is C** (Chapter 110). Galactorrhea is any inappropriate secretion of milky discharge from the breast. It often results from abnormally elevated prolactin levels. Prolactin levels can be elevated from physiologic, physical, or hormonal reasons as well as by medications, dietary supplements, and illegal drugs. Galactorrhea also occurs in some systemic diseases such as hypothyroidism, Cushing's disease or hypercortisolism, and acromegaly. ED evaluation includes an appropriate physical exam, a pregnancy test, and CT or MRI if an intracranial mass is suspected. There is no indication of an intracranial mass in this patient. A neurosurgery consult is not required, and the patient can be further evaluated and treated by her primary care physician.

10-12.   **The answer is B** (Chapter 110). Fibrocystic breast disease is the most common cause for benign breast disease in premenopausal women. It includes nodularity and tenderness that occurs as a result of breast tissue response to hormonal cycling. Fibrocystic changes do not include skin thickening, edema, discoloration, nipple retraction, or discharge. All patients with a palpable mass with or without other symptoms should be referred to a breast specialist. All women over the age of 40 with a normal exam should also be referred to a breast specialist. If the patient is under 30 with a breast mass, then an outpatient ultrasound should be performed with possible needle aspiration. For patients in their 30s, the management is not clear. It is clear that the risk factors for breast cancer in young women include the inheritance of the *BRCA1* or *BRCA2* genes, a history of childhood malignancy, and a history of childhood irradiation. For women 30 and older the risks factors also include a first-degree relative with breast cancer, increased exposure to endogenous estrogens, and biopsy-confirmed atypical hyperplasia of the breast.

10-13. **The answer is A** (Chapter 111). There are four common classifications of incontinence. They include stress, urge, total, and overflow. Stress incontinence occurs as a result of increased intra-abdominal pressure. Urge incontinence occurs with detrusor muscle instability. Total incontinence usually results from a urinary fistula and involves painless leaking of urine and recurrent infections. Overflow incontinence results from a hypotonic detrusor muscle generally seen in the setting of neuropathy. The neuropathy can be secondary to diabetes, spinal cord injury, postoperative problems, or lower motor neuron diseases. Patients complain of incomplete voiding and leaking of urine. The diagnosis is made through the history and physical exam. The postvoid residual volume is needed to determine if the patient is retaining urine.

10-14. **The answer is A** (Chapter 111). Lymphedema of the lower extremities often fol-

lows inguinal node resection and is treated supportively with elevation and support stockings. The most common oncologic complication is bleeding and requires gynecologic consultation after stabilization. Gastrointestinal obstruction is common as a progressive symptom of malignancy, especially with ovarian and uterine tumors. Viruses appear to play a role in gynecologic malignancies. Human papillomavirus is a risk factor for both cervical and vulvar cancers. Cervical cancer is an AIDS-defining illness in an HIV-positive patient.

10-15. **The answer is A** (Chapter 112). This patient presents with a delayed complication of an induced abortion. These include excessive bleeding and postabortive endometritis that can both be secondary to retained products. A pelvic ultrasound should be obtained to evaluate the uterine cavity for retained products.

10-16. **The answer is D** (Chapter 109). Pregnancy decreases the risk of PID because a mucous plug protects the cervical os. PID can occur during the first trimester and may cause fetal loss. Consistent barrier contraception is associated with lower risk of PID. Other risk factors for PID include multiple sex partners, history of other STDs, history of sexual abuse, younger age, and frequent vaginal douching.

10-17. **The answer is C** (Chapter 109). Even though culdocentesis can be performed rapidly, its utility is limited since findings of leukocytes and bacteria are nonspecific. Diagnostic guidelines for treatment include an elevated sedimentation rate and C-reactive protein level as well as the sonographic findings of fluid-filled fallopian tubes with or without free pelvic fluid. The absence of leukorrhea in saline preparations of vaginal secretions is a negative predictor for PID. Other criteria for diagnosis include uterine or adnexal tenderness and cervical motion tenderness.

10-18. **The answer is B** (Chapter 108). The use of clindamycin vaginal cream during pregnancy is not recommended because of the possibility of preterm deliveries among pregnant women with this medication. Alternatives to metronidazole are not as efficacious. All patients on oral metronidazole should avoid alcohol for 24 hours after its use because of the disulfiram-like reaction that can occur.

10-19. **The answer is B** (Chapter 107). Confirmation of true labor as opposed to false labor is an important initial step in the management of the term pregnant patient. False labor or Braxton Hicks contractions are defined as uterine contractions characterized as irregular and brief that do not lead to cervical changes. True labor is characterized by painful, repetitive uterine contractions that increase in intensity and duration and lead to cervical changes. These cervical changes are effacement and dilatation. Effacement of the cervix refers to the process of thinning that occurs during labor. Cervical dilatation describes the diameter of the internal cervical os and is an indicator of the progression of labor.

10-20. **The answer is C** (Chapter 107). SROM occurs during the course of active labor in most patients. If SROM is suspected a sterile speculum examination should be performed and digital examination should be avoided or limited because studies have shown an increased risk of infection after a single digital examination. Use nitrazine paper to test residual fluid in the fornix or vaginal vault while performing a sterile speculum examination. Amniotic fluid has a pH of 7.0–7.4 and will turn nitrazine paper dark blue. As amniotic fluid dries on a slide, ferning occurs and is also used to confirm SROM.

10-21. **The answer is B** (Chapter 104). Most women experience dyspnea during pregnancy. Since the respiratory rate is not changed, the sensation may result from the increase in tidal volume with resultant de-

crease in P_{CO_2}. Gastric reflux commonly occurs as a result of delayed gastric emptying, decreased intestinal motility, and decreased lower esophageal sphincter tone. Gallbladder emptying is delayed and less efficient, resulting in pregnancy increasing the risk of cholesterol gallstones. There is a 40–45% increase in circulating blood volume.

10-22. **The answer is D** (Chapter 102). The complications of ovarian cysts result in the typical presentation of sudden unilateral pelvic pain. These complications include rupture, hemorrhage, torsion, and infection. Ultrasonography aids in the diagnosis and can be done in the ED or during an outpatient follow-up depending on the clinical situation. Ovarian cysts that are <8 cm, unilocular, and unilateral are generally observed. The natural history of functional cysts is generally spontaneous resolution within cycles.

10-23. **The answer is A** (Chapter 102). An elevated white blood cell count is neither sensitive nor specific for an acute surgical condition. Positive findings on urinalysis are not specific for urinary pathology. Urinalysis can be falsely positive with hematuria or evidence of infection in other pelvic and abdominal organs. Testing for gonorrhea and chlamydia should be done. Positive test results have public health implications and should have a follow-up system in place. Ultrasonography is the test of choice for evaluating suspected pelvic and gynecologic pathology. Laparoscopy is the gold standard for diagnosing PID.

10-24. **The answer is D** (Chapters 103, 113). The classic triad of symptoms in ectopic pregnancy is abdominal pain with vaginal bleeding or spotting with amenorrhea. The most common symptom is abdominal pain and is reported in 90% of patients with ectopic pregnancy. The physical examination is variable and vital signs are usually normal. Dilute urine may cause a false negative urine pregnancy test and, therefore, a quantitative serum test should be performed if the diagnosis of ectopic pregnancy is still being considered. There is no single β-hCG level that can reliably distinguish between a normal and a pathologic pregnancy. The placenta secretes progesterone during pregnancy. Absolute levels of progesterone are lower in pathologic pregnancies. When ectopic pregnancy is suspected, ultrasonography should be performed even in patients with low β-hCG levels. Both transabdominal and transvaginal ultrasound examinations should be done.

10-25. **The answer is B** (Chapter 103). The treatment of ectopic pregnancy can be divided into surgical, medical, and expectant approaches. Methotrexate is the only drug currently approved for medical management. Laparotomy is the treatment of choice for hemodynamically unstable patients, and laparoscopy is the treatment of choice for hemodynamically stable patients. Both the American College of Emergency Physicians and the American College of Obstetricians and Gynecologists recommend treatment of 50 μg of anti-Rh$_0$ immunoglobulin for Rh-negative women with ectopic pregnancy.

10-26. **The answer is B** (Chapter 105). The clinical diagnosis of thromboembolism in pregnancy is similar to that in the nonpregnant patient. Impedance plethysmography and perfusion lung scans with technetium 99m pose no threat to the fetus. Iodine-125 fibrinogen scanning should not be used because unbound iodine crosses the placental barrier. Treatment is with intravenous heparin. Low-molecular-weight heparin can also be used. Warfarin is contraindicated because it crosses the placenta and is associated with embryopathy in the first trimester and CNS and ophthalmologic abnormalities in the second and third trimesters.

10-27. **The answer is D** (Chapter 107). With the fetal head at the introitus, delivery is immi-

nent. Transport to another area of the hospital or to another hospital is not practical. The providers present should prepare for delivery of the infant and control the situation as much as possible. It is important to deliver the infant systematically as outlined and to maintain control of the newborn so that inadvertent dropping does not occur.

10-28. **The answer is B** (Chapter 107). Decelerations in fetal heart rate are an indicator of fetal distress and should be treated with repositioning of the patient, hydration, and oxygen supplementation but not necessarily delivery. Breech delivery is more common in premature infants and is associated with a greater incidence of umbilical cord prolapse. If cord prolapse is noted on exam, the examiner should continue to elevate the presenting fetal parts while the patient is prepared for cesarean section. Shoulder dystocia is impaction of fetal shoulders at the pelvic outlet after delivery of the head. Fundal pressure should never be applied since this will further impact the shoulder on the pelvic rim. Instead an assistant should apply suprapubic pressure to disimpact the anterior shoulder from the pelvic rim.

10-29. **The answer is B** (Chapter 108). This is an initial presentation of genital herpes. Diagnosis is suspected by clinical presentation and confirmed by either culture or PCR. Treatment is not curative. Patients who are pregnant with life-threatening disease and those patients with severe disease need hospitalization with intravenous acyclovir therapy. All of the oral regimens listed are for initial episodes except acyclovir 400 mg bid, which is for daily suppressive therapy.

10-30. **The answer is A** (Chapter 106). Eclampsia must be ruled out in a pregnant patient who has a seizure. Repeat vital signs, obstetrics consultation, and administration of magnesium are key to appropriate management. Neurology consultation is not usually necessary.

10-31. **The answer is C** (Chapter 106). The HELLP syndrome is an important clinical variant of preeclampsia. HELLP is an acronym for hemolysis, elevated liver enzymes, and low platelets. The coagulation profile is abnormal. The blood pressure is variable and may not be initially elevated. The HELLP syndrome should be considered in any pregnant patient who presents to the ED with abdominal pain especially in the right upper quadrant. In contrast to preeclampsia, where the primagravid patient is more common, the multigravid patient more commonly develops the HELLP syndrome.

Hematologic and Oncologic Emergencies
Questions

11-1. In iron, vitamin B_{12}, or folate deficiency anemias, which of the following red blood cell (RBC) indices may change before the mean corpuscular volume (MCV)?

(A) Hematocrit.

(B) Mean corpuscular hemoglobin (MCH).

(C) Mean cellular hemoglobin concentration (MCHC).

(D) Red cell distribution width (RDW).

11-2. Paramedics bring in a 70-year-old woman with coffee-ground emesis after self-medicating with aspirin for three days to treat her osteoarthritis. Vital signs are blood pressure 130/90 mmHg, pulse 124 beats per minute, respirations 26 per minute, temperature 98.6°F, and oxygen saturation 94%. The patient has a nasal cannula delivering oxygen at 3 L/min, and an IV of Ringer's lactate. The patient is alert and complains of mild epigastric pain and shortness of breath, but she denies chest pain. Her abdomen is soft, mildly tender, and her rectal exam reveals melena. A nasogastric tube produces 300 cc of dark blood. Her hemoglobin is 9 g/dL. An electrocardiogram reveals sinus tachycardia without ST-segment elevation or depression. A chest x-ray is normal. What is the next MOST appropriate immediate action or intervention?

(A) Obtain an arterial blood gas.

(B) Administer platelets.

(C) Administer morphine 2 mg intravenously.

(D) Transfuse the patient with packed red blood cells.

11-3. Which of the following conditions is LEAST likely associated with a platelet disorder?

(A) Epistaxis.

(B) Retroperitoneal bleeding.

(C) Ecchymoses.

(D) Petechiae.

11-4. Which of the following conditions is LEAST likely to be associated with a coagulation factor deficiency?

(A) Intra-articular bleeding.

(B) Delayed bleeding.

(C) Retroperitoneal bleeding.

(D) Petechiae.

11-5. Which of the following conditions is LEAST likely to be associated with coagulation factor II, V, VII, VIII, IX, or X deficiency?

(A) Hemarthrosis.

(B) Delayed bleeding.

(C) Retroperitoneal bleeding.

(D) Arterial and venous thrombosis.

11-6. What clinical finding is MOST commonly associated with the onset of idiopathic thrombocytopenic purpura (ITP)?

(A) Ecchymoses.

(B) Purpura.

(C) Petechiae.

(D) Gingival bleeding.

11-7. Which of the following statements regarding chronic ITP is TRUE?

(A) It is more likely to develop in female children.

(B) Spontaneous remissions are typical.

(C) Underlying disease or autoimmune disorders are common.

(D) Platelet transfusions constitute initial, definitive therapy.

11-8. Which thrombocytopenia-producing condition is NOT due to increased platelet destruction?

(A) Radiation therapy.

(B) Idiopathic thrombocytopenic purpura (ITP).

(C) Thrombotic thrombocytopenic purpura (TTP).

(D) Hemolytic uremic syndrome (HUS).

11-9. Which lab finding would suggest the patient has severe liver disease and not disseminated intravascular coagulation (DIC)?

(A) Thrombocytopenia with bleeding.

(B) Prolonged prothrombin time.

(C) Hypofibrinogenemia.

(D) Normal or minimally elevated D-dimer assay.

11-10. A 50-year-old man with known cirrhosis and ascites presents with fever and abdominal pain, and is suspected of having acute spontaneous bacterial peritonitis. The patient is hemodynamically stable and not actively bleeding (negative nasogastric tube aspiration and no occult blood in rectal exam). Initial labs include a prolonged prothrombin time, increased INR, decreased platelets, and a minimally decreased fib-

rinogen level. Which of the following is indicated prior to performing a paracentesis?

(A) Cryoprecipitate.

(B) Fresh frozen plasma (FFP).

(C) Platelet transfusion.

(D) Desmopressin (DDAVP).

11-11. Which of the following is the MOST commonly observed abnormality in patients with DIC?

(A) Prolonged prothrombin time.

(B) Thrombocytopenia.

(C) Hypofibrinogenemia.

(D) Elevated fibrin degradation products and D-dimer assay.

11-12. A 60-year-old woman presents with urosepsis, hematuria, petechiae, and mucosal bleeding. She has a hemoglobin of 12 g/dL, an elevated prothrombin time, a platelet count of 76,000/µL, and a fibrinogen level of 80 mg/dL. Oxygen, intravenous fluids, pressors, antibiotics, and fresh frozen plasma are being administered. What other treatment modality is indicated next?

(A) Platelet transfusion.

(B) Packed red blood cell transfusion.

(C) Cryoprecipitate.

(D) Heparin.

11-13. Which of the following is the MOST common cause of DIC?

(A) Adenocarcinoma.

(B) Trauma due to burns, crush injury, or fat embolism.

(C) Infection due to gram-negative sepsis.

(D) Acute promyelocytic leukemia.

11-14. Paramedics bring in a 19-year-old male who was the restrained back-seat passenger in a vehicle that was rear-ended at approximately 35 miles per hour. He is on a backboard and is wearing a cervical collar. The patient states he struck his head on the front seat headrest, and though he did not lose consciousness, he does have a headache. He denies neck pain. His past medical history is significant for hemophilia B. His vital signs are stable and his physical examination is entirely normal except for a forehead contusion. What is the next MOST appropriate step in this man's care?

(A) Obtain cervical spine films.

(B) Obtain a CT scan of the head.

(C) Administer factor IX.

(D) Administer cryoprecipitate.

11-15. A 7-year-old male presents with left lower quadrant abdominal pain after being hit by a knee in his lower torso 2 hours ago while wrestling with his twin brother. The patient has severe hemophilia A. His vital signs are normal. The physical examination is notable for a contusion in the left inguinal area, above and below the inguinal crease. The patient is mildly tender to palpation in the left lower quadrant. Bowel sounds are present. The genitalia are normal and not contused. His rectal examination is negative for blood. Obturator sign is negative. The patient has pain with extension of his left lower extremity, and he walks with his trunk slightly flexed forward. What is the appropriate treatment plan?

(A) Give factor VIII and order a CT scan of the abdomen.

(B) Give factor IX and order a CT scan of the abdomen.

(C) Give desmopressin (DDAVP) and order a CT scan of the abdomen.

(D) Give fresh frozen plasma and order an ultrasound of the abdomen.

11-16. A 9-year-old female with mild type I von Willebrand's disease presents with mild gingival bleeding after her first overly vigorous attempt to use dental floss. She stopped as soon as she noticed bleeding, which is limited to the space between her upper central incisors. She is somewhat anxious, but her vital signs are normal. The physical exam is normal except for gingival bleeding between the upper central incisors. Bleeding has continued despite apply-

ing pressure to the site for 30 minutes. What is the MOST appropriate action?

(A) Subcutaneous DDAVP 0.03 µg/kg.

(B) Intravenous DDAVP 0.03 µg/kg over 30 minutes.

(C) Intranasal DDAVP 150 µg (one spray in one nostril).

(D) Cryoprecipitate.

11-17. Which of the following would be the MOST appropriate over-the-counter analgesic for a patient with type I von Willebrand's disease?

(A) Aspirin 80 mg.

(B) Aspirin 325 mg.

(C) Ibuprofen 200 mg.

(D) Acetaminophen 325 mg.

11-18. Which of the following statements regarding patients with sickle cell anemia is TRUE?

(A) Acute chest syndrome is the leading cause of death from sickle cell disease in the United States.

(B) Hydroxyurea effectively decreases the frequency and severity of painful crises in children.

(C) Infants often present at around 3 months of age with dactylitis (hand-foot syndrome).

(D) Simple or exchange transfusion is indicated for dactylitis.

11-19. Which of the following statements regarding clopidogrel is TRUE?

(A) It inhibits platelet aggregation by blocking the adenosine diphosphate (ADP) release.

(B) It is contraindicated in patients with aspirin hypersensitivity who have unstable angina or non-ST-segment elevation myocardial infarction.

(C) Thrombotic thrombocytopenic purpura can rarely occur.

(D) It is poorly tolerated due to side effects.

11-20. A transfusion of 2 units of packed red blood cells is started on a 40-year-old man with a hemoglobin of 7 g/dL, due to a bleeding gastric ulcer. Ten minutes later, he complains of low back pain and chills. Vital signs are blood pressure 95/60 mmHg, pulse 110 beats per minute, respirations 24 breaths per minute, room air oxygen saturation of 96%, and temperature 37°C. The patient appears flushed and dyspneic. The transfusion is stopped immediately, and crystalloid is infused at 300 mL/hour. The donor blood and the patient's posttransfusion blood are sent to the lab. Which laboratory findings are MOST likely?

(A) Elevated serum haptoglobin, elevated lactate dehydrogenase, elevated plasma free hemoglobin, and hemoglobinemia.

(B) Elevated serum haptoglobin, decreased lactate dehydrogenase, elevated plasma free hemoglobin, and hemoglobinuria.

(C) Decreased serum haptoglobin, decreased lactate dehydrogenase, elevated plasma free hemoglobin, and hemoglobinuria.

(D) Decreased serum haptoglobin, increased lactate dehydrogenase, elevated plasma free hemoglobin, and hemoglobinuria.

11-21. The oncology clinic refers a 7-year-old boy who is currently undergoing chemotherapy for acute lymphocytic leukemia to the ED for fever of 38°C and an absolute neutrophil count of 450/mm^3. His blood pressure is 110/70 mmHg, pulse is 110 beats per minute, respiratory rate is 20 breaths per minute, and oxygen saturation on room air is 100%. He denies headache, vision changes, oral pain, cough, shortness of breath, or abdominal pain but does report pain with defecation. The clinic reports his funduscopic examination was normal. Which of the following is the appropriate action at this time?

(A) Complete a physical examination including a digital rectal examination, then administer broad-spectrum antibiotics.

(B) Complete a physical examination but not the rectal examination, then administer broad-spectrum antibiotics.

(C) Complete a physical examination but not the rectal examination, obtain blood cultures, and administer broad-spectrum antibiotics.

(D) Complete a physical examination and the rectal examination, obtain blood cultures, and administer broad-spectrum antibiotics.

11-22. A 60-year-old man presents to the ED after accidentally cutting his left index finger with a knife while cutting onions. A 3-cm laceration through the finger pad actively bleeds if pressure is released. There is full range of motion of the DIP, good two point discrimination, and distal capillary refill. He tells you that he takes coumadin 5.0 mg every day since he had a deep venous thrombosis 5 months ago. He has not had his INR checked in 3 months. He denies chest pain, shortness of breath, or new leg swelling. You send a stat PT and INR and have the patient apply pressure while you prepare to anesthetize and clean the laceration. The INR is 6. Which of the following is the MOST appropriate action?

(A) Repair the laceration and instruct the patient to skip the next dose of coumadin.

(B) Repair the laceration and instruct the patient to contact his private provider as soon as possible.

(C) Repair the laceration and administer oral vitamin K 1–2 mg.

(D) Repair the laceration and administer intravenous vitamin K 5–10 mg slowly.

11-23. Which of the following statements regarding thrombotic thrombocytopenic purpura (TTP) is TRUE?

(A) The metalloprotease enzyme that forms von Willebrand factor multimers is qualitatively or quantitatively deficient.

(B) Microvascular platelet-fibrin thrombi shear red blood cells and cause micro-angiopathic hemolytic anemia (MAHA).

(C) Preeclampsia commonly precipitates TTP.

(D) Serum unconjugated bilirubin is elevated and the direct Coombs' test is negative.

11-24. A 65-year-old man with lung cancer who presents with a 5-day history of generalized weakness, anorexia, and constipation is found to have a serum calcium of 14 mg/dL. An electrocardiogram shows sinus tachycardia 120, a widened T wave, and a shortened QT interval. The sodium is 148 mEq/L, potassium is 3.0 mEq/L, chloride is 108 mmol/L, bicarbonate is 18, glucose is 80 mg/dL, blood urea nitrogen is 40, and creatinine is 1.8 mg/dL. The serum albumin is 4.0 g/dL. The patient is awake, diffusely weak, with diminished reflexes. Vital signs are blood pressure 140/90 mmHg, pulse 120 beats per minute, respirations 22 breaths per minute, and temperature 37°C. The first troponin is negative. After he receives 1.5 L normal saline over 1 hour, the infusion is continued at 300 mL/hour. What would be the next MOST appropriate course of action?

(A) Administer oral glucocorticoids.

(B) Administer intravenous glucocorticoids.

(C) Administer furosemide 40-80 mg IV every 2 hours.

(D) Administer calcitonin 4 IU/kg SC or IM every 6–12 hours.

Hematologic and Oncologic Emergencies
Answers, Explanations, and References

11-1. The answer is **D** (Chapter 218). The RDW may increase even before the MCV changes in deficiency anemias. The RDW, which is derived from the bell-shaped red cell size-distribution curve, will reflect both the mean and the presence of different sized cell populations outlying on the "tails" of the curve. The MCV corresponds directly to the mean of the curve. An increase in RDW indicates the presence of different sized cell populations, which occurs early in deficiency anemias. Depending on the automated counter used, hemoglobin and hematocrit are either measured directly or calculated from the RBC count and MCV or RBC size-distribution curve. The MCH and MCHC are in turn calculated values, derived from the RBC count, hemoglobin, and MCV. The RDW, MCV, and reticulocyte count are the most useful guides for classifying anemias.

11-2. The answer is **D** (Chapter 218). Although this patient is not hypotensive and has a hemoglobin higher than 7 g/dL (the standard level for transfusion), a blood transfusion is indicated, given her advanced age, tachycardia, hypoxia, and significant acute blood loss. Testing for acidosis and cardiac ischemia and providing analgesia are also indicated, but in this case, the transfusion of packed red blood cells is the foremost priority.

11-3. The answer is **B** (Chapter 218). Retroperitoneal bleeding is commonly associated with a coagulopathy rather than a platelet disorder. Mucocutaneous bleeding such as epistaxis, ecchymoses, petechiae, gastrointestinal and genitourinary bleeding, and menorrhagia are associated with platelet disorders (qualitative or quantitative).

11-4. The answer is **D** (Chapter 218). Petechiae are a form of mucocutaneous bleeding and are thus a sign of platelet disorders. Coagulation factor deficiencies are often associated with intra-articular, delayed, or retroperitoneal bleeding.

11-5. The answer is **D** (Chapter 218). A deficiency of protein C or S is associated with a hypercoagulable state, manifested by arterial and venous thromboses. Protein C and protein S normally form a complex that inactivates coagulation factors V_a and VIII_a and inhibits hemostasis. Protein C and S are vitamin K–dependent factors, as are coagulation factors II, VII, IX, and X. Coagulation factor deficiencies are often associated with intra-articular, delayed, or retroperitoneal bleeding.

11-6. The answer is **C** (Chapter 219). Petechiae are most commonly associated with the onset of ITP. Ecchymoses, purpura, gingival bleeding, epistaxis, and menorrhagia may also develop. Otherwise, the physical examination will be normal.

11-7. The answer is **C** (Chapter 219). HIV, systemic lupus erythematosus, Hashimoto's thyroiditis, Graves' disease, and antiphospholipid antibody syndrome are frequently found in patients with chronic ITP. Acute ITP affects young male and female children equally and may spontaneously resolve. Chronic ITP affects adults and, typically, females more than males. Spontaneous remissions seldom occur with chronic ITP. Steroids constitute the first-line therapy for chronic ITP. Patients with platelet counts of <20,000–30,000/µL who are not bleeding, or those without life-threatening bleeding and platelet counts <50,000/µL, are placed on a prednisone taper. Severe bleeding would require either high-dose parenteral steroids, IV immunoglobulin, or both, followed by a platelet transfusion.

11-8. **The answer is A** (Chapter 219). Radiation therapy decreases the megakaryocyte mass and overall platelet production. Other conditions that decrease platelet production include aplastic anemia; marrow infiltration; viral hepatitis; drugs such as ethanol, estrogens, thiazides, and chemotherapeutic agents; and toxins such as benzene and insecticides. ITP, TTP, and HUS are conditions associated with increased platelet destruction.

11-9. **The answer is D** (Chapter 219). A normal or minimally elevated D-dimer assay is suggestive of liver disease because D-dimer is significantly elevated in DIC. Thrombocytopenia, bleeding, prolonged prothrombin time, and hypofibrinogenemia are seen in both DIC and severe liver disease. Fibrinogen levels <100 mg/dL are usually associated with severe DIC.

11-10. **The answer is B** (Chapter 219). FFP is indicated since this coagulopathic, nonbleeding patient requires a diagnostic paracentesis. If the patient were bleeding, cryoprecipate, desmopressin, and platelet and RBC transfusion also would be indicated. FFP provides each coagulation factor, at one factor unit/mL. There is a risk of volume overload since each bag of FFP is 200–250 mL, and repeated doses may be required. Cryoprecipitate provides fibrinogen. DDAVP decreases bleeding time.

11-11. **The answer is B** (Chapter 219). Thrombocytopenia is the most commonly observed laboratory finding in DIC. The other abnormalities suggestive of DIC include prolonged prothrombin time, hypofibrinogenemia (especially if <100 mg/dL), and increased fibrin degradation products and D-dimer assays.

11-12. **The answer is C** (Chapter 219). The patient has DIC and is bleeding. Cryoprecipitate is required since the fibrinogen level is <100 mg/dL. A unit of cryoprecipitate contains 200–250 mg of fibrinogen. Ten-unit increments are given to maintain a fibrinogen level of 100–150 mg/dL. Platelets are indicated if the platelet count is <20,000/µL without bleeding or <50,000/µL with bleeding. Blood transfusions would be indicated if the patient had severe bleeding, anemia, or tissue hypoxia. Heparin is given only in the presence of thromboembolic events. All patients with DIC should receive vitamin K and folate supplementation.

11-13. **The answer is C** (Chapter 219). Infection is considered the most common cause of DIC. Gram-negative sepsis causes DIC in 10–20% of patients. Adenocarcinoma, lymphoma, and promyelocytic leukemia can cause DIC. Trauma due to burns, crush injury, fat embolism, and brain injury is frequently complicated by the development of DIC.

11-14. **The answer is C** (Chapter 220). This patient with hemophilia B has sustained a blunt head injury, has a headache, and is at severe risk of intracranial hemorrhage. The single most appropriate action is to initiate the immediate administration of factor IX prior to obtaining any imaging studies. The patient needs a minimal factor level of 100%. Each unit of factor IX per kilogram of body weight will raise the plasma level by 1% (0.01 U/mL). The calculation for the amount of factor needed is weight in kilograms × 1.0 × % change in factor activity. Fresh frozen plasma contains both factor

VIII and factor IX each in 1 U/mL concentrations. In an extreme emergency it might be the most readily available product. There would be the potential of volume overload, especially for requirements greater than 50%. Cryoprecipitate unit bags are small volume and contain high levels of factor VIII (80–100 units), vWF, and fibrinogen, but not factor IX. Ten to fifteen "unit bags" of cryoprecipitate are usually administered.

11-15. **The answer is A** (Chapter 220). A patient with hemophilia A, abdominal pain, a limp, and a history of blunt trauma to the abdomen needs factor VIII and a CT scan of the abdomen. The risk is high for intra-abdominal or retroperitoneal bleeding. The patient will require a minimum factor level of 50% for the deep muscle hematoma and may require a level of 100% if intra-abdominal or retroperitoneal bleeding is found on CT. DDAVP causes endothelial cells to release vWF, the carrier protein for factor VIII, thus increasing available levels of factor VIII two- to threefold. DDAVP is useful for mild bleeding in patients with von Willebrand's disease or mild hemophilia A. Patients with severe hemophilia A will not respond to DDAVP. Fresh frozen plasma would be a second-line therapy if factor VIII were not readily available. An ultrasound might detect free intra-abdominal fluid but would miss a retroperitoneal hemorrhage.

11-16. **The answer is C** (Chapter 220). Patients with type I von Willebrand's disease, the most common variant, have a quantitative platelet disorder, whereby vWF antigen and vWF activity are 50% below normal. DDAVP is the therapeutic agent used in type I patients, via subcutaneous, intravenous, or intranasal routes. The correct dosage of DDAVP for the subcutaneous or intravenous route is 0.3μg/kg. If given intravenously, it should be diluted in 30–50 mL saline and infused over 10–20 minutes to decrease hypotension or tachycardia. The intranasal dose of DDAVP in a child

older than 5 years would be 150 μg, the amount in a single spray in a single nostril. The adult intranasal dosage is 300 mg, one spray in each nostril. A repeat dose of DDAVP may be required in 8–12 hours, but the amount of released vWF will be less. Cryoprecipitate is also used to manage major bleeding in patients with type I von Willebrand's disease, but DDAVP would be the first-choice therapy in the patient in this case. Other adjunctive therapies in this case might include dry topical thrombin, oral epsiloaminocaproic acid (an antifibrinolytic agent), and absorbable gelatin sponges.

11-17. **The answer is D** (Chapter 219). Patients with von Willebrand's disease should avoid medications that further diminish platelet function. Acetaminophen does not affect platelet function. Aspirin in low or full dose irreversibly inhibits platelet function, and ibuprofen has a variable effect. Other medications that inhibit platelet function include penicillin G, ampicillin, ticarcillin, nafcillin, mezlocillin, moxalactam, cefotaxime, nitrofurantoin, and heparin. Ticlopidine and clopidogrel are antiplatelet drugs.

11-18. **The answer is A** (Chapter 221). Acute chest syndrome is the leading cause of death from sickle cell disease in the United States. Hydroxyurea is not approved for use in children but does effectively decrease the frequency and severity of painful crises in adults, by increasing the level of fetal hemoglobin (HbF), which inhibits sickling. Dactylitis is commonly the first manifestation of sickle cell anemia in children older than 6 months of age because protective levels of HbF have declined. Dactylitis is treated with analgesics, not transfusion. Simple or exchange transfusion is indicated for aplastic crisis, pregnancy, respiratory failure, stroke, general surgery, and priapism.

11-19. **The answer is C** (Chapter 224). Clopidogrel inhibits platelet aggregation initiated by ADP release. Specifically, clopidogrel alters the platelet membrane near the fibrinogen receptor site, thus preventing formation of an interplatelet fibrinogen bridge. Clopidogrel is indicated in patients with aspirin hypersensitivity. Other indications include unstable angina, non-ST-segment elevation myocardial infarction (MI), secondary prevention of MI or CVA, and known peripheral vascular disease. Rare cases of thrombotic thrombocytopenic purpura (TTP) have been reported following the use of clopidogrel, but there is a stronger association between ticlopidine and TTP. Most patients tolerate clopidogrel well, but side effects include dyspepsia, rash, and diarrhea.

11-20.   **The answer is D** (Chapter 223). The patient is having a transfusion reaction with acute intravascular hemolysis. The lysed red blood cells release hemoglobin and lactate dehydrogenase, raising both levels in plasma. Serum haptoglobin binds hemoglobin but is rapidly depleted, so decreased levels are a sign of hemolysis. Other proteins also bind hemoglobin, but some hemoglobin may remain free in the plasma, which will appear pink if the serum hemoglobin is 50 mg/dL or higher. Hemoglobin is excreted by the kidneys. Hemoglobinuria turns spun urine reddish brown and positive for heme (as will myoglobin). If the plasma is pink, assume that reddish brown spun urine is positive for hemoglobin. The transfusion must be stopped immediately, and the patient must be supported hemodynamically. Fluids and pressors are used to correct shock and maintain renal blood flow and urine output. Mannitol and furosemide are useful adjuncts. Acute hemolytic reactions can also activate the coagulation system and cause DIC, which is treated with fresh frozen plasma.

11-21.   **The answer is C** (Chapter 225). Cancer patients with neutropenia, or an absolute neutrophil count <500/mm^3, are vulnerable to bacteremia and other infections. Subtle signs of infection may be limited to fever, pain, and erythema—purulence will be ab-

sent due to granulocytopenia. Timely ED administration of broad-spectrum antibiotics after appropriate blood and urine cultures and chest radiograph can be life-saving for the febrile neutropenic patient. The EP must perform a careful physical examination including the nasal, oral, vaginal, and rectal areas. However, the digital rectal examination should not be performed until the patient has received empiric antibiotics, due to the risk of bacteremia. Patients with acute leukemia are especially susceptible to perirectal infections. Funduscopy may reveal fungal or bacterial endophthalmitis or signs of increased intracranial pressure. Empiric antibiotics should include coverage for aerobic gram-negative and gram-positive organisms. Typically, an aminoglycoside plus an antipseudomonal β-lactam are administered. Vancomycin is added if there are signs of mucositis, hypotension, catheter infection, methicillin-resistant *Staphylococcus aureus*, quinolone prophylaxis, or resistant gram-positive organisms.

11-22.   **The answer if C** (Chapter 224). The patient does not have major or life-threatening bleeding, but the INR is >5, so oral vitamin K, 1–2 mg, is warranted. If the INR had been above therapeutic (2–3) but <5, then stopping warfarin, and monitoring the INR sequentially would be appropriate. Follow-up with the patient's private provider is always appropriate but the patient required instruction to stop warfarin at the time of his ED visit. Intravenous vitamin K is reserved for situations involving a markedly elevated INR >20 and clinically significant, potentially life-threatening bleeding. Anaphylaxis is a rare but serious risk of intravenous vitamin K. Overcorrection or recurrent thrombosis are more likely risks.

11-23.   **The answer is D** (Chapter 222). The signs and symptoms of TTP reflect end-organ damage stemming from microvascular occlusion and hemolysis due to platelet thrombi which do not incorporate fibrin. The TTP clinical pentad includes: (1) thrombocytopenia, (2) microangiopathic hemolytic anemia (MAHA), (3) fever, (4) renal dysfunction, and (5) neurologic dysfunction. Thrombocytopenia and MAHA occur most commonly. TTP is both an acquired and a familial disorder. The common feature involves either a qualitative or quantitative deficiency in the metalloprotease enzyme that normally cleaves the vWF multimers that are formed by endothelial cells and megakaryocytes. The vWF multimers attached to the endothelium adhere to platelets and create platelet thrombi. Altered laminar blood flow shears RBCs and causes a hemolytic anemia, characterized by schistocytes and helmet cells on peripheral smear, elevated unconjugated bilirubin, elevated reticulocyte count, and decreased serum haptoglobin. The direct antiglobulin test (DAT, or Coombs' test) is negative because anti-RBC autoantibodies are not the cause of the hemolysis. In TTP, the platelet count is <20,000/μL. Coagulation studies are normal. Pregnancy is the most common trigger for TTP but preeclampsia shares many features and must be differentiated from TTP. Preeclampsia usually occurs in the third trimester, while TTP usually occurs earlier, at 23–24 weeks. Delivery is the definitive treatment for preeclampsia but will have no effect on TTP. Plasma exchange therapy has markedly decreased maternal overall TTP mortality, but fetal mortality remains high. Plasma exchange therapy has also reduced mortality in other conditions that trigger TTP including infection (especially HIV), systemic lupus erythematosus, ticlopidine or clopidogrel usage, and the post–bone marrow transplant or postchemotherapy states.

11-24.   **The answer is C** (Chapters 27, 225). Hypercalcemia occurs in 20–30% of patients with a malignancy. For serum calcium levels 14 mg/dL or higher, isotonic saline is the initial emergency treatment followed by forced saline diuresis. Use of furosemide 40–80 mg IV every 2 hours increases renal excretion of calcium. Diuretics are administered only after the patient has received enough isotonic fluid to correct dehydration and then has adequate urine output (100 mL/hour). Glucocorticoids such as prednisone and hydrocortisone are used to treat hypercalcemia due to multiple myeloma, lymphoma, leukemia, and breast cancer. Glucocorticoids are best given after hematologic consultation. Calcitonin decreases renal calcium reabsorption and inhibits bone resorption. Additional doses produce a blunted response (tachyphylaxis). Glucocorticoids diminish calcitonin-associated tachyphylaxis. Bisphosphonates (pamidronate) inhibit bone resorption and produce a prolonged decrease in calcium over 2–4 weeks. Failure to give bisphosphonates slowly (over 4–24 hours) will precipitate bisphosphonate-calcium deposits in the kidney and result in renal failure.

CHAPTER 12

Imaging
Questions

12-1. When ordering an abdominal CT scan, when should the emergency physician specifically order the CT scan without IV contrast?

(A) Abdominal trauma.
(B) Suspected appendicitis.
(C) Suspected kidney stone.
(D) Suspected diverticulitis.

12-2. When looking at a transverse ultrasound image of the aorta and inferior vena cava (IVC), where is the IVC seen on the screen?

(A) Above the aorta.
(B) To the right of the aorta.
(C) Below the aorta.
(D) To the left of the aorta.

12-3. Echocardiographic evidence of tamponade includes which of the following?

(A) Pericardial effusion >1 cm in largest diameter.

(B) Pericardial effusion with left ventricular collapse.
(C) Pericardial effusion with right ventricular collapse.
(D) Pericardial fluid collection.

12-4. An elderly patient has a suspected hip fracture despite negative AP and lateral plain films. What is the most accurate imaging technique to detect occult fracture?

(A) Oblique plain films.
(B) CT scan.
(C) MRI.
(D) Bone scan.

Imaging
Answers, Explanations, and References

12-1. **The answer is C** (Chapter 302). Contrast may obscure kidney stones in the ureter and should not be used. Other examples of the "acute abdomen" all benefit from the addition of IV contrast.

12-2. **The answer is D** (Chapter 303). Transverse ultrasound images of the abdomen are similar to CT cuts and can be thought of as looking from the feet upward toward the head. Thus, while the IVC travels up the abdomen to the right of the aorta, it is seen to the left on an ultrasound image. See Figure 303-4 in the *Study Guide*.

12-3. **The answer is C** (Chapter 303). Although not always seen, right-sided collapse (i.e., decreased filling) due to pericardial effusion is evidence of tamponade. Presence of pericardial fluid does not equate to tamponade, while the absence of fluid does exclude the diagnosis.

12-4. **The answer is C** (Chapter 305). While CT is quite good, MRI is more accurate due to its sensitivity to marrow and trabecular bone changes.

Infectious Disease Emergencies
Questions

13-1. Which of the following is acceptable antimicrobial therapy for gonorrhea?

(A) Doxycycline 100 mg by mouth twice a day for 14 days.

(B) Benzathine penicillin G 6.2 million units intramuscularly.

(C) Azithromycin 1 g by mouth.

(D) Ceftriaxone 125 mg intramuscularly.

13-2. A 19-year-old male comes to the ED with a small, indurated, painless ulcer on the glans of his penis. The base of the ulcer is clean and is starting to heal. Firm, rubbery inguinal lymph nodes are present. What is the BEST treatment plan for this patient?

(A) Obtain a culture, then call the patient back if the culture is positive.

(B) Give benzathine penicillin G 2.4 million units intramuscularly.

(C) Tell the patient to follow up with his primary care provider if the lesion does not heal.

(D) Give acyclovir 400 mg by mouth 3 times a day for 7 days.

13-3. Which of the following is TRUE of the majority of toxic shock syndrome (TSS) cases?

(A) They are unrelated to menses and cross all segments of society.

(B) They have gram-positive rods on blood culture.

(C) They have a diffuse, painful, sunburn-like rash that results in bullae.

(D) They are associated with hyperkalemia and hypercalcemia.

13-4. Which of the following is the herpes virus associated with?

(A) Meningitis.

(B) Bell's palsy.

(C) Baker's cyst.

(D) Pustular lesions of the fingers that need drainage.

13-5. What is the most common mechanism of acquired immunodeficiency syndrome (AIDS) transmission in adults and adolescents?

(A) Male homosexual contact.

(B) Injection drug use.

(C) Heterosexual contact.

(D) Blood product transfusion.

13-6. Which of the following CD4$^+$ T-cell counts and viral loads are associated with increased risk of progression to an AIDS-defining illness?

(A) CD4$^+$ T-cell count of 100 cells/μL and a viral load of 500.

(B) CD4$^+$ T-cell count of 1000 cells/μL and a viral load of 5000.

(C) CD4$^+$ T-cell count of 1000 cells/μL and a viral load of 500,000.

(D) CD4$^+$ T-cell count of 100 cells/μL and a viral load of 50,000.

13-7. Which of the following is TRUE of crypto-coccal central nervous system (CNS) infections?

(A) They can often be identified on CT scan.

(B) They are associated with elevated intracranial pressure, which should be treated by cerebrospinal fluid lumbar puncture drainage.

(C) They are initially treated with oral fluconazole.

(D) They cause meningeal signs.

13-8. Which of the following is the MOST appropriate postexposure prophylaxis (PEP) for needle stick injuries to health care workers?

(A) Begin prophylaxis within 48 hours of exposure.

(B) Use only a 1-drug regimen if the source is known to be low risk.

(C) Treat for 4 weeks.

(D) Use a 4-drug regimen if the source is known to be high risk.

13-9. A 26-year-old Hispanic male construction worker presents for evaluation of a 2-day-old puncture wound to his foot and muscle stiffness. His pulse is 112 beats per minute and temperature is 39.5°C, and he is diaphoretic. His wound does not appear infected. He has stiffness and extension of his lower extremities. He also has pain and stiffness in his masseter muscles. Which of the following should be the initial treatment of this patient?

(A) Tetanus immunoglobulin.

(B) Tetanus-diphtheria toxoid.

(C) Wound debridement.

(D) Penicillin.

13-10. Which of the following patients should receive rabies postexposure prophylaxis?

(A) A child who was found petting a stray neighborhood dog.

(B) A forestry worker who was bitten on the face by a squirrel.

(C) A spelunker who inadvertently put his hand into bat guano while caving.

(D) A homeowner who was bitten on the hand by a skunk he was chasing out of a shed.

13-11. Which species of the genus *Plasmodium* infecting humans with malaria parasites is becoming increasingly resistant to antimalarial medications?

(A) *P. ovale.*

(B) *P. malariae.*

(C) *P. vivax.*

(D) *P. falciparum.*

13-12. Which of the following parasites is most likely to cause respiratory symptoms?

(A) *Trichuris.*

(B) *Giardia.*

(C) *Ascaris.*

(D) *Leishmania donovani.*

13-13. Which of the following is TRUE of infestation with fish tapeworm?

(A) It may cause birth defects by competing with the host folic acid.

(B) It may cause liver granulomas.

(C) It may cause extremity paresthesias.

(D) It may cause a papular pruritic rash.

13-14. What is the most common cause of bacterial foodborne illnesses in the United States?

(A) *Campylobacter.*

(B) *Salmonella.*

(C) *Shigella.*

(D) *Escherichia coli.*

13-15. Normal physiologic defense mechanisms that exist to prevent disease from food and waterborne pathogens may be disrupted by which of the following?

(A) Over-the-counter vitamin use.

(B) H_2 blockers and proton-pump inhibitors.

(C) Foods treated with pesticides.

(D) Extensive exercise.

13-16. The usual incubation period for *Shigella*, *Campylobacter*, and *E. coli* 0157:H7 is:

(A) 7–14 days.

(B) >14 days.

(C) 2–6 days.

(D) 2–6 hours.

13-17. Tick removal is safely achieved by which of the following?

(A) Apply viscous lidocaine, then use gentle traction on the tick with fine forceps, ensuring that all parts are removed.

(B) Carefully apply a burning match or cautery, which causes the tick to remove its mouth parts.

(C) Crush the tick with fine forceps, then remove the tick with a quick pulling motion.

(D) Apply petroleum jelly to cause suffocation, then remove the tick with fine forceps.

13-18. What is the MOST common vectorborne zoonotic infection in the United States?

(A) Rocky Mountain spotted fever.

(B) Lyme disease.

(C) Colorado tick fever.

(D) Ehrlichiosis.

13-19. Which of the following is TRUE of Lyme disease?

(A) It is characterized by 4 stages.

(B) It is best prevented by a complete vaccination series.

(C) It can be prevented by a single 200-mg dose of doxycycline within 72 hours of tick bite.

(D) It is caused by *Rickettsia rickettsii*.

13-20. Which of these diseases follows peripheral nerve tracts after inoculation?

(A) Ehrlichiosis.

(B) Babesiosis.

(C) Rabies.

(D) West Nile virus.

13-21. Which of the following is TRUE of a Hantavirus infection?

(A) It is caused by inhalation of dried, particulate feces, contact with urine, or by rodent bite.

(B) It should be treated with fluoroquinolones or doxycycline.

(C) It causes development of a bubo followed by pneumonia and sepsis from hematologic spread.

(D) It may cause extrapulmonary manifestations involving the heart, central nervous system, and liver.

13-22. What are the two MOST common household pet sources for zoonotic infections?

(A) Small rodents and pet birds.

(B) Reptiles and aquarium fish.

(C) Dogs and cats.

(D) Ferrets and hedgehogs.

13-23. Which of the following infections can ticks and fleas inhabiting dogs and cats transmit?

(A) *Campylobacter* and *Bordetella*.

(B) *Cryptococcus* and *Giardia*.

(C) *Bartonella* and *Salmonella*.

(D) Tularemia, plague, and Rocky Mountain spotted fever.

13-24. What is the MOST important factor in preventing clostridial wound infections?

(A) Wound care at the time of initial evaluation and treatment.

(B) Hyperbaric oxygen therapy.

(C) Use of vasoconstrictors.

(D) Antibiotic therapy.

13-25. Which of the following is the MOST appropriate antibiotic therapy for gas gangrene?

(A) Potassium penicillin.

(B) Sodium penicillin.

(C) Sulfonamides.

(D) Fluoroquinolones.

13-26. Which of the following is TRUE of necrotizing fasciitis?

(A) It is characterized by widespread necrosis involving the subcutaneous tissue and fascia.

(B) It often involves underlying muscle.

(C) Treatment of choice is medical management.

(D) It is usually caused by a single organism.

13-27. Which of the following is TRUE of erysipelas?

(A) It presents in pediatric patients as a red or "slapped cheek" appearance.

(B) Toe-web intertrigo has the highest attributable risk for development of this disease.

(C) It most often presents as a rash distal to skin entry.

(D) It is diagnosed primarily by blood cultures.

13-28. Which of the following is TRUE concerning most cases of superficial and localized abscesses?

(A) Infiltration of a local anesthetic is the best way to relieve pain prior to incision and drainage.

(B) Fluctuance is always easy to identify in abscesses.

(C) Antibiotic treatment following incision and drainage speeds healing in otherwise healthy patients.

(D) The American Heart Association recommends prophylactic antibiotics for those patients in high-risk categories prior to incision and drainage.

13-29. Which of the following is a nationally reportable communicable disease?

(A) Trichomonal infections.

(B) Giardiasis.

(C) Herpes simplex type 2.

(D) Infectious mononucleosis.

13-30. Which of the following statements about rubeola is TRUE?

(A) It is the most common vaccine-preventable cause of death among children.

(B) It causes miscarriages, stillbirths, and fetal anomalies.

(C) It is primarily transmitted by bodily fluids.

(D) It is best prevented by postexposure administration of immunoglobulin.

13-31. Which of the following is TRUE of patients with possible exposure to severe acute respiratory syndrome (SARS)?

(A) They should be admitted for infection control.

(B) They should have a surgical mask applied and be kept away from other patients.

(C) They should be given immunoglobulin.

(D) They should be started on acyclovir, penciclovir, or ganciclovir.

Infectious Disease Emergencies
Answers, Explanations, and References

13-1. **The answer is D** (Chapter 141). Doxycycline, penicillin, and azithromycin are not listed by the CDC as being effective for gonorrhea. Acceptable antibiotics for gonorrhea include ceftriaxone, cefixime, ciprofloxacin, ofloxacin, levofloxacin, spectinomycin, norfloxacin, and gatifloxacin.

13-2. **The answer is B** (Chapter 141). This patient is showing signs of syphilis. It is important for the emergency physician to recognize signs of syphilis and to begin treatment in the ED when it is recognized. Contacting a patient after discharge from the ED is sometimes difficult. Primary syphilis is characterized by a painless chancre such as the one described in this case. Secondary syphilis is characterized by nonspecific constitutional symptoms and a rash and occurs 3–6 weeks after primary syphilis. Tertiary or latent syphilis is seen in about one-third of patients. Involvement of the neurologic and cardiovascular system is characteristic of this stage. Acyclovir may be prescribed for genital herpes.

13-3. **The answer is A** (Chapter 142). TSS is an acute-onset multisystem disease with symptoms, signs, and laboratory abnormalities reflecting multiple-organ involvements. The rash of TSS is a diffuse, branching erythroderma, classically described as painless "sunburn" that fades within 3 days and is followed by full-thickness desquamation. Sodium, potassium, calcium, and phosphate abnormalities are common. Hypocalcemia is out of propor-

tion to the degree of hypoalbuminemia and may be difficult to correct if there is a concomitant decrease in the serum magnesium level. Blood cultures may be positive for *Staphylococcus aureus* but are not always.

13-4. **The answer is B** (Chapter 143). Herpes simplex virus (HSV) may affect the peripheral branches of the cranial nerves and is a frequent cause of Bell's palsy. HSV has been noted to cause encephalitis but not meningitis. Herpetic whitlow is a primary or recurrent HSV infection of the finger. Incision may delay healing or allow a secondary infection to occur. There is no known association with Baker's cyst and HSV infections.

13-5. **The answer is A** (Chapter 144). While all of the answers listed are important mechanisms of AIDS transmission, male homosexual contact remains the most common method of transmission of HIV.

13-6. **The answer is D** (Chapter 144). Knowledge of recent $CD4^+$ T-cell counts and HIV viral load can be extremely helpful in placing a patient's ED presentation in an appropriate context. T-cell counts of <200 cells/μL and viral loads of >50,000 are associated with increased risk of progression to an AIDS-defining illness and often are used as indicators for initiation of antiretroviral therapy.

13-7. **The answer is B** (Chapter 144). Neuroimaging studies are usually normal and meningismus is uncommon with cryptococcal CNS infections. Elevated intracranial pressure is associated with cryptococcal meningitis. Patients with an opening pressure of >25 cm H_2O should prompt drainage of fluid until pressure is less than 20 cm H_2O or 50% of initial opening pressure. Patients with CNS cryptococcosis should be admitted for intravenous amphotericin B with oral flucytosine for 14 days. Initial therapy should be followed by 8–10 weeks of oral fluconazole, but oral therapy is not recommended initially.

13-8. **The answer is C** (Chapter 144). PEP following an occupational exposure should be initiated as quickly as possible, preferably within 1–2 hours. Animal studies suggest little benefit if PEP is started 24–36 hours after exposure. Treatment regimens vary by type of exposure. A basic regimen consists of 2 drugs, often azidothymidine and lamivudine; an expanded regimen adds a third drug, such as indinavir or nelfinavir. PEP treatment duration is 4 weeks.

13-9. **The answer is A** (Chapter 146). Tetanus is diagnosed solely on the basis of history and clinical examination. Patients with tetanus should be managed in an intensive care unit. Penicillin, a centrally acting GABA antagonist, may potentiate the effects of tetanospasmin, thus its use should be avoided. The efficacy of antibiotics is questionable, but most physicians do use them. Parenterally administered metronidazole is the antibiotic of choice. Tetanus immunoglobulin should be given before wound debridement because exotoxin may be released during wound manipulation. If the patient has not been immunized or incompletely immunized, tetanus toxoid should also be given.

13-10. **The answer is D** (Chapter 147). Postexposure prophylaxis is indicated for persons exposed to a rabid animal. The following animals very rarely have been found to be rabid and hence their bite almost never requires postexposure prophylaxis for rabies: squirrels, hamsters, guinea pigs, gerbils,

chipmunks, mice, domesticated rabbits, and other small rodents. Bites, scratches, abrasions, open wounds, or mucous membranes exposed to potentially infectious material constitute exposure. Other contact by itself, such as petting a rabid animal and contact with blood, urine, or feces (e.g., guano) of a rabid animal, does not constitute exposure and is not an indication for prophylaxis. Skunks are known to carry rabies.

13-11. **The answer is D** (Chapter 148). Annually, over 250 million persons develop malaria, and more than 2.5 million persons die. The incidence of malaria has been increasing in recent years despite aggressive worldwide attempts at control. Not only is the mosquito vector becoming less susceptible to a variety of insecticides, but *P. falciparum*, the parasite responsible for the most deadly form of malaria, is becoming increasingly resistant to antimalarial medications.

13-12. **The answer is C** (Chapter 149). *Trichuris* can cause seizures, nausea and vomiting, conjunctivitis and keratitis, diarrhea, edema, and eosinophilia. It is not known to cause pulmonary symptoms. *Giardia* causes primarily gastrointestinal symptoms and is not known to cause problems with the lungs. *Ascaris*, *Strongyloides*, and *Toxocara* may cause asthmalike symptoms since part of their life cycle involves lung tissue. *L. donovani* causes granuloma inguinale. It is not known to cause pulmonary symptoms.

13-13. **The answer is C** (Chapter 149). *Diphyllobothrium* can compete with the host for vitamin B_{12} and thus patients can present with pernicious anemia. The patients' symptoms are usually symmetrical and often include paresthesias in the extremities and impaired vibration and position sense. They may progress to abnormal gait, spastic atoxia, and quadriparesis. Psychiatric abnormalities may also exist that can be prominent and isolated. Patients infected with *Schistosoma* present in the chronic stage with granulomas in the liver. Schistosomes penetrate the skin, creating a papular pruritic rash.

13-14. **The answer is A** (Chapter 150). The most common cause of bacterial foodborne illnesses in the United States is *Campylobacter*, followed by *Salmonella*, *Shigella*, and *E. coli*.

13-15. **The answer is B** (Chapter 150). A gastric pH of 3 or less is generally found in most healthy adults and can effectively kill most foodborne pathogens. A reduction in acidity can occur secondary to antacids, H_2 blockers, and proton-pump inhibitors. Chronic underlying medical conditions such as diabetes, pernicious anemia, and gastric surgery also reduce gastric pH. Pesticides, vitamins, and good physical condition are not associated with an increased risk of foodborne or waterborne disease.

13-16. **The answer is C** (Chapter 150). Obtaining a complete history of an acute diarrheal illness is important. In a presumed foodborne illness, determining the exact time of exposure can help direct the evaluation to a particular causative agent. *Shigella*, *Campylobacter*, *E. coli* 0157:H7, *Vibrio cholerae*, *Streptococcus* group A, and *Yersinia entercolitica* all have incubation periods of 2–6 days. Foodborne illnesses from *Staphylococcus aureus* and *Bacillus cereus* present within hours.

13-17. **The answer is A** (Chapter 151). Techniques to avoid in tick removal include the use of a burning match or any action that results in crushing the tick. These attempts can cause infection by tick regurgitation into the wound site and often result in incomplete tick removal. Proper removal involves gentle traction on the tick to ensure all body parts are removed.

13-18. **The answer is B** (Chapter 151). Lyme disease is the most common vectorborne zoonotic infection in the United States with approximately 15,000 cases reported annually.

13-19. **The answer is C** (Chapter 151). Lyme disease has three stages; the first stage is characterized by erythema migrans and erythematous plaque with central clearing. The second stage is characterized by fever, adenopathy, neuropathies, cardiac abnormalities, arthritic problems, and multiple annular dematologic lesions. The third stage of illness occurs years after the initial infection and can be characterized by chronic arthritis, myocarditis, subacute encephalopathy, axonal polyneuropathy, and leukoencephalopathy. A vaccine was commercially available but has been withdrawn from the market. There was little demand for the vaccine and a concern that immunization would lead recipients to disregard physical precautions against tickborne diseases in general. Currently, the disease is best prevented by avoidance of tick bites. Lyme disease is caused by *Borrelia burgdorferi*. *R. rickettsii* causes Rocky Mountain spotted fever.

13-20. **The answer is C** (Chapter 151). Rabies follows peripheral nerve tracts after inoculation. *Ehrlichia* bacteria are gram-negative pleomorphic coccobacilli that infect circulating leukocytes. Babesiosis is a malaria-like disease transmitted by ticks with the etiologic agents being protozoan parasites. West Nile virus causes encephalitis.

13-21. **The answer is A** (Chapter 151). Hantavirus is spread to humans by infected rodents that were bitten by deer mice that act as the vector in the United States. Humans get the virus through inhalation of rodent excrement or rodent bite. Hantavirus infection treatment consists of supportive care with attention to adequate oxygenation and possibly the use of an inhalation solution of ribavirin. Antibiotics are not helpful with this viral infection, which carries with it a very high mortality. Hantavirus pulmonary infection consists of an initial flulike prodromal illness of 3–4 days' duration, rapidly followed by pulmonary edema, hypoxia, hypotension, tachycardia, and metabolic acidosis. Hepatic involvement is not listed as a usual result of Hantavirus infections. Plague from *Yersinia pestis* causes a bubo, then sepsis and pneumonia from hematologic spread.

13-22. **The answer is C** (Chapter 151). Man's best friend, the dog, and his feline friend, the cat, are the most common household pets in North America. They account for the majority of zoonotic infections. Small rodents, pet birds, reptiles, and aquarium fish account for only a fraction of the zoonotic infections in the United States.

13-23. **The answer is D** (Chapter 151). Ticks and fleas inhabit dogs and cats and can transmit the zoonotic infections of tularemia, plague, and Rocky Mountain spotted fever. Transmission is often by cat bite, tick bite, or scratch. Dogs do not directly transmit tularemia but do serve as carriers of the ticks that can transmit tularemia. *Campylobacter* is transmitted by cats and dogs. *Bordetalla* is transmitted by dogs. *Cryptococcus* is transmitted by bird droppings and cats. *Giardia* is transmitted by ingestion of infected water and by cats, dogs, and beavers. *Bartonella* is transmitted by cats. Dogs, cats, reptiles, and farm animals transmit *Salmonella*.

13-24. **The answer is A** (Chapter 152). Debridement of crushed or dead tissue and copious irrigation prior to wound closure will help prevent the development of an environment favorable to clostridial growth. Avoid the use of vasoconstrictors when possible due to the possibility of decreasing perfusion to already ischemic muscle. Hyperbaric therapy should be initiated after surgical debridement of gangrenous tissue. Antibiotic therapy is used as treatment but does not prevent gangrene.

13-25. **The answer is B** (Chapter 152). Sodium penicillin is recommended over potassium penicillin to reduce the risk of worsening hyperkalemia in patients with hemolysis and tissue necrosis. Penicillin G, clindamycin, ceftriaxone, and erythromycin are also listed as appropriate antibiotics.

13-26. **The answer is A** (Chapter 152). Necrotizing fasciitis infection does not spread through the fascial layer into the underlying muscle, as it does with the clostridial and nonclostridial myonecrosis infections. It is an infectious process that has been recognized for centuries but was brought to the world's attention in the mid-1990s when the tabloid press began reporting about an outbreak of "flesh-eating bacteria." As with gas gangrene, there is a mixed-organism form of this infection, which is the most common, and a single-organism form, which is typically caused by group A streptococci and is less common. Treatment of choice is surgical debridement, often rather extensive, along with broad-spectrum antibiotics.

13-27. **The answer is B** (Chapter 152). Erysipelas most often occurs proximal to the portal of entry into the skin. Intertrigo causes the most erysipelas, and it is estimated that 60% of lower extremity erysipelas could be prevented if toe-web intertrigo was not a factor. The diagnosis is based primarily on physical findings. Blood cultures are positive in about 5% of patients and so are not helpful. "Slapped cheek" appearance is associated with fifth disease.

13-28. **The answer is D** (Chapter 152). It is often difficult to determine clinically whether an area of fluctuance is present within an area of induration and swelling. Needle aspiration can help in the diagnosis. There is no good data to support the concept that antibiotic treatment following incision and drainage speeds infection resolution in otherwise healthy patients with localized soft tissue infections. Infiltration of a local anesthetic prior to incision and drainage often gives poor pain relief. Regional or field blocks, however, can be effective. For those patients in the high-risk and moderate-risk categories, antibiotic selection should be directed at the most likely organism causing the abscess.

13-29. **The answer is B** (Chapter 153). Of the selections listed in this question, giardiasis is the only nationally reportable communicable disease. The Centers for Disease Control and Prevention publishes a list of notifiable infectious diseases that is updated and revised routinely.

13-30. **The answer is A** (Chapter 154). Obstacles to measles eradication in the United States include increasing numbers of susceptible children and infants who are not immunized and circulation of measles virus from other geographic regions of the world. Rubella, the German measles, causes miscarriages, stillbirths, and fetal anomalies. Transmission of measles is primarily person-to-person via large respiratory droplets, although airborne transmission via aerosolized droplet nuclei has been documented in closed areas. For postexposure prophylaxis, measles vaccine provides permanent protection and may prevent disease if given within 72 hours of exposure. Any immunity conferred by immunoglobulin is temporary.

13-31. **The answer is B** (Chapter 154). Patients with SARS need admission for medical care but not for infection control, unless infection control is not possible outside of a hospital setting. SARS is thought to be a coronavirus; therefore, acyclovir, penciclovir, organciclovir, and immunoglobulin are not known to be helpful. Epidemiologic criteria for disease are travel within 10 days of onset of symptoms to an area with SARS, or close contact within 10 days of onset of symptoms with a person suspected to have SARS.

Musculoskeletal Emergencies
Questions

14-1. A 35-year-old paint factory worker presents complaining of a wound to the volar aspect of his nondominant left hand which occurred 1 hour ago while using a high-pressure device. Upon exam the patient appears to have a small puncture wound approximately 0.5 cm wide with trace surrounding erythema and swelling 2 cm distal to the hypothenar eminence. He is neurovascularly intact on exam, and an x-ray reveals no fractures or obvious foreign body. What is the MOST appropriate next step in management?

(A) Irrigate the wound, update his tetanus, and suture.

(B) Irrigate, update tetanus, and do not suture but prescribe prophylactic antibiotics.

(C) Irrigate, update tetanus, and arrange outpatient follow-up with his primary care provider.

(D) Irrigate, update tetanus, and consult an orthopedist immediately.

14-2. Which of the following statements is TRUE regarding compartment syndromes of the hand?

(A) Patients may complain of intense pain but have little if any physical findings.

(B) Paresthesias occur as a prominent feature.

(C) Pain is not a prominent feature.

(D) Patients prefer to maintain their hand in 45-degree flexion at the MCP and PIP joints, the "cupping position."

14-3. Which of the following fractures may not be radiologically apparent on the first day of injury, necessitating repeat x-rays on a follow-up visit?

(A) Nondisplaced radial head fracture.

(B) Clavicular fracture.

(C) Calcaneus fracture.

(D) Scapula fracture.

14-4. A 56-year-old man presents after an industrial accident where the patient's chest was pinned between heavy machinery. On exam you note an obese man; blood pressure is 150/80 mmHg, heart rate is 90 beats per minute, and respiration rate is 24 breaths per minute. He is complaining of left anterior neck and chest discomfort as well as dysphagia. On exam, the patient has swelling and tenderness along the left clavicular area and over the sternum, with pain exacerbated upon movement of the left shoulder. A chest x-ray (CXR) reveals no fractures or pneumothorax, but the patient continues to complain of pain and difficulty swallowing. What is the MOST appropriate next diagnostic step?

(A) Oral challenge and discharge with appropriate follow-up.

(B) Left shoulder radiographs.

(C) CT of the chest.

(D) End-expiratory CXR.

14-5. What is normal two-point discrimination in the fingertips?

(A) <2 mm.

(B) <4 mm.

(C) <6 mm.

(D) <12 mm.

14-6. Which of the following is TRUE regarding gamekeeper's thumb?

(A) The mechanism of injury is usually forced adduction at the MCP joint.

(B) Delaying surgery as long as 1 month for an acutely ruptured ligament will help preserve future function.

(C) More than 40 degrees of radial angulation on stress testing indicates complete rupture.

(D) Injury to the dorsal capsule and volar plate are rare.

14-7. Which of the following is TRUE regarding perilunate and lunate dislocations?

(A) All require emergent orthopedic consultation.

(B) Associated carpal bone fractures are rare.

(C) Complications of these injuries include avascular necrosis and median nerve compression.

(D) Patients present with obvious hand deformity.

14-8. A 20-year-old female complains of right wrist pain after a fall onto an outstretched hand. Radiographs appear completely normal, but the patient has significant snuffbox tenderness on exam. You suspect a scaphoid fracture. Which of the following is TRUE regarding this injury?

(A) A fat pad sign is insensitive for detecting fracture in obese patients.

(B) Avascular necrosis can occur if the blood supply to the distal portion of the scaphoid is compromised by the fracture.

(C) Clinically suspected scaphoid fractures should be splinted in a short arm thumb spica splint in a dorsiflexed and ulnar-deviated position.

(D) Unstable scaphoid fractures (rotated, comminuted, or displaced fractures) should be splinted in a long arm spica splint.

14-9. Which of the following is TRUE regarding carpal fractures?

(A) Carpal bone fractures account for the majority of all hand injuries.

(B) Carpal bone fractures are usually readily apparent on the first set of radiographs obtained on the day of injury.

(C) Lunate fractures can result in avascular necrosis.

(D) Pisiform fractures should be splinted in an ulnar gutter splint and have a very poor prognosis due to ulnar nerve compromise.

14-10. A 35-year-old man presents with left wrist pain following a fall off a snowboard. A radiograph reveals a Colles' fracture of the distal radius. Which of the following is TRUE regarding Colles' fractures?

(A) Stable Colles' fractures can be treated with a wrist splint for 6 weeks.

(B) The goals of reduction are to restore the dorsal tilt, radial inclination, and proper length to the radius.

(C) Associated ulnar styloid fractures may indicate disruption of the cartilaginous structures stabilizing the wrist.

(D) The x-ray demonstrates volar angulation of the distal radius.

14-11. A 22-year-old woman presents to the ED complaining of right elbow pain and swelling after falling off her motor scooter. On exam, she is holding the right arm in 45 degrees of flexion, and you palpate a prominent olecranon posteriorly. Radiographs reveal a posterior elbow dislocation. Which of the following statements is TRUE?

(A) The preferred method of reduction involves hyperflexion and internal rotation until a palpable reduction occurs.

(B) If full, smooth, passive range of motion (ROM) is not possible postreduction, the postreduction film should be examined for entrapment of the medial epicondyle.

(C) A long arm plaster splint should be applied in full extension and appropriate orthopedic follow-up arranged.

(D) An intact radial pulse postreduction rules out any possibility of vascular compromise.

14-12. Which of the following is TRUE regarding supracondylar fractures?

(A) An anterior fat pad may be the only visible sign of a nondisplaced fracture on radiographs.

(B) Refusal to open the hand, pain with passive finger extension, and forearm tenderness are commonly found with this injury and should be treated with analgesics.

(C) Volkmann's ischemic contracture results from postischemic swelling in the forearm compartment, leading to compromised capillary perfusion and eventual fibrosis of the affected tissues.

(D) Most supracondylar fractures are displaced anteriorly.

14-13. Which of the following is suggestive of a radial head fracture?

(A) Abnormality of the capitellum.

(B) Anterior fat pad.

(C) Lack of pain on exam.

(D) Swelling on the medial aspect of the elbow.

14-14. Which of the following is TRUE regarding the injury shown in Figure 14-1?

(A) Associated radial head dislocations are rare.

(B) These types of fractures are classified according to the location of the ulnar fracture and the direction of the radial head dislocation.

(C) Most of these fractures are treated with closed reduction and prolonged cast immobilization.

(D) All of the above.

14-15. Which of the following is TRUE regarding distal interphalangeal joint dislocations?

(A) They are often associated with neurologic deficits.

(B) They usually are displaced in a volar direction.

(C) Irreducible cases may indicate an entrapped volar plate.

(D) They all require surgical repair.

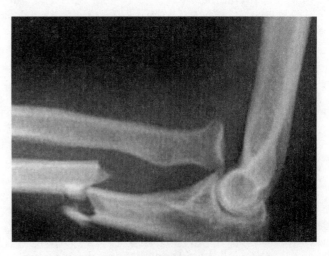

Figure 14-1.

14-16. An 8-year-old football player is brought to your ED with an anxious set of parents and right shoulder pain. Radiographs reveal a minimally displaced midshaft fracture of the right clavicle. The parents ask you to tell them everything they need to know about the injury. Which of the following statements is TRUE?

(A) This is an uncommon place for a clavicular fracture to occur.

(B) A figure-of-eight harness is necessary for proper healing.

(C) The patient will likely have chronic shoulder pain as an adult.

(D) This fracture may be associated with intrathoracic injury.

14-17. Which of the following is TRUE regarding scapular fractures?

(A) They are seldom associated with other injuries.

(B) Most require surgical fixation to ensure long-term shoulder function.

(C) They are usually the result of severe trauma.

(D) Fractures of the acromion and the scapular spine are the most common.

14-18. A 26-year-old man is brought to the trauma room after a high-speed motorcycle accident. He has suspected injuries to the abdomen and head as well as an obvious deformity of the left ankle. The left foot is dusky and cool, and pulses are difficult to palpate. What is the MOST appropriate next step in the management of this injury?

(A) Obtain ankle films immediately as other trauma radiographs are obtained.

(B) Call the orthopedist on call immediately to request assistance for the reduction.

(C) Perform immediate reduction prior to obtaining radiographs.

(D) Attempt reduction only after films and ankle-brachial indices have been obtained for both lower extremities.

14-19. Which of the following is TRUE regarding acromioclavicular joint injuries?

(A) It is difficult to diagnose them clinically.

(B) Most injuries occur in the elderly.

(C) Shoulder radiographs are needed.

(D) Treatment of most injuries consists of analgesia, rest, and immobilization in a simple sling.

14-20. For which of the following patients can the cervical spine be clinically "cleared" by NEXUS criteria?

(A) The 18-year-old woman complaining of severe left leg pain with an obvious deformity after a motor vehicle accident.

(B) The 65-year-old man with tenderness to palpation along the lateral cervical musculature but no midline tenderness along the bony prominences.

(C) The 48-year-old man with a Glasgow Coma Scale score of 14 and repetitive questioning after a motor vehicle accident who insists, "Nothing is wrong with me, let me go!"

(D) The 33-year-old football player with tingling in his left fingers but no neck pain after being tackled to the ground during practice.

14-21. Which of the following is TRUE regarding cervical spine injuries?

(A) Fanning or widening of the spinous processes may indicate an injury to the anterior ligamentous structures.

(B) Injuries to the transverse ligament of the odontoid can occur without bony fracture and should be considered unstable injuries.

(C) The flexion-teardrop fracture is considered mechanically stable.

(D) A bilateral interfacetal dislocation ("locked facets") is considered mechanically stable.

14-22. A 76-year-old female with a history of a right hip replacement presents after a fall from standing with right hip pain. Initial radiographs reveal a dislocated prosthesis. Which of the following is the next MOST appropriate step in management?

(A) Perform immediate closed reduction under conscious sedation.
(B) Obtain immediate orthopedic consultation.
(C) Obtain additional radiographs of the hip to better delineate the dislocation.
(D) Obtain an AP pelvic film to detect associated occult pelvic injuries.

14-23. Which of the following is TRUE regarding rhabdomyolysis?

(A) Symptoms relating to the musculoskeletal system are almost always present in clinically significant rhabdomyolysis.
(B) Complications of rhabdomyolysis include hyperkalemia, DIC, and renal failure.
(C) Patients who present with oliguric acute renal failure (ARF) secondary to rhabdomyolysis need IV mannitol therapy immediately to promote diuresis.
(D) The degree of creatine kinase (CK) elevation correlates with the severity of illness and the development of renal failure.

14-24. A 30-year-old factory worker presents after a crush injury to the left leg. You suspect compartment syndrome and obtain compartment pressures immediately. The pressures consistently read as 35 mmHg. How do you interpret this reading?

(A) Normal.
(B) Mildly elevated but likely safe.
(C) Moderately elevated and should be repeatedly measured.
(D) Severely elevated and grounds for emergent fasciotomy.

14-25. Which of the following is a common cause of compartment syndrome?

(A) Femur fracture.
(B) Metacarpal fracture.
(C) Radius fracture.
(D) Tibia fracture.

14-26. A 35-year-old man presents after jumping from a 3-story building in a suicide attempt. He is unconscious on arrival and immediately intubated. His feet are swollen and appear deformed, and radiographs are obtained to rule out calcaneal fractures. Which of the following is TRUE regarding calcaneal injuries?

(A) Boehler's angle measured at 10 degrees rules out the possibility of occult fracture.
(B) Management is primarily supportive care, and surgery is rarely necessary.
(C) Associated vertebral fractures are classic but not commonly found.
(D) The patient is at risk for developing a compartment syndrome.

14-27. A 50-year-old woman presents after a bicycle accident complaining of right midfoot tenderness. You are concerned about an injury to the Lisfranc's joint. Which of the following is TRUE regarding this injury?

(A) A fracture noted at the base of the first metatarsal is pathognomonic.
(B) Plantar ecchymosis may be an occult sign of injury.
(C) A gap of <3 mm between the bases of the first and second metatarsals is considered normal.
(D) Most injuries require prolonged casting for up to 12 weeks.

14-28. A 42-year-old man presents complaining of severe, sudden left leg pain and weakness that occurred while playing tennis earlier that day. You suspect an Achilles tendon rupture. Which of the following is the next MOST appropriate step in management?

(A) Immediate orthopedic consultation.

(B) Splinting in neutral position and orthopedic follow-up within 1 week.

(C) Immediate MRI to confirm the diagnosis.

(D) Splinting in plantar flexion and orthopedic follow-up within 3–4 weeks.

14-29. A 55-year-old woman presents after a high-speed motor vehicle accident. She complains of right hip pain, and on exam you appreciate a shortened, rotated right leg. Which of the following statements is TRUE regarding this patient?

(A) If her leg is internally rotated and adducted, she most likely has an anterior hip dislocation.

(B) If her leg is externally rotated and abducted, she most likely has a posterior hip dislocation.

(C) Closed reduction can wait until radiographs are obtained.

(D) Closed reduction should not be attempted unless an orthopedic specialist is available to perform the reduction.

14-30. A 29-year-old man is brought in by ambulance after a high-speed motorcycle accident. The paramedics state that when they arrived on the scene, the patient's left knee appeared severely deformed, and a splint was immediately applied. Upon removal of the splint in the ED, you do not appreciate any obvious deformity but do note severe swelling of the joint. The patient is in severe pain at the knee, and you appreciate severe instability of the knee in multiple directions. Which of the following is TRUE regarding this patient?

(A) He most likely has a quadriceps tendon rupture and should be splinted in a knee immobilizer.

(B) Any effusion present should be immediately aspirated.

(C) This patient is at high risk for neurovascular injuries and should be admitted regardless of the neurovascular exam.

(D) Radiographs should be ordered to rule out a fracture, and the patient should receive prompt outpatient follow-up to evaluate potential ligamentous injuries.

14-31. In what region are the majority of epidural cord compressions found?

(A) Cervical spine.

(B) Thoracic spine.

(C) Lumbar spine.

(D) Sacral nerve roots.

14-32. What is the MOST appropriate imaging modality in a patient with neck and arm pain worsening over the last week who has triceps weakness with no history of trauma?

(A) No imaging is necessary; attempt conservative therapy.

(B) Obtain plain films of the neck.

(C) Perform MRI

(D) Perform CT myelography.

14-33. What is the MOST common systemic disease affecting the spine?

(A) Multiple sclerosis.

(B) Rheumatoid arthritis.

(C) Amyotrophic lateral sclerosis.

(D) Malignancy.

14-34. A 35-year-old male with a 1-week history of progressive pain radiating from the lumbar spine down the back of the leg presents to the ED. His physical examination is normal except for complaints of back pain with movement. What is the MOST appropriate imaging test?

(A) No imaging is necessary; attempt conservative therapy.

(B) Obtain plain films of the lumbar spine.

(C) Perform MRI.

(D) Perform CT.

14-35. What is the MOST common finding in cauda equina syndrome?

(A) Urinary retention.

(B) Decreased anal sphincter tone.

(C) Weakness or numbness in the lower extremities.

(D) Saddle anesthesia.

14-36. What is the MOST specific radiologic sign of a rotator cuff tear?

(A) Sclerosis of the humeral head.

(B) Obliteration of the peribursal fat plane.

(C) Narrowing of the acromiohumeral space.

(D) Osteophytic changes of the acromion and/or clavicle.

14-37. In Figure 14-2, the examiner is attempting to examine which muscle?

(A) Teres minor.

(B) Teres major.

(C) Infraspinatus.

(D) Supraspinatus.

14-38. In which of the following rheumatic diseases is pulmonary fibrosis rarely found?

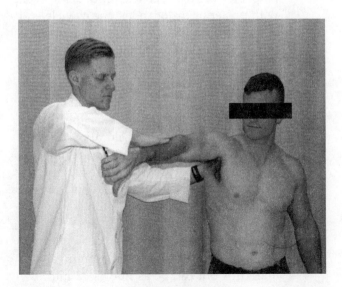

Figure 14–2.

(A) Systemic lupus (SLE).

(B) Rheumatiod arthritis (RA).

(C) Spondylarthropathies.

(D) Scleroderma.

14-39. Temporal arteritis is MOST commonly associated with which of the following diseases?

(A) Systemic lupus (SLE).

(B) Polyarteritis nodosa (PAN).

(C) Wegner's granulomatosis.

(D) Polymyalgia rheumatica (PMR).

14-40. What is the MOST frequently used approach for the drainage of felon?

(A) A J-type or "hockey stick" incision.

(B) Through and through lateral incision.

(C) "Fishmouth" incision.

(D) Unilateral longitudinal incision.

14-41. An erythematous, swollen knee is aspirated, yielding cloudy yellow fluid that has a white blood cell count of 8000, 70% PMNs, and no crystals. Of the following, which is the MOST likely disorder causing this effusion?

(A) Traumatic arthritis.

(B) Gonoccocal arthritis.

(C) Lyme arthritis.

(D) Rheumatic fever.

14-42. An erythematous, inflamed olecranon bursa is aspirated. The aspirate shows straw-colored fluid, white blood cell count of 20,000, predominantly PMNs. Of the following, which is the MOST likely disorder causing this effusion?

(A) Septic bursitis.

(B) Traumatic bursitis.

(C) Idiopathic bursitis.

(D) Crystal-induced bursitis.

CHAPTER 14

Musculoskeletal Emergencies
Answers, Explanations, and References

14-1. **The answer is D** (Chapter 268). High-pressure injection injuries of the hand are considered high-risk injuries, although the benign appearance may mislead the clinician. Both the kinetic energy inherent to the wound and the chemical irritation that can result from frequently injected materials lead to tissue edema and resulting ischemia. Compartment syndrome may result and thus this injury is a surgical emergency, necessitating immediate orthopedic consultation. Neither suturing nor prophylactic antibiotics are indicated in this injury, nor is outpatient follow-up appropriate.

14-2. **The answer is A** (Chapter 268). Compartment syndromes of the hand differ from those of other sites and can be more elusive to diagnose. Hand compartment syndromes may lack typical paresthesias, and "pain with passive stretch" is difficult to assess due to the difficulty of isolating muscles in each compartment. Pain, however, is the most consistent clinical sign and is often described as deep and out of proportion to clinical findings. Patients may demonstrate the "intrinsic minus" position of the involved hand at rest (MCP extended and PIP slightly flexed). Compartment pressures are needed to make the diagnosis, and the suspicion of compartment syndrome of the hand warrants emergent orthopedic consultation.

14-3. **The answer is A** (Chapter 267). Nondisplaced radial head and scaphoid fractures are classic examples of fractures that may not be apparent on the first day of injury.

Often, the clinician must use historical features such as the mechanism of injury and physical findings such as joint effusions or point tenderness to make a clinical diagnosis of a fracture. In such cases, the injury is splinted and treated as a fracture, and follow-up is arranged for 7–10 days later, when enough bony resorption has occurred at the fracture site to reveal a lucency on x-ray.

14-4. **The answer is C** (Chapter 271). The patient described in this scenario has sustained a blunt injury to the chest and has a posterior sternoclavicular dislocation. Sternoclavicular dislocations are uncommon, with anterior dislocations more frequently encountered. Patients with sternoclavicular joint dislocations usually have severe pain, exacerbated by arm movement. On exam, anterior dislocations may have a prominent palpable medial clavicle end. However, with posterior dislocations, the clavicle end is not palpable. Patients with posterior dislocations can have impingement of mediastinal contents and potentially life-threatening injuries to the great vessels, trachea, or esophagus. Routine radiographs are often not conclusive, and CT is the test of choice if a posterior dislocation is suspected. Additional shoulder radiographs or an end-expiratory CXR would not be of use in diagnosing this injury. This patient should be kept NPO.

14-5. **The answer is C** (Chapter 268). Normal two-point discrimination is <6mm at the fingertips but can be as fine as <2 mm. Because patients often guess correctly, repeat testing should be performed on each side of the digit. Less than 80% accuracy is suggestive of digital nerve injury.

14-6.   The answer is C (Chapter 268). Gamekeeper's thumb occurs when forced radial deviation at the MCP joint occurs, rupturing the ulnar collateral ligament. The injury often includes significant damage to the dorsal capsule and volar plate. Stress testing of the ulnar collateral ligament at the MCP joint may be needed to elucidate the injury in the case of normal radiographs. More than 40 degrees of radial angulation indicates complete rupture and requires prompt orthopedic follow-up within 1 week. Hand surgery referral is recommended for all patients with any laxity of the ligament on stress testing, with point tenderness at the volar-ulnar aspect of the MCP joint, or with weakness of pincer function. Immediate treatment in a thumb spica splint is indicated.

14-7.   The answer is A (Chapter 269). Lunate and perilunate dislocations generally result from forced dorsiflexion and impact on the outstretched hand. These injuries generally require a significant amount of force to disrupt the intrinsic and extrinsic ligaments of the midcarpal region. The amount of force needed to produce these injuries frequently results in associated fractures of the carpal bones in an arc around the lunate. Clinically, the patients have a significant amount of swelling but may lack an obvious gross deformity. Radiographs reveal a disruption in the linear arrangement of the distal radius, the lunate, and the capitate. If the lunate bone retains contact with the radius on radiographs, the injury is classified as a perilunate dislocation. If the lunate is completely displaced off the radius and no longer articulates with the capitate as well, the injury is termed a lunate dislocation. All patients with these injuries require emergency orthopedic consultation. Open reduction and internal fixation are required for unstable, open, or irreducible injuries.

Closed reduction and long arm splint immobilization may be appropriate if the injury is reducible, but some orthopedists prefer to operate on all perilunate and lunate dislocations. Because the lunate is dislocated in a volar direction into the carpal tunnel, median nerve compression is sometimes an associated complication of these injuries. Early degenerative arthritis, malunion, nonunion, and avascular necrosis are also possible complications if associated carpal fractures have occurred.

14-8.   The answer is D (Chapter 269). Scaphoid fractures result from falls onto an outstretched hand or axial loads directed along the thumb. The scaphoid acts to stabilize the carpal bones and transmits compression forces from the hand to the forearm, increasing its propensity for injury. Patients may complain of pain along the radial aspect of the wrist and have tenderness to palpation in the anatomic snuffbox. Standard wrist and special scaphoid view radiographs should be examined for fractures. Occasionally, a distorted fat stripe adjacent to the scaphoid may suggest an otherwise nonapparent fracture. Because initial radiographs may fail to detect up to 10% of scaphoid fractures, clinical suspicion of a fracture based on historical and physical findings should guide immediate management. Patients should receive a thumb spica splint with dorsiflexion and radial deviation and have prompt orthopedic follow-up arranged. The vascular supply of the scaphoid enters the distal segment of the bone, thus the proximal segment is at risk for avascular necrosis if the injury is not properly treated. The main complications of improperly healed scaphoid fractures are avascular necrosis, delayed union or malunion, and early arthritis.

14-9.   The answer is C (Chapter 269). Carpal bone fractures account for 7–10% of all hand injuries; however, they are commonly missed. A high index of suspicion and a focused exam is necessary to recognize carpal bone injuries. Carpal bone fractures are often not visualized on the initial set of radiographs. Triquetrum fractures should be suspected if the patient has focal tenderness over the dorsum of the wrist just distal to the ulnar styloid. Lunate fractures generally occur in association with other carpal injuries but should be suspected with tenderness along the dorsal aspect of the wrist. Flexing the wrist causes the lunate to rise and become easily palpable in this location. The lunate is similar to the scaphoid and has its blood supply enter through the distal portion, placing it at similar risk for avascular necrosis (Kienböck's disease). Trapezium fractures should be suspected if focal tenderness is present or if the patient has painful thumb movement and/or a weak pinch. Thumb spica splinting is appropriate. Pisiform fractures usually result from a direct blow and lead to focal tenderness over the pisiform itself in the hypothenar eminence. It is necessary to exclude associated ulnar artery or nerve involvement. Compression dressings or splinting in 30-degree flexion and ulnar deviation are appropriate. Pisiform fractures have an excellent prognosis. Hamate fractures should be splinted and referred to an orthopedist for follow-up. Nonunion of hamate hook fractures is common. Capitate fractures usually occur in conjunction with a scaphoid fracture and are most often in the neck. The capitate shares the risk for avascular necrosis with the lunate and the scaphoid. Splinting and referral are appropriate; however, due to the high incidence of associated injuries, capitate fractures usually require surgical reduction. Trapezoid fractures are very rare and should be treated in a thumb spica splint.

14-10. **The answer is C** (Chapter 269). Colles' fractures are common injuries of the distal radius and result in a dorsally angulated fracture with dorsal and proximal displacement of the distal fragment. Any degree of comminution may be seen, and the fracture line may involve the radioulnar or radiocarpal joint. An associated fracture of the ulnar styloid suggests injury to the triangular fibrocartilage complex. Closed reduction should be attempted in stable fractures. The goals of closed reduction are to restore the volar tilt, radial inclination, and full length to the radius in order to ensure complete function of the wrist. Volar tilt should ideally be restored to normal, but neutral or zero degrees of angulation is acceptable. All fractures should receive prompt orthopedic follow-up.

14-11. **The answer is B** (Chapter 270). The vast majority of elbow dislocations are posterior. Severe swelling may obscure bony landmarks. It is especially important to assess neurovascular status, with particular attention paid to the brachial artery and the ulnar, median, and radial nerves, since associated injuries to these structures are fairly common. Examinations both before and after reduction are important. Reduction is generally accomplished with slow longitudinal traction applied to the wrist and forearm. As distal traction continues, the elbow is flexed and a palpable clunk is felt as reduction occurs. The elbow is then moved through its full ROM. If full, smooth ROM is not possible, the postreduction film should be examined for entrapment of the medial epicondyle, especially in children. A long arm splint in 90 degrees of flexion at the elbow is applied. Cylindrical casts must be avoided secondary to swelling. A follow-up neurovascular exam is necessary the following day to rule out any neurovascular compromise. Prompt orthopedic referral is necessary. Any patients with potential neurovascular compromise, irreducible fractures, open fractures, or joint capsule disruption should have emergent orthopedic consultation. Vascular complications occur in 5–13% of these patients. The brachial artery is the most common vessel injured. Absence of a radial pulse before reduction, open dislocation, or concomitant systemic injuries are associated with arterial injuries.

14-12. **The answer is C** (Chapter 270). Supracondylar fractures are common, especially in children. Radiographs that do not reveal an obvious fracture should be inspected for the fat-pad sign. A visible posterior fat pad is not normal and indicates that hemarthrosis is present; it should be considered evidence of fracture in the setting of trauma. Anterior fat pads are normally thin stripes, and any enlargement of such should be considered abnormal. Abnormal fat pads may also be seen in joint capsule disruption with extravasation of intra-articular fluid. Most supracondylar fractures are displaced posteriorly. There are numerous complications of supracondylar fractures, including neurovascular injuries and delayed union, malunion, or nonunion. Both radial and median nerve injuries have been described. Acute vascular injuries should always be sought in the patient with a supracondylar fracture. Absence of the radial pulse is concerning for vascular injury, although it may reflect transient arterial spasm in children. Repeated exams are necessary to exclude intimal injury or entrapment of the brachial artery. The most serious complication of supracondylar fractures is Volkmann's ischemic contracture. Ischemic tissue in the forearm leads to increased swelling and pressures within the osteofascial forearm compartment. This reduces capillary blood flow and can result in muscle and nerve necrosis. Eventually, the necrotic tissue is replaced with fibrotic tissue and a contracture results. Any signs of impending compartment syndrome in the forearm (forearm tenderness, pain with passive movement, or refusal to open the hand in children) should be considered signs of impending ischemia. Emergency orthopedic consultation is warranted for irreducible fractures or fractures with signs of neurovascular compromise.

14-13. **The answer is D** (Chapter 270). Radial head fractures are among the most common fractures of the elbow. Although the fracture may not be radiographically apparent on the day of injury, subtle clues exist that should lead the clinician to suspect fracture. Any tenderness with palpation of the radial head laterally or pain with pronation and supination of the forearm is suggestive of fracture. Radiographically, a posterior fat pad sign or disruption of the radiocapitellar line (a line drawn from the center of the radial shaft that should transect the radial head and capitellum) are helpful in diagnosing this fracture, especially in children whose epiphysis has not fused.

14-14. **The answer is B** (Chapter 270). The injury shown consists of an ulnar shaft fracture with an associated radial head dislocation. This injury is known as Monteggia's fracture-dislocation. In Monteggia's fracture, the apex of the ulna fracture points in the direction of the radial head dislocation, which is often missed on initial radiographic interpretation. Orthopedists use a classification system for these fractures, but generally these fractures are treated with open reduction and internal fixation. Galeazzi's fracture (or reverse Monteggia's fracture) is a fracture of the distal third of the radius, which is often associated with a distal radioulnar joint dislocation.

14-15. **The answer is C** (Chapter 268). Distal interphalangeal joint dislocations are usually produced by an axial load with hyperextension. The firm attachments of the skin and subcutaneous tissue to the underlying bone make these injuries fairly uncommon. Dorsal dislocations are the most common and occur when the volar plate ruptures. Reduction is performed with longitudinal traction and application of direct dorsal pressure. Irreducible cases may indicate entrapment of an avulsion fracture, profundus tendon, or the volar plate. These injuries should be splinted in full extension and referred for follow-up within 1 week.

14-16. **The answer is D** (Chapter 271). Clavicle fractures are the most common fracture of childhood and account for nearly half of significant injuries to the shoulder girdle.

nized for evidence of fracture. Compression fractures may be subtle, and the Boehler's angle measurement helps to discern an otherwise nonapparent fracture (see Figure 14-3). A Boehler's angle of <20 degrees indicates a likely fracture. Calcaneal fractures, especially comminuted fractures, are at high risk of developing compartment syndrome of the foot. Calcaneal injuries caused by such a mechanism are frequently associated with injuries to the axial spine, and a thorough radiologic investigation must be undertaken in this patient to exclude such associated injuries.

14-27.   **The answer is B** (Chapter 277). The tarsal-metatarsal complex of the first 3 digits of the foot is known as the Lisfranc's joint. Injuries to this joint are frequently missed in the ED. Clues to a Lisfranc's injury include the plantar ecchymosis sign and tenderness about the joint on palpation. A fracture of the base of the second metatarsal is pathognomonic of Lisfranc's joint disruption, as

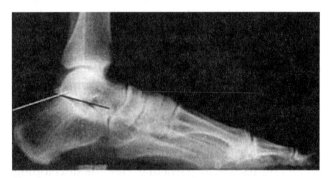

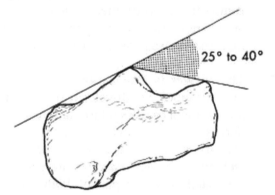

Figure 14-3. Boehler's angle.

well as a separation of >1 mm between the first and second metatarsals. CT scanning is recommended to further elucidate the injury once suspected. Lisfranc's joint injuries require immediate orthopedic consultation, and the majority need operative repair.

14-28.   **The answer is B** (Chapter 275). Achilles tendon ruptures are common in sports settings. Poorly conditioned individuals, persons with a history of rheumatoid arthritis or lupus, and those with a history of steroid injections to the tendon or quinolone use are at higher risk for injury. Clinical signs of rupture include a palpable defect in the tendon and no plantar flexion response when the gastrocnemius is squeezed (the Thompson-Doherty test). Correct management of this injury in the ED includes splinting in neutral position, crutches, instructions to avoid weight bearing, and early orthopedic referral.

14-29.   **The answer is C** (Chapter 273). This patient has a dislocated hip. Hip dislocations are true orthopedic emergencies. Posterior dislocations account for the majority of hip dislocations, and the patient presents with an adducted, shortened, and internally rotated leg. Anterior dislocations can occur in either an inferior or superior direction and present with an abducted, externally rotated leg. Treatment for all dislocations is early closed reduction under conscious sedation. Radiographs should be obtained prior to reduction to rule out acetabular or femoral fractures, which can have a similar clinical appearance on exam. Closed reduction should then be performed as soon as possible to reduce the risk of avascular necrosis, which increases in direct proportion to the delay in adequate reduction.

14-30.   **The answer is C** (Chapter 274). A severe mechanism of injury and a knee that is unstable in multiple directions indicates tremendous ligamentous disruption. This patient has most likely dislocated his knee. Spontaneous reduction of knee dislocations often occurs, and patients may not have an obvious deformity upon presentation. Knee dislocations have a high incidence of associated complications, including injuries to the popliteal artery and peroneal nerve. A detailed neurovascular exam is important to document pre- and postreduction (if reduction is required). All patients with knee dislocation should be admitted. Whether and when patients with knee dislocations require arteriography is controversial and should be determined in conjunction with the orthopedic consultant.

14-31. **The answer is B** (Chapter 281). The thoracic spine is the level where the majority of epidural cord compression syndromes occur. Approximately 70% of epidural cord compressions are located at the thoracic spine level and 10% at the cervical level.

14-32. **The answer is C** (Chapter 281). MRI is indicated for those patients with neurologic signs or symptoms regardless of the plain film findings.

14-33. **The answer is D** (Chapter 282). Malignant neoplasm is the most common systemic disease affecting the spine, 80% of which occurs in patients 50 years of age or older.

14-34. **The answer is A** (Chapter 282). No imaging is necessary; attempt conservative therapy. If the patient has no risk factors in the history and physical examination for serious disease other than sciatica, treat conservatively and do not perform any diagnostic tests in the ED.

14-35. **The answer is A** (Chapter 282). Urinary retention with overflow incontinence is the most common symptom of cauda equina syndrome, with a sensitivity of 90% and a specificity of about 95%.

14-36. **The answer is C** (Chapter 283). Narrowing of the acromiohumeral space, <7 mm, is the most specific radiologic sign for large rotator cuff tears.

14-37. **The answer is D** (Chapter 283). Figure 14-2 demonstrates the "empty beer can position," which isolates the supraspinatus muscle. The other muscles are in the rotator cuff but are not specifically isolated by this maneuver.

14-38. **The answer is A** (Chapter 284). Pulmonary fibrosis is rare in SLE, common in scleroderma, and infrequent but not rare in RA and the spondylarthropathies.

14-39. **The answer is D** (Chapter 284). Temporal arteritis occurs in up to 30% of patients with PMR.

14-40. **The answer is D** (Chapter 285). The unilateral longitudinal incision, distal to the distal interphalangeal crease, is most commonly used and spares the sensate volar pad.

14-41. **The answer is C** (Chapter 286). This is consistent with an inflammatory arthritis, differential to include gout, pseudogout, spondylarthropathies, rheumatoid arthritis, Lyme disease, and SLE. The absence of crystals makes Lyme the most likely of the choices listed.

14-42. **The answer is A** (Chapter 286). Although the white blood cell count is below the mean of 75,000 for septic bursitis, the count is high enough with the predominance of PMNs to make septic bursitis the most likely choice.

CHAPTER 15

Neurologic Emergencies
Questions

15-1. Which patient has the highest likelihood of a carotid artery dissection?

(A) A 20-year-old male complaining of severe headache immediately after a physical therapy treatment followed by right-sided weakness 2 days later.

(B) A 60-year-old hypertensive male presenting with painless right-sided weakness after he was out rowing.

(C) An 8-year-old boy with a history of recurrent headaches associated with vomiting and right-sided weakness who comes from school with these symptoms and has family members with a similar history.

(D) A 5-year-old male with sickle cell disease who presents with focal weakness and a headache following a hike.

15-2. What is the recommended treatment for a previously hypertensive patient with subarachnoid hemorrhage, normal swallowing, and a mean arterial pressure of 150 mmHg?

(A) Intravenous antihypertensive medication to lower the mean arterial pressure to 90 mmHg.

(B) Nifedipine by mouth.

(C) Immediate neurosurgery.

(D) Prophylactic phenytoin loading.

15-3. Which of the following is TRUE of Bell's palsy?

(A) Sudden onset is common.

(B) Preservation of motor function in the upper face is seen.

(C) Associated pain generally rules out the diagnosis.

(D) Steroids are indicated and should be started at any phase of the disease.

15-4. Which clinical finding or findings would be caused by a complete paralysis of cranial nerve III?

(A) Dilated pupil with downward and outward deviation and ptosis.

(B) Afferent pupillary defect.

(C) Impaired corneal reflex.

(D) Difficulty abducting the globe.

15-5. A 40-year-old previously healthy female presents with sudden onset of a severe occipital and nuchal headache following a coughing fit. Vital signs and physical examination are normal. Which of the following is indicated?

(A) Contrast CT scan of the brain followed by lumbar puncture if negative.

(B) Noncontrast CT scan of the brain followed by lumbar puncture if negative.

(C) MRI scan of the brain.

(D) Trial of pain medication and CT scan of the head and lumbar puncture only if headache is unrelieved.

15-6. Which is considered an indication for emergent neuroimaging?

(A) Headache after lumbar puncture.

(B) A cluster headache in a patient with a prior history of them.

(C) New headache in an HIV-positive patient.

(D) Headache, isolated fever, stiff neck, and photophobia.

15-7. Which is a recommended sequential treatment for migraine?

(A) Dihydroergotamine (DHE), then metoclopramide.

(B) Sumatriptan, then dexamethasone.

(C) Metoclopramide, then meperidine.

(D) DHE, then sumatriptan.

15-8. Which finding is MOST suggestive of a lesion in the dominant cerebral cortex?

(A) Right-sided lesion on CT scan.

(B) Inattention by the patient to a person approaching from the left.

(C) Difficulty with naming common objects.

(D) Inability to identify by touch a coin placed in the patient's hand.

15-9. Which clinical scenario is MOST suspicious for temporal arteritis?

(A) An obese 16-year-old female on tetracycline and birth control pills with 1 month of headache, nausea, and visual disturbances.

(B) A 26-year-old female with frequent facial pains lasting for seconds at a time.

(C) A 60-year-old female with new-onset throbbing frontal headache and a sedimentation rate of 90 mm/hour.

(D) A 30-year-old male with 1 week of severe, daily, unilateral temporal headache and rhinorrhea relieved with high-flow oxygen.

15-10. Which of the following is TRUE of the condition depicted in Figure 15-1?

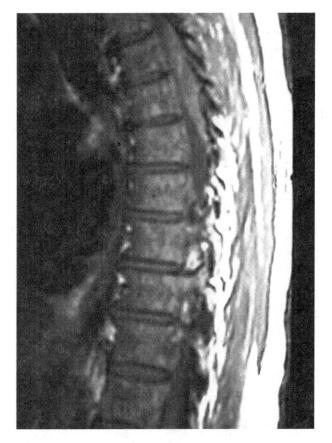

Figure 15-1.

(A) Postvoid residual urine volume of 50 mL is suggestive.

(B) Normal reflexes generally rule out this diagnosis.

(C) Injection drug use is a risk factor.

(D) A narrow-based shuffling gait is common.

15-11. Which clinical picture is MOST consistent with the findings on the CT image shown in Figure 15-2?

(A) Contralateral leg greater than arm weakness.

(B) Contralateral weakness and numbness affecting the face and arm more than the legs.

(C) No weakness noted, but reduced contralateral sensation to pinprick and light touch.

(D) Diplopia with contralateral limb weakness.

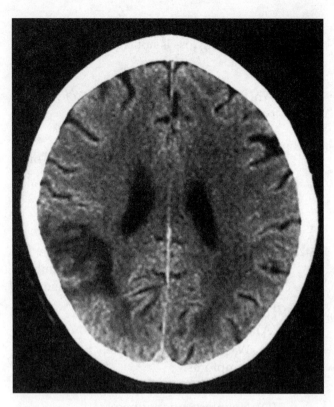

Figure 15-2.

(C) Hypotension and tachycardia classically accompany this finding.

(D) The increased intracranial pressure may lead to cerebral ischemia.

15-14. In a patient with possible coma, which finding is correctly linked with its etiology?

(A) Pinpoint pupils and uncal herniation.

(B) Lack of pupillary response and toxic-metabolic coma.

(C) Nystagmus with caloric vestibular testing and pseudocoma.

(D) Localizing signs and hypoxia.

15-15. Which is TRUE of cerebrospinal fluid shunts?

(A) A lumbar puncture performed by the emergency physician is indicated when a shunt infection is suspected.

(B) Shunt infections are more common the longer the shunt has been in place.

(C) *Staphylococcus epidermidis* is the pathogen responsible for half of all shunt infections.

(D) Vomiting is the cardinal sign of a shunt malfunction.

15-16. Which of the following is the MOST common sign or symptom of brain abscess?

(A) Neck stiffness.

(B) Fever.

(C) Increased intracranial pressure.

(D) Headache.

15-17. Which of the following is TRUE of encephalitis caused by herpes simplex virus (HSV) type 1?

(A) It spreads to the central nervous system hematogenously after invasion and replication elsewhere in the body.

(B) Psychiatric symptoms can predominate.

(C) It is typically seen in neonates.

(D) Prednisone is the treatment of choice.

15-12. Which of these scenarios is MOST consistent with delirium?

(A) An alert patient with acute onset of auditory hallucinations and delusions.

(B) An alert patient who has lost short-term memory over the past several years.

(C) A patient who for several days has been more somnolent during the day and confused and agitated at night.

(D) An unarousable patient with hypothermia.

15-13. Which of the following statements is TRUE regarding a patient with increased intracranial pressure?

(A) Paralysis and sedation should not be used after such a patient is placed on a ventilator as they will obscure the neurologic exam.

(B) Ketamine is a good choice for rapid sequence intubation.

15-18. Which is TRUE concerning chemoprophylaxis for high-risk contacts of patients with *Neisseria meningitidis?*

(A) All health care providers who cared for the patient should be treated.

(B) Four doses of rifampin are first-line treatment.

(C) School contacts for the last month should be treated.

(D) Anyone who was exposed to the patient in the last week should be treated.

15-19. Which of the following is TRUE regarding the workup and treatment of suspected bacterial meningitis?

(A) Steroids should always be given.

(B) A CT scan must always precede the lumbar puncture.

(C) Empiric antibiotic therapy should always be given in the ED.

(D) Lumbar puncture results should always guide initial antibiotic choice.

15-20. Which clinical scenario is correctly linked with the neuroimaging modality?

(A) A 69-year-old male with an AICD in whom a basilar skull fracture is suspected and plain skull films.

(B) An otherwise well-appearing 2-year-old male with a broken arm in whom child abuse is suspected and CT scan of the brain.

(C) A 69-year-old female with a pacemaker, difficulty breathing, and a suspected posterior fossa lesion and MRI of the brain.

(D) A 3-month-old female with focal neurologic signs and ultrasound of the brain imaging through the open fontanels.

15-21. Which is TRUE of Meniere's disease?

(A) It usually occurs in patients aged 65 and older.

(B) The duration of vertigo is short.

(C) Attacks usually occur daily.

(D) Hearing loss is not an associated finding.

15-22. Which finding is suggestive of benign paroxysmal positional vertigo?

(A) It is worse in the evening.

(B) Attacks are precipitated by rolling over in bed.

(C) Hearing loss can be associated.

(D) Nausea is generally not associated.

15-23. A 1-year-old child is brought to the ED with ataxia 7 days after the onset of chicken pox. Which of the following management plans is appropriate?

(A) Administer acyclovir.

(B) Warn the parents of likely residual symptoms.

(C) Perform a lumbar puncture.

(D) No intervention is necessary.

15-24. Which treatment of benign paroxysmal positional vertigo associated with nausea is unlikely to be effective?

(A) Diphenhydramine intramuscularly.

(B) Ondansetron intravenously.

(C) Scopolamine transdermal patch.

(D) Intramuscular promethazine followed by the Epley maneuver.

15-25. Which of the following is the appropriate management for an uncomplicated seizure of 2 minutes duration?

(A) Intravenous lorazepam.

(B) Bag-valve-mask ventilation.

(C) Insertion of a bite block.

(D) Observation and monitoring.

15-26. Which is TRUE of seizures in pregnancy?

(A) All previously prescribed anticonvulsants should be stopped due to the risk of teratogenic effects.

(B) Eclampsia is a serious cause of seizures as early as the 16th week of pregnancy.

(C) MRI or CT of the head with shielding of the abdomen are considered acceptable.

(D) Phenytoin is the first-line anticonvulsant in a 32-week pregnant patient with new-onset seizures.

15-27. Which is TRUE of alcohol withdrawal seizures?

(A) Phenytoin loading is indicated.

(B) Patients should be admitted to the hospital.

(C) Seizures usually occur between 6 and 48 hours after stopping or reducing alcohol intake.

(D) Workup of first-time alcohol withdrawal seizure can be less complex than the workup for other first-time seizures.

15-28. Which of the following is TRUE of carpal tunnel syndrome?

(A) It is worse at the end of the workday.

(B) Generally it is unilateral.

(C) It is exacerbated by pregnancy.

(D) Numbness is localized to the hand.

15-29. Which of the following is TRUE of Guillain-Barré syndrome?

(A) The only danger of death is from respiratory failure.

(B) It is more common in HIV-infected patients.

(C) In classic cases, sensation on exam is usually abnormal.

(D) It is easily distinguished from Lyme disease.

15-30. A 30-year-old male presents with normal mentation, sensation, and reflexes but a complaint of proximal limb weakness. Besides weakness, extraocular movements are abnormal, and there is an absence of the pupillary light reflex. What is the MOST likely diagnosis?

(A) Botulism.

(B) Myasthenia gravis.

(C) Acute intermittent porphyria.

(D) Tick paralysis.

15-31. A patient with known myasthenia gravis and a normal airway anatomy presents with weak respirations. Which of the following drugs would be preferred for intubation?

(A) Pancuronium.

(B) Tubocurarine.

(C) Succinylcholine.

(D) Propofol.

15-32. Which of the following is TRUE of multiple sclerosis?

(A) Central visual loss is a common presenting complaint.

(B) MRI is normal in most cases of multiple sclerosis.

(C) The majority of patients have a reduction in life expectancy.

(D) Relapses are more common in pregnancy.

15-33. Which disease has the lowest incidence of respiratory failure?

(A) Parkinson's disease.

(B) Lambert-Eaton myasthenic syndrome.

(C) Myasthenic crisis.

(D) Amyotrophic lateral sclerosis.

15-1. **The answer is A** (Chapter 228). Arterial dissection accounts for 20% of all ischemic strokes in patients between the ages of 15 and 50 years. Stroke symptoms may come several days after headache begins; precipitants as mild as sharp turning of the head can cause dissection. Although hypertension is a risk factor for dissection, other causes of stroke would be much more likely in an older patient. Recurrent symptoms in a patient with a family history would signal a possible complex migraine. The sickle cell patient is at highest risk for ischemic stroke or, less likely, cerebral aneurysm with subarachnoid hemorrhage.

15-2. **The answer is D** (Chapters 227, 228). The mean arterial pressure should be maintained at prehemorrhage levels or approximately 110 mmHg. Nimodipine reduces the incidence and severity of vasospasm and therefore the amount of cerebral ischemia; nifedipine would be contraindicated due to unpredictable effect and possible hypotension. Neurosurgical consultation (but not necessarily surgery) and phenytoin loading are appropriate.

15-3. **The answer is A** (Chapters 226, 233). Sudden onset is typical of Bell's palsy. Bell's palsy is due to a peripheral abnormality of cranial nerve VII, and the upper face is involved. A cortical lesion (often stroke) results in weakness of the lower and mid face with motor function preserved in the forehead because of bilateral upper motor neuron innervation of the upper face. Pain is variably seen and is often around the ear.

Use of steroids is controversial; they should not be given if there is a high risk of complications from them or if the patient is seen more than a week after weakness begins.

15-4. **The answer is A** (Chapter 226). Cranial nerve III controls extraocular muscles that adduct, elevate, and depress the globe. It also controls pupilloconstriction and levator function. An afferent pupillary defect may indicate optic nerve (cranial nerve II) dysfunction. The corneal reflex is controlled by cranial nerves V (sensory) and VII (motor). Cranial nerve VI innervates the lateral rectus muscle, and defects in abduction would be seen if it were paralyzed.

15-5. **The answer is B** (Chapter 227). A sudden, severe onset of an occipitonuchal headache is a common presentation of subarachnoid hemorrhage. Physical exam may be entirely normal, yet 12% of those presenting to the ED with the sudden onset of a severe headache have subarachnoid hemorrhage despite a normal exam. Exertion as minor as coughing or defecating at the onset of a headache is also suggestive of this diagnosis. Noncontrast-enhanced CT scan is the best neuroimaging test for diagnosing subarachnoid hemorrhage, although a negative scan alone does not exclude the diagnosis. Lumbar puncture would be indicated as a follow-up test. Contrast scans are not considered more diagnostic. MRI scanning is equally or less sensitive than CT scanning in the first few days following a bleed, and it can be a more costly and difficult test to obtain. Response to pain medications does not rule out the diagnosis.

15-6.   The answer is C (Chapters 227, 237). Acute, sudden onset of headache, new headache in HIV-positive patients, and new focal neurologic deficit are considered level B recommendations in the 2002 ACEP Clinical Policy on Acute Headache. (There were no level A recommendations.) Typical headache after lumbar puncture and typical headaches of the migraine, tension, or cluster type generally do not need emergent neuroimaging. In the absence of papilledema, decreased level of consciousness, or focal neurologic findings (evidence of increased intracranial pressure), CT is not required prior to obtaining a lumbar puncture to rule out meningitis. Chapter 237 states, however, that "despite the absence of scientific validation, it has become the standard of care to precede lumbar puncture with non-contrast-enhanced CT of the head."

15-7.   The answer is B (Chapter 227). Dexamethasone is effective in reducing the rate of recurrent migraine following standard treatment. Pretreatment with an antiemetic prior to DHE use is recommended due to the high incidence of vomiting with DHE. Meperidine is less effective than other agents, and the frequent use of opioids for recurrent headaches may lead to adverse effects or exacerbate headaches. Sumatriptan should not be given within 24 hours of DHE or other ergot use because both cause vasoconstriction.

15-8.   The answer is C (Chapter 226). Aphasias including difficulty naming objects represent lesions in the dominant hemisphere where language function resides. The left hemisphere is dominant in most people whether right- or left-handed. Impairments of sensory discrimination or visual perception involve the nondominant (usually right) hemisphere.

15-9.   The answer is C (Chapter 227). Temporal arteritis is more common in women and is almost exclusively seen in patients over the age of 50. The headache is severe, throbbing, and in the frontotemporal region. Diagnosis is made when 3 out of 5 of these criteria are met: age over 50 years, new-onset localized headache, temporal artery tenderness or decreased pulsation, erythrocyte sedimentation rate greater than 50 mm/hour, and abnormal artery biopsy findings. The first scenario suggests pseudotumor cerebri (benign intracranial hypertension). The second patient presented has symptoms of trigeminal neuralgia, and the last patient's story is suspicious for cluster headaches.

15-10.   The answer is C (Chapters 226, 282, 306). The MRI scan shows a lesion compressing the spinal cord. In an injection drug user with fever and back pain, an epidural abscess must be considered. A postvoid residual volume of >75 mL can suggest a neurogenic bladder, which can be seen with spinal cord compression. Although abnormal reflexes are a cardinal sign of spinal cord compression, reflexes can take up to several days to become hyperactive, and normal reflexes should not keep the physician from pursuing the diagnosis. A narrow-based gait with small, shuffling steps suggests Parkinson's disease.

15-11.   The answer is B (Chapter 228). A middle cerebral artery infarction is shown in the CT image by the area of edema, which causes contralateral weakness affecting the face and arm more than the legs. Findings of contralateral leg greater than arm weakness are more common in anterior cerebral artery problems. Reduced contralateral sensation to pinprick and light touch without weakness is found in patients with posterior cerebral artery abnormalities. The hallmark of vertebrobasilar (posterior circulation) stroke is crossed deficits: ipsilateral deficits of the cranial nerves with contralateral motor weakness.

15-12. **The answer is C** (Chapter 229). Delirium involves dysfunction of the arousal system and shows fluctuating confusion and changes in behavior. It is often worse at night. Alert patients with rapid onset of hallucinations and delusions should be suspected of having a psychiatric illness. Dementia is usually of more gradual onset; consciousness is usually preserved, but short-term memory is often impacted. Coma best describes the unarousable patient.

15-13. **The answer is D** (Chapters 19, 229). Cerebral perfusion pressure is equal to the mean arterial pressure minus the intracranial pressure. Therefore, ischemia will develop as the intracranial pressure approaches the mean arterial pressure. Noxious stimuli such as distress from being ventilated can increase intracranial pressure. Paralysis and sedation are indicated in these cases. Modification of intubation protocols are indicated with suspected increased intracranial pressure. Ketamine is contraindicated as it can further raise the intracranial pressure. Hypertension and bradycardia caused by increased intracranial pressure is a classic finding referred to as the Cushing reflex.

15-14. **The answer is C** (Chapters 226, 229). Nystagmus found with caloric testing can be a sign of a nonphysiologic coma. Pinpoint pupils are a hallmark of pontine hemorrhage; a unilateral dilated pupil that is poorly or not reactive to light may suggest uncal herniation. Pupillary response is generally present in toxic-metabolic coma, and with systemic causes of coma such as hypoxia, localizing findings are seldom seen.

15-15. **The answer is C** (Chapter 236). *S. epidermidis* is the most commonly cultured agent in shunt infections, followed by *S. aureus*. A traditional lumbar puncture has no role in evaluating potential shunt infection as it has a low sensitivity. A neurosurgeon should be consulted regarding a shunt tap. Eighty percent of all shunt infections occur within 6 months of placement, most in the first 2 weeks. No single sign or symptom can predict shunt malfunction, and presenting complaints may be vague. A decreasing level of consciousness has the highest correlation with shunt malfunction, however.

15-16. **The answer is D** (Chapter 235). Presenting features of brain abscess are nonspecific, but headache is present in almost all cases. Meningeal signs like neck stiffness are uncommon. Focal neurologic signs are seen in about 33–60% of cases, and symptoms of increased intracranial pressure such as vomiting, confusion, and obtundation are seen about half of the time.

15-17. **The answer is B** (Chapter 235). HSV involves areas of the brain causing psychiatric features, memory disturbance, and aphasia. Three important viruses—rabies, herpes simplex, and herpes zoster—reach the brain by traveling backward through nerves, not hematogenously. Although HSV type 2 is seen in neonates following perinatal transmission, HSV type 1 tends to be a reactivation disease in older children and adults. It is responsive to antiviral therapy, and acyclovir is the agent of choice.

15-18. **The answer is B** (Chapter 235). The first-line treatment for high-risk contacts of patients with *N. meningitidis* is rifampin every 12 hours for 4 doses. Only health care workers who performed mouth-to-mouth resuscitation or who intubated the patient without wearing a face mask need treatment. School contacts for the previous *week* and those with direct contact with the patient's secretions (e.g., kissing or sharing utensils or toothbrushes) need treatment.

15-19. **The answer is C** (Chapter 235). Beginning empiric antibiotic treatment promptly for suspected bacterial meningitis is critical. Steroid use is not clearly proven to be beneficial in all cases of bacterial meningitis. A lumbar puncture can be performed safely without a preceding CT scan if mass lesion is not suspected on historical and clinical grounds. Local resistance patterns and patient demographic information are best used to guide initial antibiotic choice by more rapidly determining the likelihood of different pathogens.

15-20. **The answer is D** (Chapter 237). In infants with a patent fontanelle, ultrasound is the study of choice for intracranial assessment. CT shows bony abnormalities unseen on MRI and is superior to plain films in assessing the base of the skull, but plain films are still used as part of the skeletal survey for children. Although MRI is superior to CT scanning in imaging the posterior fossa, MRI is contraindicated in the presence of devices such as pacemakers. It also prevents monitoring of critically ill patients.

15-21. **The answer is A** (Chapter 231). The first attack of Meniere's disease is usually in patients aged 65 and older. Attacks typically last 2–8 hours. Attacks usually occur several times a week to several times a month. Tinnitus or hearing loss may be associated with this condition.

15-22. **The answer is B** (Chapter 231). Different movements, including rolling over in bed, can precipitate attacks. The symptoms of benign paroxysmal positional vertigo fatigue tend to be worse in the morning. Although nausea may be associated, there is no associated hearing loss.

15-23. **The answer is D** (Chapter 230). Little workup of ataxia is needed when it occurs in the convalescent phase of varicella. Recovery is uniformly excellent, and antivirals are not indicated.

15-24. **The answer is B** (Chapter 231). Ondansetron has not been shown to be effective in treating nausea associated with motion. Scopolamine patch, antihistamines, and the Epley maneuver all may be helpful.

15-25. **The answer is D** (Chapter 232). During a seizure, little needs to be done besides protecting the patient from injury. A bite block risks damage to the teeth if it can be inserted at all. Although suction and airway equipment should be available and the patient turned to one side to reduce aspiration risk if possible, it is seldom necessary or possible to ventilate a patient during a seizure. There is no indication for intravenous anticonvulsant medications during an uncomplicated seizure.

15-26. **The answer is C** (Chapter 232). MRI or head CT with abdominal shielding are considered safe in pregnancy when indicated. Despite risks of fetal effects from anticonvulsants, the risk to mother and fetus of uncontrolled seizures warrants the continuation of use (although sometimes on a modified regimen) of anticonvulsants during pregnancy. Eclampsia occurs between 20 weeks' gestation and up to 3 weeks postpartum. Seizures are best treated with magnesium sulfate rather than with phenytoin or diazepam when there is a high suspicion of eclampsia. Magnesium sulfate is the drug of choice for eclampsia until the fetus is delivered or an alternative etiology for the seizure in a pregnant woman is made.

15-27. **The answer is C** (Chapter 232). Classic alcohol withdrawal seizures tend to occur within 6–48 hours of reducing or stopping alcohol use. It is not thought that acute or chronic treatment with phenytoin is useful in this scenario. Generally, patients have 1 or 2 seizures within 6 hours; if presentation and evaluation are consistent with this diagnosis and workup is negative, the patient can be discharged and referred for detoxification. Generally, a first seizure in an alcohol-abusing patient should be worked up like any first-time seizure, with the addition of evaluating potential intracranial bleeding and toxic-metabolic abnormalities.

15-28. **The answer is C** (Chapters 233, 285). Carpal tunnel syndrome is often exacerbated by conditions causing fluid retention like congestive heart failure and pregnancy.

It tends to be worse at night and often wakes the patient. It is often bilateral, and numbness may be poorly localized and felt up to the elbow.

15-29. **The answer is B** (Chapter 233). Guillain-Barré syndrome is more common in the early stage of HIV infection. This etiology as well as lupus and lymphoma should be considered when there is a CSF pleocytosis. Both respiratory failure and autonomic instability can cause death with this disease. In classic cases there may be subjective sensory loss, but objective sensory testing is usually normal. Lyme disease can present with a similar clinical picture.

15-30. **The answer is A** (Chapter 233). Botulism can present in adults who ingest botulinum toxin. It can also rarely be transmitted through a wound. Like myasthenia gravis, it is a disorder of the neuromuscular junction, but it is distinguished from myasthenia gravis by the absence of the pupillary light reflex. Lyme disease and acute intermittent porphyria are acute peripheral neuropathies. Both tend to show diminished reflexes and may have abnormal mentation; in acute intermittent porphyria, weakness is usually more pronounced in the legs.

15-31. **The answer is D** (Chapter 234). Patients with myasthenia gravis should not receive either depolarizing or nondepolarizing paralytic agents if it can be avoided. These patients are extremely sensitive to paralytics, and their effects can last 2–3 times longer than in healthy individuals. Smaller than usual doses of etomidate, fentanyl, or propofol are preferred.

15-32. **The answer is A** (Chapter 234). Optic neuritis usually causes central vision loss, and it is the initial sign of multiple sclerosis in up to 30% of patients. MRI shows some pathology in almost all multiple sclerosis patients. The majority of multiple sclerosis patients do not have a reduction in overall life expectancy. Exacerbations are less common in pregnancy.

15-33. **The answer is B** (Chapter 234). Respiratory failure is rarely seen in cases of Lambert-Eaton myasthenic syndrome. The most common cause of death in severe Parkinson's disease is respiratory failure. Myasthenic crisis is characterized by respiratory failure. Amyotrophic lateral sclerosis eventually leads to complete respiratory failure in 80% of patients.

Pediatric Emergencies
Questions

16-1. A female pediatric patient is brought to the ED for evaluation of a swollen left arm. She is otherwise well, and your exam reveals that she is able to walk well, she speaks in phrases, and she demonstrates stranger anxiety. What is the MOST likely developmental stage of this female?

(A) Early infancy.
(B) Late infancy.
(C) Toddler.
(D) Preschool.

16-2. A 15-year-old female presents to the ED with crampy abdominal pain and brisk vaginal bleeding. She states that her last menstrual period was "about 3 months ago." Vital signs at triage include a heart rate of 150 beats per minute, respiratory rate of 36 respirations per minute, and blood pressure of 90/60 mmHg. She appears pale, with dry lips. She is with a friend who drove her to the ED. She states that her mother is at work and can't be disturbed. She has no other guardian. What is the MOST appropriate next step?

(A) Call her mother at work to obtain permission to treat, since the patient is only 15 years of age.
(B) Tell the patient to call her mother and request that she come to the ED. Refrain from any treatment until the patient's mother arrives.

(C) Ask the patient if there is any "next of kin" who can be contacted for permission to treat.
(D) Begin treatment immediately while the nurse is trying to contact the patient's mother.

16-3. The greatest incidence of bacteremia occurs in children in which age group?

(A) Neonates.
(B) Young infants.
(C) Older infants.
(D) Adolescents.

16-4. A 2-month-old infant is brought to the ED by his young parents, who says he is "very sick." He cried most of the night, and this morning he seemed very sleepy and wouldn't wake up to take his bottle. His vital signs include a temperature of 35.4°C, respiratory rate of 72 respirations per minute, and heart rate of 192 beats per minute. His feet and hands are quite cool, and his radial pulse is not palpable. What is the MOST likely diagnosis?

(A) Pneumonia.
(B) Urinary tract infection.
(C) Sepsis.
(D) Gastroenteritis.

16-5. A 3-week-old infant was brought to the ED by his mother and grandmother with a concern of vomiting. He was fine yesterday, but this morning he was fussy and started crying a lot. About 2 hours prior to presentation to the ED he started vomiting, and at triage he was noted to have an episode of bilious emesis. He is awake and alert on exam, but his lips are dry and he is tachycardic with a heart rate of 190. What is the MOST likely diagnosis?

(A) Intussusception.
(B) Feeding intolerance.
(C) Malrotation and volvulus.
(D) Pyloric stenosis.

16-6. What is the MOST common reason for reevaluation and admission to the hospital as a result of early discharge from the newborn nursery?

(A) Jaundice.
(B) Vomiting.
(C) Rash.
(D) Crying.

16-7. A 1-week-old infant is brought to the ED by his mother with concern of poor feeding for the past 12 hours and blood in his stool this morning. The mother states the infant was born 1 month early and weighed almost 6 pounds. He seemed well when he was discharged home from the nursery on his third day of life, but yesterday he cried more than usual and ate less than half his usual amount of formula. On exam, the infant is lethargic with a distended abdomen. Stools are guaiac positive, and demonstrates pneumatosis intestinalis. What is the MOST likely diagnosis?

(A) Intussusception.
(B) Necrotizing enterocolitis.
(C) Hirschsprung's disease.
(D) Anal fissure.

16-8. Which of the following congenital heart lesions will MOST likely cause cyanosis in an infant?

(A) Patent ductus arteriosus.
(B) Coarctation of the aorta.
(C) Tetralogy of Fallot.
(D) Atrial septal defect.

16-9. A 3-month-old infant is brought to the ED by his parents with a concern of difficult feeding. The mother says the baby seems to get tired when eating, and for the past 3 days he has been sweaty after feeds. On physical exam in the ED, the infant is acyanotic, irritable, and tachypneic, with a respiratory rate of 68. When assessing circulation, you note that his femoral pulses are markedly diminished, although his brachial pulse is easy to feel. Cardiac exam reveals a systolic ejection murmur at the cardiac base, with interscapular radiation. What is the MOST likely diagnosis?

(A) Coarctation of the aorta.
(B) Patent ductus arteriosus.
(C) Ventricular septal defect.
(D) Tetralogy of Fallot.

16-10. Of the following, which is the MOST common cardiac dysrhythmia in the pediatric age range?

(A) Complete atrioventricular block.
(B) Atrial flutter.
(C) Ventricular tachycardia.
(D) Supraventricular tachycardia.

16-11. What is the drug of choice for the treatment of acute otitis media in children?

(A) Ceftriaxone.
(B) Amoxicillin.
(C) Azithromycin.
(D) Amoxicillin-clavulanate.

16-12. Of the following, what is the MOST frequent cause of infectious conjunctivitis in the neonate?

(A) *Chlamydia trachomatis.*
(B) *Streptococcus pneumoniae.*
(C) *Staphylococcus aureus.*
(D) *Haemophilus influenzae.*

16-13. A 9-year-old child is brought to the ED by her mother with a concern of a "swollen left eye." The mother says that the child is usually well, although she had a mild cough and cold last week. Yesterday she had some mild redness around her eye, and this morning it looked swollen. She has had no fever and no change in vision. The child denies recent trauma or injury. On exam, she has some moderate erythema and swelling of the periorbital area. She has proptosis and some mild limitation of extraocular muscle function. What is the MOST likely diagnosis?

(A) Allergic reaction.

(B) Periorbital cellulitis.

(C) Trauma.

(D) Orbital cellulitis.

16-14. A 4-week-old infant is brought to the ED for "cold in the eye" and cough. The mother says the infant developed some drainage from her right eye 2 days ago and she had a little cough. Now the cough seems worse, and she is breathing faster than usual. She is still eating fairly well and has had no fever. On physical exam in the ED she is awake and looking about; she does not appear to be systemically ill. She has moderate injection of the conjunctiva and a mild mucopurulent discharge. She is also noted to have intermittent episodes of a short, abrupt cough (stamLato cough), and auscultation of the chest reveals diffuse rales. A chest radiograph shows hyperexpansion and diffuse alveolar interstitial infiltrates. What is the MOST likely diagnosis?

(A) *Bordetella pertussis.*

(B) *Staphylococcus aureus.*

(C) *Mycobacterium tuberculosis.*

(D) *Chlamydia trachomatis.*

16-15. Most children with uncomplicated bacterial pneumonia can be safely treated as outpatients. The choice of antibiotic should be based on the most likely etiologic organism given the age of the child and clinical presentation. For children between 3 months and 5 years of age, which is the preferred antibiotic?

(A) Amoxicillin.

(B) Trimethoprim sulfate.

(C) Amoxicillin-clavulanate.

(D) Cephalexin.

16-16. Asthma is a common childhood disease, affecting 4.8 million children younger than 18 years of age. Which of the following is a risk factor that contributes to the deaths of children with asthma?

(A) Age younger than 2 years.

(B) Limited access to health care.

(C) History of pneumonia.

(D) Medication allergies.

16-17. A 7-year-old male with asthma is brought to the ED because "he can't breathe." He is breathless while talking and is using short phrases. He is somewhat agitated but seems to be alert. On exam, heart rate is 114 beats per minute, respiratory rate is 46 breaths per minute, and he has increased work of breathing with suprasternal retractions. He has audible wheezing throughout the lung fields. Based on NIH Expert Panel Report 2 guidelines classifying the severity of asthma exacerbation, what is the severity of this child's exacerbation?

(A) Mild.

(B) Moderate.

(C) Severe.

(D) Respiratory arrest imminent.

16-18. A 3-month-old female is brought to the ED with noisy breathing. The mother says the child has never had difficulty breathing before. She developed a runny nose and low-grade fever 2 days ago, and yesterday she developed a "hard cough." On exam, she is tachypneic with a respiratory rate of 72 breaths per minute. She has coarse wheezes heard throughout the lung fields and a coarse wheezy cough. She has moderate intercostal retractions and an oxygen saturation of 94% on room air. What is the MOST likely etiologic agent?

(A) Influenzavirus.
(B) Parainfluenzavirus.
(C) Rhinovirus.
(D) Respiratory syncytial virus.

16-19. A 20-month-old child is brought to the ED by paramedics who were called to the home for "a seizure." The child is usually well and has no history of medical problems. He had a cough and runny nose yesterday, and while he was taking a nap today the mother heard a funny noise. When she went to his room he was shaking all over and his eyes were "rolled back in his head." She called 911, but the movements had stopped by the time paramedics arrived. Temperature was noted to be 39.8°C and the child was "lethargic." He was transported to the ED and began to wake up en route. At the time of your exam in the ED, he is awake and alert, sitting on the mother's lap looking somewhat frightened. Vital signs include a temperature of 39.4°C, heart rate of 138 beats per minute, and respiratory rate of 32 breaths per minute. Oxygen saturation is 98% on room air. What is the MOST likely diagnosis?

(A) Idiopathic seizure.
(B) Rigors.
(C) Febrile seizure.
(D) Reaction to over-the-counter cold medicine.

16-20. A 5-year-old child with seizures was started on a new anticonvulsant medication approximately 1 month ago. He is brought to the ED today because of changes in his behavior and increasing lethargy. He has been vomiting for 2 days. Laboratory tests in the ED include elevated liver enzymes and hyperammonemia. Which of the following is MOST likely the anticonvulsant?

(A) Valproic acid.
(B) Phenobarbital.
(C) Lorazepam.
(D) Diazepam.

16-21. You are seeing a 19-month-old infant who has had diarrhea for 3 days. The child has had a low-grade fever. Stools are not bloody. The parent is uncertain about urine output as there is so much stool on the diapers. The infant is otherwise still active and willing to drink. On exam he is afebrile, heart rate is 124 beats per minute, respiratory rate is 24 breaths per minute, and when you examine his ears he cries and has tears. His lips and tongue are dry. Skin turgor is normal, and capillary refill is 1–2 seconds. What is the MOST appropriate therapy at this point?

(A) Place an IV bolus with 20 mL/kg of normal saline, check electrolytes, and reassess.
(B) Place an IV with 20 mL/kg of normal saline, and reassess.
(C) Order oral rehydration solution 50 mL/kg over 4 hours, and reassess.
(D) Order oral rehydration solution 20 mL/kg over 24 hours, and reassess.

16-22. A 6-week-old infant presents with non-bloody, watery diarrhea for 2 days. The parent states the stools are now occurring every 15–30 minutes. The infant has become progressively lethargic and now won't drink. He has a temperature of 37.0°C, heart rate is 198 beats per minute, and respiratory rate is 40 breaths per minute. The infant is listless and does not cry with needle sticks. He has a sunken fontanel and dry mouth. Capillary refill is 4 seconds, and there is tenting of the skin.

The nurses have been unable to place a peripheral IV. What should you do next?

(A) Place an intraosseous line and administer a 20 mL/kg bolus of normal saline over 5–10 minutes, then reassess.

(B) Consult a surgeon for a saphenous vein cutdown.

(C) Order oral rehydration solution 50 mL/kg over 4 hours, and reassess.

(D) Place an intraosseous line and administer a 20 mL/kg bolus of D_5 ¼ normal saline over 1 hour, then reassess.

16-23. You are evaluating a 3-year-old child who presents with diarrhea, lethargy, and decreased urination. The last stool had blood streaks. On exam her blood pressure is 122/76 mmHg, heart rate is 150 beats per minute, and she is pale. Pertinent laboratory studies include BUN of 36 mg/dL, Cr of 3.4 mg/dL, hemoglobin of 7.1 g/dL, and platelet count of 60,000. The urinalysis shows blood and protein. The manual review of her blood smear shows signs of hemolysis. What is the MOST likely diagnosis?

(A) Rotavirus.

(B) Bacteremia secondary to *Streptococcus pneumoniae*.

(C) Henoch-Schönlein purpura.

(D) Hemolytic uremic syndrome.

16-24. A 12-year-old boy with type 1 diabetes presents with 12 hours of vomiting. He has eaten nothing today and is unable to keep fluids down. He did not take his morning insulin. He feels weak and light-headed. Vitals are a heart rate of 130 beats per minute, blood pressure of 96/60 mmHg, respiratory rate of 32 breaths per minute, and temperature of 36.8°C. Initial labs include blood glucose of 840 mg/dL, 3+ ketonuria, and a venous pH of 7.22. His nurse asks if you want to give bicarbonate. Which of the following is a TRUE statement about the administration of bicarbonate in this patient?

(A) It is indicated in the management of the acidosis seen in DKA.

(B) It is dangerous in this patient and should not be used.

(C) It will increase his serum potassium level.

(D) It will cause alkalosis in the central nervous system.

16-25. You are evaluating an 18-month-old infant for acute onset of lethargy. He was well yesterday and had no fever, and there is no history of trauma. He was found sleeping on the floor in the family room, and the parents were unable to wake him up. The parents had a party last night, and numerous unfinished drinks were left out. His vital signs are unremarkable, there are no external signs of trauma, and he moves symmetrically to deep pain. Upon placing an IV and drawing initial screening labs, the nurse reports that his glucose is 24. Which of the following is the MOST likely cause of this child's hypoglycemia?

(A) Amoxicillin ingestion.

(B) Sepsis.

(C) Ethanol ingestion.

(D) Child abuse.

16-26. You are seeing a patient with a ventriculoperitoneal shunt (VPS) that was placed at age 3 months for congenital hydrocephalus. The patient has been vomiting for 2 days and today has become progressively more lethargic. You suspect a problem with the shunt. What is the appropriate study to specifically evaluate this diagnosis?

(A) Complete blood count (CBC).

(B) Measurement of the head circumference.

(C) Lumbar puncture.

(D) Brain CT.

16-27. A 10-year-old girl was riding on her friend's handlebars and fell off onto her outstretched arm. She was transported by paramedics with her arm splinted. Which of the following possible bone injuries is MOST commonly associated with acute vascular compromise?

(A) Midshaft clavicular fracture.
(B) Nondisplaced fracture of the distal radius and ulna.
(C) Supracondylar fracture of the humerus.
(D) Scaphoid fracture.

16-28. A 15-year-old adolescent presents with a chief complaint of near syncope. What historical information makes you most concerned for a serious etiology?

(A) The dizziness occurred when the patient got up off the sofa after watching TV for 2 hours.
(B) The patient skipped breakfast and felt light-headed in front of her locker.
(C) The patient is a varsity starter on the basketball team and had chest pain during warmups.
(D) The patient was standing still for a prolonged period of time under spotlights during a chorus performance at school.

16-29. You are treating a 25-kg child with presumed acute appendicitis. The patient is mildly dehydrated, has normal electrolytes, and needs to be NPO until he goes to the OR. Which of the following fluid orders is MOST appropriate?

(A) Initial bolus of 500 mL normal saline followed by D_5 ½ NS plus 20 mEq KCl/L at 67 mL/hour.
(B) Initial bolus of 500 mL D_5 ½ NS plus 20 mEq KCl/L followed by D_5 ½ NS plus 20 mEq KCl/L at 67 mL/hour.
(C) Initial bolus of 100 mL normal saline followed by D_5 ½ NS plus 20 mEq KCl/L at 67 mL/hour.
(D) Initial bolus of 500 mL normal saline followed by D_{10} ½ NS plus 20 mEq KCl/L at 67 mL/hour.

16-30. You are seeing a child with chronic renal insufficiency managed with daily peritoneal dialysis. The child was at his father's home over the weekend and missed 2 days of dialysis. The patient is complaining of weakness, and his serum potassium is 8.1 mEq/L. Which of the following is the MOST ominous manifestation of hyperkalemia?

(A) Weakness.
(B) Peaked T waves.
(C) Widening of QRS complex.
(D) Paresthesias.

16-31. You are seeing a 12-month-old, previously well, fully immunized child with stridor. The patient had upper respiratory track infection symptoms for 2–3 days and then developed fever that has progressed to a maximum of 104°F over the past 2 days. The patient is alert and appears nontoxic. She has a muffled voice, is drooling, and is not interested in drinking. A soft tissue film of the neck is obtained (see Figure 16-1). What is the MOST likely diagnosis in this patient?

(A) Bronchiolitis.
(B) Epiglottitis.
(C) Croup.
(D) Retropharyngeal abscess.

16-32. You are seeing an 18-month-old child with signs and symptoms of viral laryngotracheobronchitis. Recent prospective clinical trials have shown that which of the following medications will decrease the need for hospital admission in patients with this disease?

(A) Levoalbuterol.
(B) Dexamethasone.
(C) Humidified oxygen.
(D) Albuterol.

16-33. Which of the following pain assessment scales is designed to objectively measure pain in infants and nonverbal toddlers?

(A) CRIES scale.

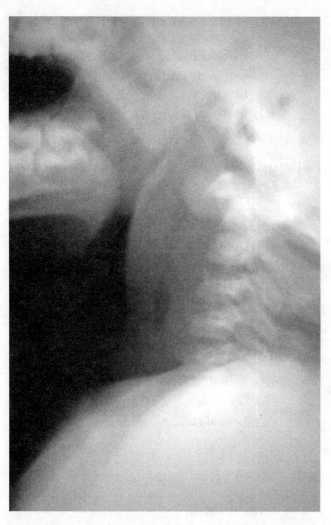

Figure 16-1. Lateral neck film of a 12-month-old infant with fever, muffled cry, and drooling.

(B) FACES pain scale.

(C) OUCHER.

(D) Visual analog scale.

16-34. You are caring for an 8-year-old child with a significantly angulated distal radius and ulna fracture (i.e., a bayonet appearance). You are asked by your orthopedic consultant to provide procedural sedation for closed reduction of the injury. The patient has a past medical history of poorly controlled seizures but is otherwise well. Which drug or combination of drugs would be MOST appropriate in this patient?

(A) Ketamine and midazolam.

(B) Midazolam.

(C) Fentanyl and midazolam.

(D) Oxycodone.

16-35. What is the MOST common cause of death in children with sickle cell disease?

(A) Acute splenic sequestration.

(B) Aplastic crisis.

(C) Acute chest syndrome.

(D) Sepsis.

16-36. A 5-month-old female infant presents with a fever to 39.6°C rectally, but she is vigorous, and her parents say she is feeding well without vomiting. She was born full-term without complications and has no other medical problems. Laboratories reveal a catheterized urinalysis with 121 WBCs/hpf and negative leukocyte esterase. What is the MOST appropriate management?

(A) Hospitalize and administer intravenous antibiotics.

(B) Hospitalize but don't administer antibiotics, pending urine culture results.

(C) Administer parental antibiotics in the ED and discharge on oral antibiotics.

(D) Discharge home and don't administer antibiotics, pending culture results.

16-37. Which of the following is NOT a diagnostic criterion for Kawasaki disease (mucocutaneous lymph node syndrome)?

(A) Rash.

(B) Leukocytosis.

(C) Conjunctivitis.

(D) Strawberry tongue.

16-38. Radial head subluxation (nursemaid's elbow) is suspected in a toddler. The supination and flexion technique is attempted without success. What is an alternative technique to supination and flexion?

(A) Hyperpronation.

(B) Longitudinal traction.

(C) Hypersupination.

(D) Hyperflexion.

16-39. A teenage female presents with acute right hip pain that began while running during a soccer game. Physical exam reveals tenderness in the right hip in the area of the iliac spine. What is the MOST likely diagnosis?

(A) Slipped capital femoral epiphysis.

(B) Hip dislocation.

(C) Pelvic avulsion fracture.

(D) Femoral neck fracture.

16-40. An adolescent male complains of acute left testicular pain for 6 hours' duration. Which of the following physical exam findings is MOST consistent with testicular torsion?

(A) Blue-dot sign.

(B) Absent cremasteric reflex.

(C) Prehn's sign.

(D) Vermiform mass in the superior testicle.

16-41. A 2-year-old toddler is brought in by her mother for refusal to walk. No fevers or other constitutional symptoms are reported, and there is no history of trauma. Physical examination reveals localized tenderness and swelling of the left knee without erythema. Synovial fluid reveals 60,000/µL polymorphonuclear neutrophil leukocytes (PMN) and low glucose, but with no organisms seen on Gram stain. What is the MOST appropriate management?

(A) Obtain emergent orthopedic consultation and admission for intravenous antibiotics.

(B) Start nonsteroidal anti-inflammatory medications, and refer to a pediatric rheumatologist as an outpatient.

(C) Start oral amoxicillin, and send Lyme titers.

(D) Initiate high-dose aspirin, and admit for evaluation of carditis.

16-42. Which of the following is the MOST common associated medical condition in infants and children with Down syndrome?

(A) Gastrointestinal atresia.

(B) Congenital heart disease.

(C) Seizure disorder.

(D) Atlantoaxial instability.

16-43. A 5-year-old boy falls on an outstretched hand and is complaining of elbow pain. Where is the MOST likely fracture site?

(A) Radial head.

(B) Olecranon.

(C) Lateral condylar.

(D) Supracondylar.

16-44. Which of the following skin infections is NOT effectively treated with penicillin or its derivatives?

(A) Impetigo contagiosa.

(B) Erysipelas.

(C) *Mycoplasma* infections.

(D) Scarlet fever.

Pediatric Emergencies
Answers, Explanations, and References

16-1. **The answer is C** (Chapter 114). It is important for the emergency physician to master the skill of differentiating critically ill pediatric patients from the larger number of less ill children who present to the ED. The key to mastering this skill is a strong knowledge base of child development. Developmental stages are described with associated age ranges, and the toddler stage (18–36 months) is characterized by the ability to walk well, scribble, and speak in phrases. Toddlers may demonstrate stranger anxiety, as do children in the late infancy stage (6–18 months), but children in late infancy can usually say only a few words or use jargon; they can sit well and are beginning to walk. In early infancy (0–6 months), a baby will often coo and smile responsively, as he/she has not yet developed stranger anxiety. Children in the preschool stage can usually walk and run well and speak in full sentences.

16-2. **The answer is D** (Chapter 114). State laws vary regarding the age at which a person may provide his or her own consent for treatment, varying between 18 and 21 years of age. In the case of minor children, consent must be obtained from the legal guardian (typically a parent unless custody has been removed) before initiation of treatment. This does not apply to triage and examination, that is, children should be evaluated without delay to determine the nature of the illness or injury. Treatment can be initiated without consent in the following situations: (a) life- or limb-threatening emergency; (b) state-protected right to

treatment, as in the setting of child abuse, pregnancy-related complaints, sexually transmitted disease, and substance abuse; and (c) state-defined "emancipated minor" status, that is, married, a member of armed forces, or self-supporting and living independently.

16-3. **The answer is A** (Chapter 114). Children between the ages of birth and 3 years are at relatively increased risk for bloodborne bacterial disease due to immaturity of the reticuloendothelial system. The risk of bacteremia decreases with age, with the greatest incidence in the first 3 months of life. Neonates with fever have a 5% risk for bacteremia, predominantly due to pathogens encountered at the time of birth. Infants 29–90 days of age are at progressively lesser risk for neonatally acquired infections but are increasingly susceptible to community-acquired pathogens. Children 3 months and older are susceptible to infection from community-acquired pathogens and are at relatively less risk for bacteremia in comparison with younger infants.

16-4. **The answer is C** (Chapter 116). The sepsis syndrome may present with a subtle or obvious, rapidly progressive clinical picture. Neurologic symptoms most frequently include altered mental status with irritability or lethargy. Poor feeding and hypotonia are common findings. Hyperpyrexia may occur, but hypothermia may also be seen in sepsis, particularly in infants younger than 3 months, and is a grave prognostic finding. Tachypnea may be present, and signs of early shock may include resting tachycardia and a widened pulse pressure. In the compensated phases of shock, the distal pulses are weak and distal extremities cool. Ultimately, these are followed by signs of decompensation with decreased sensorium and hypotension. Pneumonia and urinary tract infection may progress to full sepsis, but initially these infections do not present with findings of shock. Gastroenteritis may lead to dehydration and hypovolemic shock, but initial symptoms usually include vomiting and diarrhea.

16-5. **The answer is C** (Chapter 117). Malrotation with midgut volvulus usually presents in the first month of life with sudden onset of bilious vomiting. The incidence is 1 in 500 live births, and 50% are diagnosed in the first month of life. Bilious vomiting should always be considered a surgical emergency. Pyloric stenosis usually presents between 2 and 6 months of age, with projectile, nonbilious vomiting. Feeding intolerance is a common cause of nonbilious vomiting that can occur within the first month of life. Intussusception classically presents between 6 and 18 months of age with "currant jelly stools" and nonbilious vomiting.

16-6. **The answer is A** (Chapter 117). Jaundice is the most common reason for reevaluation and admission to the hospital as a result of earlier discharge from the newborn nursery. Physiologic jaundice is due to the hemolysis of fetal red blood cells and is characterized by bilirubin rising at a rate of less than 5 mg/dL per 24 hours. Most infants with hyperbilirubinemia can be monitored and treated with phototherapy in the outpatient setting, but those with levels approaching exchange transfusion levels must be admitted. Vomiting, rash, and crying are common concerns for which parents bring neonates to the ED, but these amount to fewer admissions within the first days of life than jaundice.

16-7. **The answer is B** (Chapter 117). Necrotizing enterocolitis is the result of inflammation or injury to the bowel wall that has been associated with infectious causes and hypoxic-ischemic insults. There is a higher incidence in premature infants than term babies, and the initial symptoms may include feeding intolerance, abdominal distention, bloody stools, apnea, and shock. The classic x-ray findings include pneumatosis intestinalis (intramural air) and hepatic portal air. Free air in the abdomen may also be seen if perforation has already occurred. Intussusception may cause bloody stools, classically described as "currant jelly stools." Hirschsprung's disease leads to constipation, sometimes resulting in blood on the stool. Anal fissures can cause blood on the stool or in the diaper and is diagnosed by physical exam.

16-8. **The answer is C** (Chapter 120). The 6 common presentations of congenital heart disease are cyanosis, congestive heart failure, pathologic murmur in an asymptomatic patient, abnormal pulses, hypertension, and syncope. The most common lesions that cause cyanosis are tetralogy of Fallot, transposition of the great arteries, tricuspid atresia, total anomalous venous return, and truncus arteriosus.

16-9. **The answer is A** (Chapter 120). Coarctation of the aorta is characterized by a localized narrowing of the aortic lumen, most often distal to the origin of the left subclavian artery and in close proximity to the ductus arteriosus or its postnatal remnant, the ligamentum arteriosus. In infancy, symptomatic infants present with congestive heart failure and feeding difficulty. Pulses are decreased in the lower extremities, and hypertension is noted in the upper extremities. With patent ductus arteriosus, pulses in both the upper and lower extremites are often brisk or bounding. Large ventricular septal defects may cause congestive heart failure in young infants, but there is no marked discrepancy in upper and lower extremity pulses. Tetralogy of Fallot is a cyanotic congenital heart lesion.

16-10. **The answer is D** (Chapter 120). Supraventricular tachycardia (SVT) is the most common dysrhythmia in the pediatric age group. Electrocardiogram shows an unvarying ventricular rate between 220 and 360 beats/minute, as opposed to a range of 150 to 200 beats/minute in adults with SVT. SVT must be distinguished from sinus tachycardia, which is the most common tachyarrhythmia in children.

16-11. **The answer is B** (Chapter 121). All drugs listed in this question are treatment options for acute otitis media in children. Despite the approval of 16 antibiotics by the U.S. FDA for the treatment of acute otitis media and the changing antibiotic susceptibility patterns that have emerged over the past few years, amoxicillin remains the drug of choice. However, due to the prevalence of drug-resistant *Streptococcus pneumoniae*, the Centers for Disease Control and Prevention working group has developed a new management scheme. There are now 2 doses of amoxicillin: the standard dose (40–45 mg/kg/day) and the high dose (80–90 mg/kg/day).

16-12. **The answer is A** (Chapter 122). The etiology of infectious conjunctivitis differs between the neonate and the older child. In the neonate, pathogens that reside in the birth canal play a major role in ocular infections. *C. trachomatis* is the most frequent, but *Neisseria gonorrhoeae* poses the greatest threat to the integrity of the eye. Later in childhood, the respiratory tract pathogens predominate.

16-13. **The answer is D** (Chapter 122). Orbital and periorbital cellulitis cause the periorbital area to appear red and swollen. The periorbital edema is usually more prominent with preseptal infections. Proptosis or limitation of extraocular muscle function indicates orbital involvement. Fever is more common with periorbital cellulitis. CT should be performed when orbital involvement is likely. An inflammatory mass is easily demonstrated when present using this modality.

16-14. **The answer is D** (Chapter 123). The clinical presentation of pneumonia in a child may sometimes be suggestive of the etiologic agent. Pneumonia due to *S. aureus* is notorious for being particularly rapid in the progression of clinical findings. Patients with *B. pertussis* typically develop prodromal symptoms including mild cough, conjunctivitis, and coryza, which lasts 1–2 weeks. A severe, paroxysmal cough is characteristic of the catarrhal phase, and the inspiratory whoop is generally present in older children. An infant with a chlamydial infection is usually afebrile and has a distinct stamLato cough with diffuse rales on auscultation. A history of maternal pelvic or conjunctival chlamydial infection is present in up to 50% of cases in which the infant develops *C. trachomatis* pneumonia.

16-15. **The answer is A** (Chapter 123). Amoxicillin is the preferred treatment for uncomplicated pneumonia in young children, age 3 months to 5 years. Alternatively, daily intramuscular injections of ceftraxone can be given. After 5 years of age and in penicillin-allergic children, erythromycin or tetracycline is the preferred initial treatment.

16-16. **The answer is B** (Chapter 124). Risk factors that contribute to the death of a child with asthma include socioeconomic background, limited access to health care, improper medication administration, unrecognized severe disease, extreme lability of disease, nocturnal asthma, and history of respiratory failure with previous intubation.

16-17. **The answer is B** (Chapter 124). To avoid delays in treatment of asthma, a brief physical exam should be performed before a detailed history is obtained. The NIH Expert Panel Report 2 is a consensus document for assessing severity of an acute asthma episode. With a mild exacerbation, the child can speak in sentences and is not short of breath at rest. Respiratory rate may be increased, but there is usually no increased work of breathing. A child with a moderate exacerbation is short of breath while talking and speaks in short phrases. Respiratory rate and heart rate are increased, and loud wheezes are heard throughout the expiratory phase. In severe exacerbations, the child is short of breath at rest and is usually very agitated, sitting upright and not speaking, or using only individual words. Wheezes are heard throughout both inspiration and expiration. If the child becomes drowsy and wheezes are absent because of decreased air movement, respiratory arrest is imminent.

16-18. **The answer is D** (Chapter 124). Bronchiolitis, or inflammation of the bronchioles, is the term applied to the clinical syndrome of wheezing, chest retractions, and tachypnea in children younger than 2 years of age. It causes more significant illness in infants younger than 6 months of age. Respiratory syncytial virus (RSV) causes 50–70% of clinically significant bronchiolitis. Non-RSV bronchiolitis is caused by influenzavirus, parainfluenzavirus, echovirus, and rhinovirus.

16-19. **The answer is C** (Chapter 125). Febrile seizure is a unique and common form of seizure in childhood. A febrile seizure is associated with fever but without evidence of intracranial infection or defined cause, usually occurring between 6 months and 5 years of age. Typically, these are generalized seizures that last less than 15 minutes, and there is no postictal focal neurologic deficit. Rigors can occur with a spike in fever, but typically they do not cause a change in mental status. Cough and cold medicines can cause irritability or lethargy in young children, but they do not typically cause tonic-clonic movements.

16-20. **The answer is A** (Chapter 125). Unwanted features of anticonvulsants may be seen soon after the drug is initiated or may develop weeks, months, or years later. With valproic acid use, hepatic failure may occur within days or up to 2 years after first use. The drug reaction results in behavior alterations, increasing lethargy, and vomiting. Levels of liver enzymes may be minimally to markedly elevated, and hyperammonemia with or without symptoms of hepatic failure may be found. Immediate cessation of valproate, hospitalization, and observation are necessary when symptomatic hepatic reaction is evident. Phenobarbital can cause lethargy but not liver failure. Lorazepam and diazepam are short-acting anticonvulsants and are not used to treat seizures long term.

16-21. **The answer is C** (Chapter 126). This child has signs and symptoms of uncomplicated diarrhea likely secondary to viral gastroenteritis. The vital signs and your exam indicate that the patient is mildly dehydrated. The appropriate treatment is rehydration using an oral rehydration solution like Pedialyte. The appropriate amount is 50 mL/kg over 4 hours plus an additional 10 mL/kg for each additional loose stool the patient has. IV rehydration is not indicated in this patient. IV rehydration is appropriate for severely dehydrated patients and moderately dehydrated patients who are unable to take or tolerate oral rehydration solutions. Electrolytes are rarely useful in the initial management of acutely dehydrated patients who require IV therapy.

16-22. **The answer is A** (Chapters 21, 126). This patient is severely dehydrated based on history, vital signs, and physical exam. The heart rate of 198 beats per minute indicates that this child is at the limit of compensated shock and is at risk for cardiovascular collapse. Immediate vascular access is needed. An intraosseous line can be lifesaving in this situation where peripheral access has been unsuccessful. An intraosseous needle can be inserted into the proximal tibia in seconds. Normal saline 20 mL/kg should be infused ("pushed") rapidly using a syringe and stopcock. Immediately reassess the patient and continue fluid resuscitation as indicated. Such patients may require 60–100 mL/kg before vital signs are improved. Consulting a surgeon for access for a saphenous cutdown would take too long in this situation. Oral rehydration therapy is not appropriate for a severely dehydrated patient in shock. Using glucose-containing solutions for IV boluses is contraindicated because of the excessive amount of glucose administered, which will lead to hyperglycemia and osmotic diuresis.

16-23.   The answer is D (Chapter 127). The constellation of bloody diarrhea, renal failure (decreased urination, hypertension, elevated BUN and Cr, and abnormal urinalysis), thrombocytopenia, and hemolysis defines the hemolytic uremic syndrome. Patients with rotavirus gastroenteritis typically have frequent voluminous but nonbloody stools and neither renal nor hemolytic disease. Serious invasive *S. pneumoniae* infections include bacteremia, pneumonia, meningitis, osteomyelitis, septic arthritis, sinusitis, otitis media, and bacteremia. Henoch-Schönlein purpura (HSP) can cause gastrointestinal bleeding and kidney disease. However, most patients with HSP present with palpable purpura, usually of the legs and buttocks. The platelet count and coagulation studies in HSP patients are usually normal.

16-24.   The answer is B (Chapter 128). This patient has diabetic ketoacidosis (DKA), as indicated by the history of diabetes, elevated glucose, ketonuria, and acidosis. The use of bicarbonate therapy in DKA is not recommended and is associated with a fourfold increase in the development of cerebral edema. In addition, bicarbonate can lead to accelerated hypokalemia and paradoxical central nervous system acidosis. Acidosis in DKA is addressed by reversing the root problems in DKA of insulin deficiency and dehydration. Careful fluid resuscitation, administration of insulin, and appropriate electrolyte replacement will correct the acidosis.

16-25.   The answer is C (Chapter 129). This patient has altered mental status caused by hypoglycemia. Prompt correction with a 0.5 g/kg bolus of glucose is indicated and will likely lead to immediate improvement in this patient's mental status. Attention then needs to turn to causes of hypoglycemia. Numerous medications can cause hypoglycemia, and toxic ingestions should always be considered high on the differential in curious toddlers presenting with altered mental status in the absence of fever or known trauma. Ethanol depresses mental status primarily and, in large doses, causes hypoglycemia, compounding central nervous system depression. Amoxicillin causes many side effects, but most are gastrointestinal and dermatologic. Sepsis can cause altered mental status but is unlikely in the absence of fever, prodromal symptoms, and abnormal vital signs. Nonaccidental head trauma can present with altered mental status; however, it would not account for the hypoglycemia.

16-26.   The answer is D (Chapter 130). Lethargy and vomiting are common signs of increased intracranial pressure in children with VPSs that are not functioning correctly. Evaluation of a VPS requires plain films of the shunt tubing (looking for kinks or disconnections) and a head CT looking for dilatation of the ventricles. A patient with a malfunctioning VPS may or may not have an increased head circumference, depending on the age and whether the sutures and fontenelles are still open. A normal head circumference does not rule out VPS malfunction, and an increased head circumference must be interpreted in the context of previous measurements to be useful. While a CBC and electrolytes may be indicated preoperatively in a patient who requires surgical repair of a VPS, they are of no use in diagnosing the malfunction. Lumbar puncture is contraindicated in patients with potential hydrocephalus and increased intracranial pressure due to the risk of herniation. VPS reservoirs can be tapped emergently in order to remove cerebrospinal fluid in patients with rapidly deteriorating neurological status due to VPS malfunction. This is optimally done with neurosurgical consultation when it is readily available.

16-27.   The answer is C (Chapter 270). Any fracture can potentially cause vascular compromise, so a careful neurovascular exam distal to the injury is always important. Falling on an outstretched arm is a very common injury mechanism in children, and all of the listed fractures can potentially occur as a result. Clavicular and nondisplaced fractures of the radius and ulna rarely result in vascular compromise. Scaphoid fractures are associated with avascular necrosis and nonunion over time but not acute vascular compromise. However, 7% of supracondylar fractures have concomitant neurologic complications resulting from traction, direct trauma, or nerve ischemia, typically of the median or radial nerves. Vascular injuries must always be suspected in these fractures. Absence of the radial pulse is common. Most frequently it is due to arterial spasm and not partial or complete transection of the brachial artery.

16-28.   The answer is C (Chapter 131). Syncope is a common cause of pediatric visits to the ED, especially in adolescents. The majority of events are due to neurally mediated syncope. Several factors increase the possibility of a serious cause of syncope. These include exertion preceding the event, recurrent episodes, occurrence while recumbent, prolonged loss of consciousness, associated chest pain and/or palpitations, past medical history of cardiac disease or use of drugs that can alter cardiac conduction, or a family history of sudden death, early cardiac disease, or deafness. The three other choices are all common stories that are more suggestive of neurally mediated syncope, a generally benign condition.

16-29.   The answer is A (Chapter 132). This patient is best treated with an initial bolus of

isotonic fluid followed by appropriate maintenance fluids preoperatively. A 20 mL/kg bolus for a 25-kg child would require 500 mL of either normal saline or lactated Ringer's solution. Maintenance fluids are calculated as follows: (100 mL × 10 kg) + (50 mL × 10 kg) + (20 mL × 5 kg) = 1600 mL per day. This daily total is divided by 24 to give an hourly infusion rate of 67 mL/hour. Glucose-containing fluids should not be used for boluses as this will lead to hyperglycemia. Fluids containing 5% dextrose, rather than 10%, are typically used for maintenance fluid in children.

16-30.   The answer is C (Chapter 132). Hyperkalemia can cause weakness and paresthesias; however, it is the effect on cardiac conduction that is most dangerous. Peaked T waves are the earliest cardiac manifestation of hyperkalemia, followed by prolongation of the PR interval. If potassium levels reach approximately 8 mEq/L or more, ST-segment depression and widening of the QRS complex occurs. This ominous finding may precede bradycardia, arterioventricular block, ventricular dysrhythmias, and asystole. Any patient with electrocardiogram changes requires emergent therapy to reverse cardiac conduction toxicity.

16-31.   The answer is D (Chapter 133). Stridor, muffled voice, and drooling indicate upper airway obstruction, and the presence of fever suggests an infectious etiology. The soft tissue film of the neck is abnormal (see Figure 16-1a in the Questions section). Retropharyngeal abscesses occur in children between 6 months and 3–4 years, with most occurring at or before 12 months. There is typically an antecedent upper respiratory infection followed by increasing fever. The location of the abscess in the posterior pharyngeal region leads to muffling of the voice, stridor, and drooling secondary to dysphagia. The diagnosis is suggested by a widening of the prevertebral soft tissue space seen on soft tissue films of the neck (see Figures 16-2 and 16-3). Epiglottitis can also cause high fever, drool-

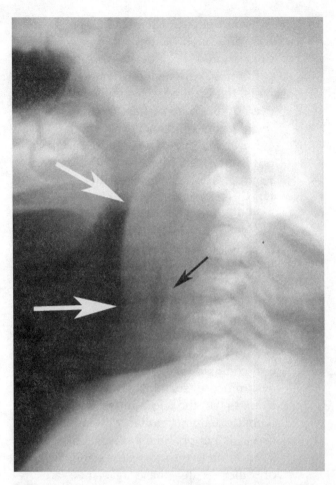

Figure 16-2. Lateral neck film of a 12-month-old infant with fever, muffled cry, and drooling. The white arrows show the prevertebral area that is significantly increased in width. The black arrow shows an area of air within the infected region, suggestive of abscess formation.

with croup require no specific treatment other than reassurance and supportive care with fluids and antipyretics. Stridor at rest is an indication for treatment in the ED. Medications that decrease edema in the epithelial lining of the upper airway will improve symptoms. Epinephrine and dexamethasone are both effective. Nebulized epinephrine often provides immediate improvement in stridor. However, the effects typically wear off after 2–3 hours and do not alter the natural course of the disease. In contrast, dexamethasone, a potent steroid, takes 0.5–2 hours to take effect, but its anti-inflammatory effects last up to 1–2 weeks. Multiple clinical trials have demonstrated that dexamethasone decreases the need for hospital admission and overall duration of symptoms in patients with croup. Bronchodilators such as albuterol and levoalbuterol have no effect on upper airway edema and thus have no role in the management of croup. Though commonly used (e.g., croup tents), humidified oxygen

ing, and stridor. However, the onset of epiglottitis is typically abrupt. This child is also fully immunized, making *Haemophilus influenzae* type B infection unlikely. Croup is the most common cause of stridor in infants and young children. It often begins with upper respiratory symptoms before the classic barking cough and stridor develop. Fever in croup is usually low grade. Bronchiolitis is a lower respiratory tract infection that causes cough, tachypnea, crackles, and wheezes rather than stridor.

16-32. **The answer is B** (Chapter 133). Croup (laryngotracheobronchitis) is the most common cause of acute stridor in children between 6 months and 3 years. Most children

Retropharyngeal Abscess

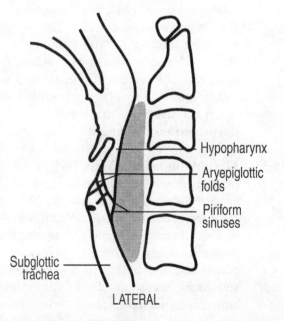

Figure 16-3. Diagram of a retropharyngeal abscess. The grey area represents the area of lymphatic tissue that becomes infected and enlarged. This results in the increased width of the prevertebral space and compression of the upper airway.

has not been shown to significantly alter the course of croup.

16-33. **The answer is A** (Chapter 134). The CRIES scale is a non-self-report tool that was developed to assess pain in infants. It takes into account cry quality, need for oxygen, changes in heart rate and blood pressure, expression, and state of sleepiness. The FACES, OUCHER, and visual analog scales are all self-reported, subjective scales commonly used to rate pain in children. The FACES scale can be used in children 3 years and older. The OUCHER pain scale becomes reliable at age 4 years and up. Visual analog scales are particularly useful in the repeated evaluation of pain over time in response to treatment.

16-34. **The answer is C** (Chapter 134). Ketamine and midazolam are commonly used for painful procedures in children. However, poorly controlled seizures are a contraindication to the use of ketamine. There is also no data to support the coadministration of midazolam with ketamine to prevent unpleasant emergence reactions from ketamine. Midazolam alone would not be appropriate as it provides anxiolysis and sedation but no analgesia. Oxycodone is a potent oral analgesic and might be appropriate for home use in this patient after discharge. However, titration of sedation and analgesia is more difficult using oral medications, so oral opiates are used less often when the degree of pain and duration of the procedure are unpredictable.

16-35. **The answer is D** (Chapter 137). Sepsis, particularly from encapsulated organisms such as *Streptococcus pneumoniae,* is the most common cause of death in children with sickle cell disease. Acute splenic sequestration is the second most common cause and occurs due to a drop in hemoglobin and resultant hypovolemic shock. Other important causes include aplastic crisis, usually precipitated by human parvovirus B19, and acute chest syndrome with resultant hypoxia.

16-36. **The answer is C** (Chapter 140). This patient has presumed acute pyelonephritis and thus should be treated with antibiotics, pending culture results. In neonates and infants, the presence of leukocyte esterase or even pyuria may be falsely negative due to their limited leukocytic response. Urine cultures are mandatory in suspected cases of urinary tract infection in this age group regardless of urinalysis results. In patients who are older than 3 months of age, appear well without comorbidities, and have good follow-up, outpatient management with oral antibiotics after IV or IM antibiotic administration is recommended.

16-37. **The answer is B** (Chapters 135, 136). The diagnostic criteria for Kawasaki disease is fever of at least 5 days' duration with the presence of at least 4 of the following: bilateral conjunctivitis, changes of the lips and oral mucosa such as strawberry tongue, changes of the extremities such as erythema or edema, polymorphous rash, and cervical lymphadenopathy. Leukocytosis, in addition to thrombocytosis and elevation of other acute phase reactants, are frequently seen but are not part of the diagnostic criteria for Kawasaki disease.

16-38. **The answer is A** (Chapter 136). The classic supination technique is supination followed by flexion of the elbow with the child's elbow at 90 degrees initially. The hyperpronation technique is an alternative procedure and is performed by holding the elbow at 90 degrees with one hand followed by firm pronation at the wrist. Some report a better success rate with hyperpronation compared with supination.

16-39. **The answer is C** (Chapter 136). Avulsion-type injuries of the pelvis are usually seen in adolescents during athletic events and are caused by sudden contraction of muscles attaching to the pelvis, commonly the rectus femoris and sartorius muscles. Femur fractures and hip dislocations usually occur with more significant trauma. Slipped capital femoral epiphysis can present acutely but more typically presents with chronic hip pain.

16-40. **The answer is B** (Chapter 139). Signs of testicular torsion include an enlarged and tender testicle that may have a transverse lie or may ride higher in the scrotum. The cremasteric reflex is usually absent. The blue-dot sign is a bluish skin discoloration at the superior aspect of the testicle and is seen in torsion of the appendix testis. Prehn's sign is relief of pain with elevation or support of the testicle and indicates epididymitis in adults but is a less reliable sign in children. A varicocele is described as a vermiform mass of dilated veins in the superior-posterior testicle and is usually on the left side.

16-41. **The answer is A** (Chapter 136). Septic arthritis should be assumed in this patient given the presentation and synovial fluid PMN count, which typically exceeds 50,000/μL after the earliest stages. Approximately one-third of septic arthritis cases fail to identify a specific pathogen, so a negative Gram stain result does not exclude septic arthritis. Juvenile rheumatoid arthritis is a consideration but only after septic arthritis has been definitively excluded. Lyme disease causing monoarticular arthritis should be treated similar to septic arthritis initially. Acute rheumatic fever can cause a migratory polyarthritis associated with carditis, subcutaneous nodules, erythema marginatum, or chorea.

16-42. **The answer is B** (Chapter 138). Congenital heart defects are seen in up to 60% of pa-

tients with Down syndrome. Abnormalities include septal defects, atrioventricular canal defects, patent ductus arteriosus, and tetralogy of Fallot. Atlantoaxial (C1–C2) instability affects up to 1 in 5 children with this syndrome; thus, cervical spine injury should be considered following motor vehicle or sporting injuries. Gastrointestinal atresias are seen in up to 12% of these patients and include esophageal and duodenal atresia, tracheoesophageal fistula, and Hirschsprung's disease. Other associated medical conditions include seizures, otitis media, thyroid disease, and cataracts.

16-43. **The answer is D** (Chapter 136). Supracondylar fractures are the most common elbow fractures in children and typically the result of a hyperextension mechanism. Radial head fractures are uncommon in children and more common in adults. Olecranon fractures are usually the result of direct elbow trauma after falls. Lateral condylar fractures comprise about 10% of pediatric elbow fractures.

16-44. **The answer is C** (Chapter 135). *Mycoplasma* infections can cause an erythematous maculopapular rash on the trunk and can also cause erythema multiforme and Stevens-Johnson syndrome. Treatment is with a macrolide such as erythromycin or azithromycin, fluoroquinolones, or doxycycline. Scarlet fever and erysipelas are usually responsive to penicillin. Impetigo contagiosa is usually treated with amoxicillin-clavulanate, dicloxacillin, erythromycin, or cephalosporins.

Prehospital Care and Disaster Preparedness
Questions

17-1. Which of the following is one of the 15 elements of an EMS system as defined by Public Law 93-154?

(A) Security.
(B) Access to care.
(C) Funding.
(D) Research.

17-2. What is the only Class I intervention (useful and effective) for the MAST garment as categorized by the National Association of EMS Physicians?

(A) Penetrating abdominal trauma.
(B) Penetrating extremity trauma.
(C) Ruptured abdominal aortic aneurysm.
(D) Pelvic fracture.

17-3. Which one of the following helmets should be removed in the field prior to the transport of a patient with a potential spine injury?

(A) Motorcycle helmet.
(B) Football helmet.
(C) Lacrosse helmet.
(D) Hockey helmet.

17-4. Which one of the following statements regarding the clinical use of helicopters in the prehospital setting is TRUE?

(A) The use of a helicopter for transport is indicated when ground transport to the tertiary care center exceeds that of the helicopter by >20 minutes.

(B) Penetrating thoracic trauma patients who are in cardiac arrest have a greater chance of survival when transported to a tertiary care center by helicopter.

(C) Helicopter transport of high-risk obstetric patients in an urban area is a viable option given prolonged ground transport times secondary to traffic congestion.

(D) Drowning is the largest nontrauma diagnostic category for the use of helicopter transport.

17-5. Mass gatherings have been defined as any voluntary and temporary collection of greater than how many people at one site or location for a common purpose?

(A) 10.
(B) 100.
(C) 1000.
(D) 10,000.

17-6. Which one of the following is a component of the Hospital Emergency Incident Command System?

(A) Incident command.
(B) Operations.
(C) Planning.
(D) Accountability of position function.

17-7. Which one of the following is a patient category as defined by the secondary assessment of victim endpoint (SAVE) system of triage?

(A) Those who are ambulatory.

(B) Those who will die unless they receive rapid airway intervention.

(C) Those who will die unless they receive definitive trauma care within 1 hour.

(D) Those who will benefit significantly from austere field interventions.

17-8. You are working a night shift as the emergency physician at a large academic medical center when the local airport calls to notify you of a major plane crash at its facility. What is the MOST appropriate next step?

(A) Verify the information.

(B) Notify the hospital administrator.

(C) Conduct an initial needs assessment.

(D) Activate the emergency department disaster plan.

17-9. You are the physician performing the triage function for a large ED that is receiving patients from a disaster scene where a high-rise building collapsed. You evaluate a patient with an amputated arm that has been placed in a tourniquet by paramedics and treated with IV opiate pain medications. The patient's pain is relatively well controlled. The patient's vitals are blood pressure 150/80 mmHg, pulse 90 beats per minute, respirations 12 breaths per minute, and pulse oximetry 98% on room air. This patient should be assigned to which triage category?

(A) Red.

(B) Yellow.

(C) Green.

(D) Black.

17-10. Which one of the following infectious biological organisms is classified as a class A agent of concern by the Centers for Disease Control and Prevention?

(A) *Coxiella burnetii.*

(B) *Chlamydia psittaci.*

(C) *Clostridium botulinum.*

(D) *Brucella.*

17-11. Which one of the following statements is TRUE regarding decontamination of a patient who has experienced a significant chemical exposure?

(A) The critically ill, nonambulatory patient requires advanced airway maneuvers and intravenous line insertion prior to gross decontamination.

(B) Ocular exposures take precedence and should be treated immediately.

(C) Whole-body decontamination should proceed from the center of the body to the extremities.

(D) Wounds should be irrigated fully during the shower decontamination process.

17-12. Which one of the following types of radiation is LEAST likely to cause whole-body irradiation?

(A) Alpha.

(B) Beta.

(C) Neutron.

(D) Gamma.

17-13. Which one of the following statements is TRUE regarding acute radiation syndrome?

(A) Whole-body beta irradiation is the primary cause of acute radiation syndrome.

(B) The toxic effects of radiation are discrete.

(C) The integumentary system is the first system to manifest injury from irradiation.

(D) The earliest laboratory indicator of acute radiation syndrome is lymphocytopenia.

CHAPTER 17

Prehospital Care and Disaster Preparedness

Answers, Explanations, and References

17-1. **The answer is B** (Chapter 1). The 15 elements of an EMS system as defined by Public Law 93-154, signed in 1973, include: (1) personnel, (2) training, (3) communications, (4) transportation, (5) facilities, (6) critical care units, (7) public safety agencies, (8) consumer participation, (9) access to care, (10) transfer of care, (11) standardization of patients' records, (12) public information and education, (13) independent review and evaluation, (14) disaster linkage, and (15) mutual aid agreements.

17-2. **The answer is C** (Chapter 2). The MAST garment has fallen into considerable disfavor because there is little evidence that it improves survival in hemorrhagic shock after trauma, and it may even be detrimental in penetrating thoracic trauma with short transport times. A position paper from the National Association of EMS Physicians categorizes possible indications for using the MAST garment into class I (useful and effective), class IIA (weight of evidence favors usefulness and efficacy), class IIB (may be helpful, probably not harmful), and class II (not indicated). The only class I intervention for MAST garments is hypotension due to ruptured abdominal aortic aneurysm.

17-3. **The answer is A** (Chapter 2). A properly fitted football helmet with shoulder pads holds the head in a position of neutral spine alignment; hence, the National Athletic Trainer's Association does not recommend field removal of these devices. Stud-

ies with standard lacrosse and ice hockey helmets also support the principal of maintaining spinal immobilization by leaving the helmet on and securing the patient to a rigid spine board for transport from the field to the hospital. Because motorcycle helmets do not fit snugly on the head and are not worn with shoulder pads, they do not maintain a neutral spine position when the patient lies down on a flat surface. Therefore, motorcycle helmets should be removed in the field.

17-4. **The answer is C** (Chapter 3). Experience has provided some reassurance that the use of helicopters to transport high-risk obstetrics patients did not result in increased out-of-hospital deliveries. Importantly, neonatal outcomes are not adversely impacted by helicopter transport. Helicopter transport of obstetric patients in an urban area is a viable solution to the problem of traffic congestion, and helicopters reduce response time for patient transport. As a rule of thumb, helicopter use is indicated when ground vehicle transport time to the local hospital exceeds the time required for helicopter transport to the tertiary care center. Patients in traumatic cardiac arrest have a near-zero survival rate regardless of method of transport. The largest single nontraumatic diagnostic criterion for helicopter transport is cardiac. Transport for primary or rescue coronary intervention is a frequent indication for helicopter use.

17-5. **The answer is C** (Chapter 5). Mass gatherings have been defined as any voluntary and temporary collection of >1000 people at one site or location for a common purpose. Gatherings can be short-term (hours) or longer (days to weeks). The event may be held in a single location or spread over several sites.

17-6. **The answer is D** (Chapter 6). The Hospital Emergency Incident Command System (HEICS) was designed to mitigate the confusion that often accompanies a hospital's response to disaster. The HEICS employs a clear management structure with defined responsibilities and mechanisms of reporting that allow clear communication and understanding between hospitals and emergency responders. It includes the following components: (1) common language, (2) defined and predicable chain of command, (3) flexible response, (4) prioritized response, (5) accountability of position function, and (6) documentation guidelines for accountability and cost recovery. The other options listed for this question are components of the Incident Command System (ICS). The ICS is a standard emergency management system used throughout the country by rescue agencies at a specific disaster site. The ICS provides a management system that is adaptable to incidents involving the response of multiple agencies and at the most basic level consists of the following 5 main components: (1) incident command, (2) operations, (3) planning, (4) logistics, and (5) finance.

17-7. **The answer is D** (Chapter 6). The SAVE triage system is designed to identify patients who are most likely to benefit from the care available under austere field conditions. The SAVE triage methodology divides patients into three categories: (1) those who will die regardless of how much care they receive, (2) those who will survive whether or not they receive care, and (3) those who will benefit significantly from austere field interventions.

17-8. **The answer is A** (Chapter 6). When a call is made to a hospital informing of a disaster, the receiver of the call must have a procedure to follow for verification of the incident. The appropriate hospital administrator is then given the information so that the external disaster plan can be put into effect including needs assessment, discharge of minor illness patients from the ED, and recall of medical personnel.

17-9. **The answer is B** (Chapter 6). The most common triage classification in the United States involves assigning patients to 1 of 4 color-coded categories depending on injury severity and prognosis.
- RED: First priority. Most urgent. Life-threatening shock or hypoxia is present or imminent, but the patient can likely be stabilized and, if given immediate care, will probably survive.
- YELLOW: Second priority. Urgent. The injuries have systemic implications or effects, but the patient is not yet in life-threatening shock or hypoxia. Although systemic decline may ensue, if given appropriate care the patient can likely withstand a 45–60-minute wait without immediate risk.
- GREEN: Third priority. Nonurgent. Injuries are localized without immediate systemic implications, with a minimum of care; these patients generally are unlikely to deteriorate for several hours, if at all.
- BLACK: Dead. Any unresponsive patient who has no spontaneous ventilation or circulation belongs in this category. Some place catastrophically injured patients who have a poor chance of survival regardless of care in this triage category.

17-10. **The answer is C** (Chapter 7). The Centers for Disease Control and Prevention have ranked selected agents in 3 categories based on their overall potential for adverse public health impact. Class A agents have the most severe potential and include viruses and bacteria such as *Clostridium bot-*

ulinum, variola major, *Bacillus anthracis*, *Yersinia pestis*, *Francisella tularensis*, and Filovirus and arenaviruses. Class B agents are considered to have less potential for causing widespread illness and death and include *Coxiella burnetii*, *Brucella*, *Burkholderia pseudomallei*, alphaviruses, *Rickettsia prowazekii*, *Chlamydia psittaci*, food safety threats such as *Salmonella* and *Escherichia coli*, and water safety threats such as *Cryptosporidium*. Class C agents are those that as technology improves could emerge as future threats.

17-11.   **The answer is B** (Chapter 8). Ocular exposures take precedence and should be treated first with immediate eye irrigation. The critically ill, nonambulatory contaminated patient should have a patent airway ensured, the cervical spine immobilized, oxygen administered, ventilation assisted, and pressure maintained on arterial bleeding. Further medical care such as intubation or intravenous line insertion is delayed until gross decontamination has been completed. Wounds are the second step in the decontamination process and should be debrided of gross contaminants, then covered with a water occlusive dressing to prevent recontamination during showering. Whole-body decontamination should begin with the head and proceed downward.

17-12.   **The answer is A** (Chapter 10). Alpha radiation possesses a significant biological hazard only when internalized. Alpha radiation is easily shielded and cannot penetrate paper or the keratin layer of skin. Beta particles can cause significant skin burns and, like alpha particles, are hazardous if internally deposited. Neutron radiation, gamma radiation, and x-rays all pose significant whole-body irradiation hazards.

17-13.   **The answer is C** (Chapter 10). A whole-body gamma dose in excess of 2 Gy (200 rad) is the primary cause of acute radiation syndrome. The signs and symptoms of radiation toxicity are not discrete and manifest as injury to the hematopoietic, gastrointestinal, cardiovascular, and central nervous systems. The hematopoietic system is the first organ system to manifest injury from radiation. The earliest laboratory indicator of biological damage is a reduction in peripheral lymphocytes.

Psychosocial Disorders Emergencies
Questions

18-1. Using the DSM multiaxial classification system, a broken wrist in an intoxicated patient would be noted in which of the following axes?

(A) Axis I.
(B) Axis II.
(C) Axis III.
(D) Axis IV.

18-2. An 18-year-old patient presents to the ED, brought by his mother after about 2 months of worsening paranoid delusions and hearing voices. On exam he is found to be alert without signs of depression and has disorganized speech and auditory hallucinations. Screen for drugs of abuse is negative. What is the MOST appropriate diagnosis?

(A) Schizophrenia.
(B) Schizophreniform disorder.
(C) Brief psychotic disorder.
(D) Delirium.

18-3. Which of the following is MORE characteristic of an organic than a functional disorder?

(A) Paranoid delusions.
(B) Auditory hallucinations.
(C) Memory impairment.
(D) Visual hallucinations.

18-4. Among patients who attempt suicide, which of the following characteristics when present is associated with a successful suicide attempt?

(A) Substance abuse.
(B) Personality disorder.
(C) Male sex.
(D) Wrist cutting.

18-5. The agent droperidol was "black boxed" by the FDA due to which of the following?

(A) Hypotension.
(B) Torsades de pointes.
(C) Ventricular fibrillation.
(D) Severe dystonic reactions.

18-6. A newly psychotic patient receives a dose of haloperidol and begins to undergo spasms of the neck. Which of the following is the MOST desirable medication to counteract this problem?

(A) Benztropine.
(B) Lorazepam.
(C) Propanolol.
(D) Bromocriptine.

18-7. Of the following antipsychotics, which would be most likely to cause cardiovascular side effects?

(A) Chlorpromazine (Thorazine).
(B) Thioridazine (Mellaril).
(C) Haloperidol (Haldol).
(D) Droperidol (Inapsine).

18-8. Which of the following physiologic changes is associated with eating disorders?

(A) Elevated serum insulin levels.

(B) Elevated T3.

(C) Elevated sedimentation rate.

(D) Hypercholesterolemia.

18-9. Which of the following medical disorders has the MOST well-documented association with panic attacks?

(A) Asthma.

(B) Fibromyalgia.

(C) Hypertension.

(D) Irritable bowel syndrome.

18-10. A patient presents with mild recurrent panic attacks. Of the medications listed below, which is the MOST appropriate outpatient treatment?

(A) Lorazepam.

(B) Trazodone.

(C) Venlafaxine.

(D) Sertraline.

18-11. A patient who presents repeatedly with intermittent total blindness despite a full workup eliminating physical causes would best be categorized as which of the following?

(A) Somatization disorder.

(B) Conversion disorder.

(C) Hypochondriasis.

(D) Depersonalization disorder.

18-12. How long does the normal grieving process typically last?

(A) 2–4 weeks.

(B) 2–4 months.

(C) 6–8 months.

(D) 1 year or more.

18-13. What is the MOST appropriate time to request organ donation from a family after the death of a loved one?

(A) As part of the conversation informing them of the death.

(B) Before taking them in to view the deceased.

(C) After viewing the deceased.

(D) When the patient's personal physician can discuss it.

18-14. Which of the following persons exceeds the National Institute on Alcohol Abuse and Alcoholism (NIAAA) definitions for at-risk drinking?

(A) A 40-year-old woman who has 2 glasses of wine 3 nights a week.

(B) A 50-year-old man who drinks a 6-pack of beer every Sunday.

(C) A 64-year-old man who drinks 3 vodka tonics 4 times per week.

(D) A 22-year-old woman who drinks 3 beers every Saturday night.

18-15. What is the MOST important type of sleep for psychological well-being?

(A) Slow wave sleep.

(B) Delta wave sleep.

(C) Alpha wave sleep.

(D) Rapid eye movement sleep.

Psychosocial Disorders Emergencies
Answers, Explanations, and References

18-1. **The answer is C** (Chapter 288). Axis III denotes general medical conditions. Axis I includes substance abuse and mood disorders, and Axis II covers personality disorders. Axes IV and V are psychosocial stressors.

18-2. **The answer is B** (Chapter 288). Psychosis not attributable to a medical condition that exceeds 1 month but is <6 months consistent with schizophreniform disorder.

18-3. **The answer is D** (Chapter 289). Delusions, hallucinations, and memory problems may occur in both organic (medical) and functional (psychiatric) disorders. Visual hallucinations, however, almost always occur from organic disease.

18-4. **The answer is C** (Chapter 289). While males are less likely to attempt suicide, they are more likely to complete it. People who have the other factors listed have higher rates of completed suicide than the general population, but they are at relatively low risk of completion within the population of suicide attempters.

18-5. **The answer is B** (Chapter 290). Although recent reports suggest that droperidol is safe when appropriate doses are used, QT prolongation and torsades de pointes have been noted to occur, resulting in the warning. Preexisting QT prolongation should caution the physician against IV haloperidol or droperidol before checking an electrocardiogram for conduction abnormalities.

18-6. **The answer is A** (Chapter 290). The scenario described is consistent with an acute dystonic reaction, for which either benztropine (1–2 mg IV) or diphenhydramine (25–50 mg IV) are good choices.

18-7. **The answer is A** (Chapter 290). Chlorpromazine is a low-potency antipsychotic. Low-potency antipsychotics, almost exclusively, are associated with cardiovascular side effects.

18-8. **The answer is D** (Chapter 291). Physiologic changes associated with eating disorders include lower insulin levels, low T3, low sedimentation rate, and hypercholesterolemia.

18-9. **The answer is D** (Chapter 292). Asthma and mitral valve prolapse have the most well-documented association with panic attacks. Hypertension and irritable bowel syndrome, as well as others, also have been associated with panic attacks.

18-10. **The answer is D** (Chapter 292). SSRIs, such as sertraline, are the pharmacologic treatment of choice for panic attacks. Benzodiazepines may be effective for acute control of panic attacks in the ED but may be habit forming and are best avoided as outpatient treatment unless attacks are situational or severe.

18-11. **The answer is B** (Chapter 293). While this diagnosis should rarely if ever be made on the basis of an ED workup, a patient with symptoms (usually functional neurologic symptoms) for which a physical cause has been clearly eliminated is termed to have a conversion disorder.

18-12. **The answer is C** (Chapter 294). Normal grieving typically lasts 6–8 months.

18-13. **The answer is C** (Chapter 294). The most appropriate time to request organ donation is after the body has been viewed, allowing for an interval after notification. Waiting for the patient's personal physician may lose valuable time.

18-14. **The answer is B** (Chapter 295). This exceeds the NIAAA limit of 4 drinks per occasion, although it is less than the 14 per week for men. Women are at risk if they drink over 3 drinks per occasion or 7 drinks per week.

18-15. **The answer is D** (Chapter 296). Rapid eye movement (REM) sleep is most important for psychological well-being, while slow or delta wave sleep is most important for physical well-being.

Pulmonary Emergencies
Questions

19-1. Which of the following conditions does not necessarily warrant a chest radiograph when the patient presents with shortness of breath and wheezing?

(A) Chronic obstructive pulmonary disease (COPD).

(B) Congestive heart failure.

(C) Asthma.

(D) Lung transplant.

19-2. Which of the following medications is FDA-approved for the treatment of hiccups?

(A) Droperidol.

(B) Chlorpromazine.

(C) Metoclopramide.

(D) Nifedipine.

19-3. Which of the following sites is MOST sensitive for the detection of cyanosis?

(A) Sublingual area.

(B) Earlobes.

(C) Conjunctivae.

(D) Nail beds.

19-4. Which of the following imaging techniques is MOST useful for the detection of a non-loculated pleural effusion?

(A) Supine chest radiograph.

(B) Upright chest radiograph.

(C) Ultrasound.

(D) Lateral decubitus chest radiograph.

19-5. Which of the following choices is MOST commonly associated with acute uncomplicated bronchitis?

(A) Influenza.

(B) *Bordetella pertussis.*

(C) *Chlamydia.*

(D) *Streptococcus pneumoniae.*

19-6. In which of the following patients with chronic bronchitis should a short course of antibiotics be considered?

(A) A 50-year-old female with COPD who smokes 2 packs per day with increased cough.

(B) A 45-year-old afebrile male with cough and persistent clear rhinorrhea.

(C) A 70-year-old afebrile male with emphysema on home oxygen therapy with increased dyspnea.

(D) A 65-year-old male with chronic bronchitis who presents with increased dyspnea and purulent sputum.

19-7. Patients with HIV can have clinical symptoms similar to those of immunocompetent patients when presenting with community-acquired pneumonia. Which of the following statements is TRUE regarding pneumonia in HIV patients?

(A) HIV patients are less likely to develop pleural effusions because of a decreased inflammatory response from impaired cell-mediated immunity.

(B) A bacterial cause for pneumonia is more likely in patients with a higher $CD4^+$ T-cell count.

(C) The incidence of bacteremia in HIV patients is similar to that of immunocompetent patients.

(D) *Pseudomonas aeruginosa* is an uncommon cause of pneumonia in HIV patients.

19-8. The Pneumonia Patient Outcomes Research Team (PORT) score classifies patients with pneumonia according to their increased risk of mortality based on clinical parameters and comorbidities. Which of the following PORT classifications is associated with an 8.2% mortality?

(A) Class I.
(B) Class II.
(C) Class III.
(D) Class IV.

19-9. Which of the following conditions is LEAST likely to increase a patient's risk for aspiration pneumonia?

(A) Periodontal disease.
(B) Intoxication.
(C) Dementia.
(D) Schizophrenia.

19-10. Which of the following antibiotics is recommended for empiric therapy for suspected community-acquired aspiration pneumonia?

(A) Clindamycin.
(B) Azithromycin.

(C) Ceftriaxone.
(D) Amoxicillin-clavulanic acid.

19-11. Which of the following clinical feature sets is present in patients with tuberculosis?

(A) Fever, cough, and prostration.
(B) Asymptomatic.
(C) Weight loss and hemoptysis.
(D) Nausea, vomiting, and diarrhea.

19-12. An otherwise healthy nurse who is employed in a suburban community clinic presents to your ED fast-track area because of concerns about a possible positive PPD test placed 48 hours ago after routine health care testing. She has had no known tuberculosis (TB) exposure. Which of the following criteria apply to confirm a positive PPD test?

(A) Induration >5 mm.
(B) Induration >7.5 mm.
(C) Induration >10 mm.
(D) Induration >15 mm.

19-13. A 21-year-old male presents with sudden onset of pleuritic chest pain. A chest radiograph identifies a 10–15% pneumothorax. Which of the following choices is the LEAST compelling treatment option?

(A) Discharged home with analgesics.
(B) Catheter aspiration of pneumothorax.
(C) Observation for a period of 6 hours.
(D) Insertion of a 14-French tube thoracostomy.

19-14. Which of the following conditions is LEAST likely to present with the x-ray shown in Figure 19-1?

(A) Pneumonia in an intravenous drug user.
(B) Cavitary tuberculosis.
(C) Transplant patient.
(D) Community-acquired pneumonia.

19-15. The x-ray findings on the radiograph shown in Figure 19-2 are MOST consistent with which of the following conditions?

(A) Community-acquired pneumonia.
(B) Viral pneumonia.
(C) *Pneumocystis* pneumonia.
(D) Miliary tuberculosis.

19-16. A 50-year-old man with a history of smoking complains of hemoptysis for two weeks. He reports a chronic productive cough but denies fever. He reports the hemoptysis was initially blood-tinged sputum but now is bright red with a frothy appearance. Which of the following diagnostic tests will likely lead to this patient's diagnosis?

(A) Sputum for culture and stain.
(B) Complete blood cell count.
(C) Chest radiograph.
(D) Coagulation studies.

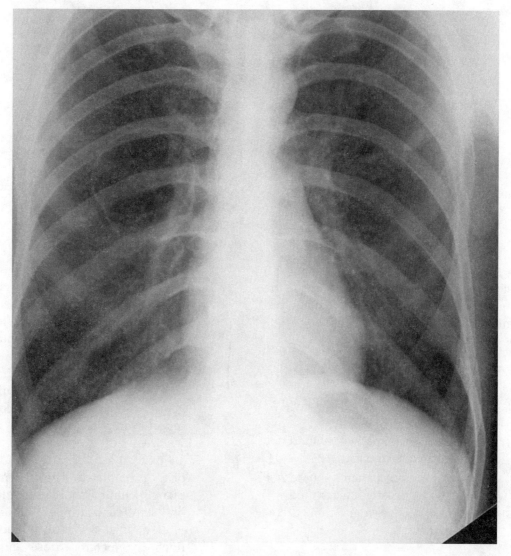

Figure 19-1.

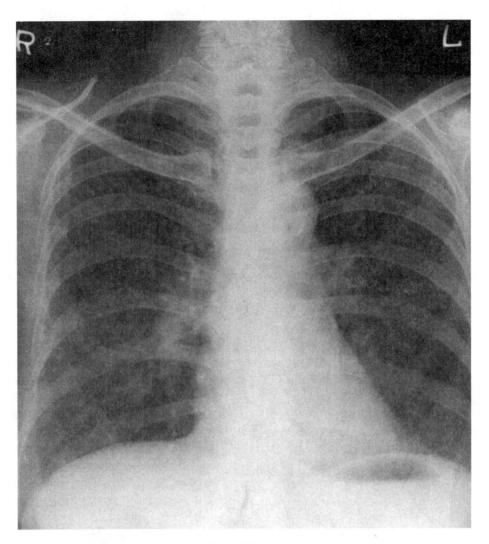

Figure 19-2.

19-17. Which of the following is TRUE about the diagnosis and treatment of pregnant patients with asthma exacerbations?

(A) Pregnant asthmatic patients should not receive oral or intravenous corticosteroids.

(B) Pregnant asthmatic patients with a PaO_2 of 65 are severely hypoxemic.

(C) Pregnant asthmatic patients should not receive inhaled β_2-agonists.

(D) Pregnant asthmatic patients should not use inhaled corticosteroids for mild persistent or more severe asthma during pregnancy.

19-18. A 45-year-old male with a history of asthma since childhood presents to the ED for treatment of an asthma exacerbation. He has an initial peak expiratory flow rate (PEFR) of <50% predicted, and an oxygen saturation of 91% on room air. He received three doses of albuterol and ipatropium by nebulization and oral corticosteroids. On repeat exam, the patient has a few scattered wheezes with good air movement, a room air oxygen saturation of 96%, and a PEFR of 65% predicted. The patient's discharge plans include a short burst of nontapering oral steroids, continued self-administration of β_2-agonist and anticholinergic medications by metered dose inhaler with a spacer, and close follow-up with his primary care provider. Which of the following additional historical elements make it MORE appropriate to admit this patient to the hospital or an observation unit instead of discharging him home?

(A) The patient has a past history of sudden severe exacerbations.

(B) The patient currently smokes tobacco.

(C) The patient reports use of a nontapering burst course of oral steroids 3 months ago.

(D) The patient uses 1 canister of albuterol per month.

19-19. Which of the following interventions is more commonly indicated for a patient with an exacerbation of chronic obstructive pulmonary disease (COPD) than a patient with an exacerbation of asthma?

(A) Measure a peak expiratory flow rate or forced expiratory volume in 1 second.

(B) Administer inhaled β_2-agonist.

(C) Obtain a chest radiograph.

(D) Administer oxygen to achieve a SaO_2 of ≥90%.

19-20. A 70-year-old female presents to the ED with an acute exacerbation of longstanding COPD. She is given oxygen by face mask and inhaled β_2-agonist and anticholinergic agents. Despite these therapies the patient is noted to have minimal improvement in her respiratory status and is being evaluated for possible noninvasive positive pressure ventilation (NIPPV) therapy. Which of the following findings would make intubation a better choice for this patient?

(A) Worsening respiratory acidosis.

(B) Rapidly deteriorating mental status.

(C) A PaO_2 of >50 mmHg on arterial blood gas despite supplemental oxygen therapy.

(D) Evidence of respiratory muscle fatigue.

19-21. What is the MOST common complication to occur in the first 3 months after a patient receives a lung transplant?

(A) Bacterial respiratory infection.

(B) Acute rejection.

(C) Airway stenosis.

(D) Bronchiolitis obliterans.

19-22. A 2-year-old girl is brought to the ED after her parents discovered that she was playing with a box of loose buttons and had several in her mouth. She has a slight cough on presentation but otherwise has a normal examination with normal vital signs and normal oxygen saturation. Which of the following pulmonary imaging studies should be undertaken first in establishing the presence of a foreign body aspiration?

(A) Chest CT.

(B) Ventilation-perfusion scan.

(C) Inspiratory and expiratory chest radiographs.

(D) Thoracic ultrasonography.

19-23. A patient with a low pretest probability of pulmonary embolism receives a ventilation-perfusion scan in the ED that is interpreted as normal. Is it necessary for this patient to undergo further diagnostic imaging to effectively rule out pulmonary embolism as a diagnosis?

(A) This patient should undergo pulmonary angiography to exclude the diagnosis of pulmonary embolism.

(B) This patient should undergo helical CT of the chest and contrast venography of the lower extremities to exclude the diagnosis of pulmonary embolism.

(C) This patient has a pulmonary embolism, and no further diagnostic imaging is necessary to confirm the diagnosis.

(D) This patient does not have a pulmonary embolism, and a different diagnosis should be entertained.

19-24. A 45-year-old female presents to the ED with a temperature of 38.8°C, heart rate of 105 beats per minute, blood pressure of 140/75 mmHg, oxygen saturation of 92% on room air, pleuritic chest pain, and cough with purulent sputum. Which of the following chest radiographs is MOST appropriate for the evaluation of possible pneumonia in this patient?

(A) Lateral decubitus views.

(B) Posterior-anterior (PA) and lateral views.

(C) Anterior-posterior (AP) view.

(D) Inspiratory and expiratory views.

Pulmonary Emergencies
Answers, Explanations, and References

19-1. **The answer is C** (Chapter 62). In patients with uncomplicated acute asthma, treatment should be based on history and physical findings. Chest radiographs are not necessary. Monitoring peak expiratory flow may be helpful to correlate physical findings of severity. The clinician may consider obtaining a chest radiograph in patients with wheezing who do not have a history of asthma. Patients with COPD may have complications such as bullae or pneumothoraces, which can be assessed on chest radiograph. In patients with acute heart failure, clinical examination and chest radiographs can help quantify the degree of decompensation. Due to the patient's immunocompromised state, a heightened clinical suspicion for infection or complication related to immunosuppression warrants investigations such as a chest radiograph.

19-2. **The answer is B** (Chapter 62). Only chlorpromazine has an FDA indication for the treatment of hiccups. Droperidol is a potent antiemetic that has recently received a "black box" warning due to associated QT prolongation. Metoclopramide is a gastrointestinal motility agent used for nausea, vomiting, and occasionally for hiccups, but it has not received an FDA indication. Nifedipine is a calcium channel blocker occasionally used for persistent hiccups, but it has not received formal FDA approval for this indication.

19-3. **The answer is A** (Chapter 62). Cyanosis represents a pathologic condition that manifests as a blue hue to the skin or mucosal membranes. Causes of cyanosis include reduced hemoglobin or hemoglobin derivatives. Beneath the tongue is considered the most sensitive location for detecting central cyanosis, probably due to its well-vascularized location. Earlobes, conjunctivae, and nail beds may demonstrate cyanosis with varying degrees of sensitivity.

19-4. **The answer is D** (Chapter 62). A lateral decubitus chest radiograph is useful for detecting moderate to large effusions, which layer out when the patient is lying on his or her side. A supine chest radiograph may demonstrate a hazy appearance of fluid posteriorly. An upright chest radiograph detects only large effusions. Ultrasound can be used to detect a pleural effusion, but it is user dependent and may not always detect small effusions or effusions in obese patients.

19-5. **The answer is A** (Chapter 63). The respiratory viruses, influenza, parainfluenza, and respiratory syncynctial virus, are the agents most commonly associated with acute uncomplicated bronchitis. *B. pertussis* and *C. pneumoniae* are also associated with bronchitis but generally present with a more prolonged or persistent course of cough. *S. pneumoniae* is associated with community-acquired pneumonia as well as being part of normal oral flora, and its impact on the overall incidence of acute bronchitis is unclear.

19-6. **The answer is D** (Chapter 63). The 65-year-old male with bronchitis who presents with increased dyspnea and purulent cough has two of the signs of an acute exacerbation of chronic bronchitis. His advanced age and comorbidities make it possible for him to benefit from a short course of an extended-spectrum antibiotic such as doxycycline. Persistent rhinorrhea may be found with viral sinusitis or early influenza. The cough may be due to postnasal drip. Antibiotics are not recommended for these conditions, which may be ameliorated with decongestants and supportive therapy. Increased dyspnea in a patient on home oxygen therapy may be caused by a multitude of reasons, including infection. If physical findings and chest radiograph do not define an infectious etiology, a progression of his presumptive emphysema may be the cause of his dyspnea. Antibiotics will probably not help this patient's condition.

19-7. **The answer is B** (Chapter 63). Bacterial pneumonia is the most common cause of pneumonia in HIV patients. *Streptococcus pneumoniae* is the leading cause of bacterial pneumonia in HIV patients. Pleural effusions occur in 60% of patients with acquired immunodeficiency syndrome (AIDS). Patients with HIV have acquired a deficiency in cell-mediated immunity. The incidence of bacteremia is significantly higher (60%) in HIV patients as compared to immunocompetent patients (15–30%). *P. aeruginosa* is a common cause of pneumonia in patients with HIV and tends to occur when CD4+ T-cell counts are low.

19-8. **The answer is D** (Chapter 63). In the study by Fine et al, patients with the diagnosis of pneumonia were assigned points based on various clinical and historical parameters. A higher score correlates with a higher mortality and consequently classification into a higher risk group. A PORT score of greater than 130 is associated with 29.2% mortality. Patients with a PORT score greater than 90 fall into the category of patients with an associated mortality of 8.2%.

Due to the higher risk of death and the need for ICU admission, it is recommended that these patients be admitted to the hospital. Class I patients have a mortality incidence of 0.1%, and it is felt that these patients can be safely managed in an outpatient setting. Class II patients have an associated mortality of 0.6% and can also be managed as outpatients. Class III patients have an associated mortality of 2.8%. These patients can be admitted for a short hospital stay or alternatively observed in an observation unit if available.

19-9. **The answer is D** (Chapter 64). It is unlikely that schizophrenia has a direct link to an increased risk of aspiration pneumonia. One might assume that schizophrenia when uncontrolled can predispose an individual to certain behaviors that are deemed high risk. Not infrequently, patients with schizophrenia may use illicit drugs or alcohol or be displaced from their homes, which can increase the risk of aspiration pneumonia. Neurologic conditions including stroke or dementia have a high association with aspiration pneumonia. Intoxication can impair normal gag reflexes and thus predispose individuals to aspiration pneumonia. Patients with periodontal disease often have latent colonization and overgrowth of oral flora, which if delivered to the distal airway can cause an aspiration pneumonia.

19-10. **The answer is C** (Chapter 64). Ceftriaxone or levofloxacin are the agents of choice because they cover gram-positive and gram-negative bacteria that are potential pathogens. Clindamycin covers gram-positive and anaerobic bacteria but is currently not recommended as monotherapy. Azithromycin has suitable coverage for several gram-positive and atypical pathogens but is not the currently recommended first-line agent for aspiration pneumonia syndromes. Amoxicillin-clavulanic acid provides excellent coverage for gram-positive and anaerobic bacteria. It has very good bioavailability, and oral dosing is usually sufficient for most infections, but amoxicillin-clavulanic acid has not been endorsed as first-line therapy for aspiration pneumonia.

19-11. **The answer is B** (Chapter 65). Primary infection with tuberculosis is commonly clinically silent. Patients may have a self-limited pneumonitis, and chest radiographs may identify a Ghon's complex. Although fever may be present in primary infection, prostration, hemoptysis, and pneumonia are usually seen when tuberculosis is reactivated. Nausea, vomiting, and diarrhea are not part of the constellation of symptoms associated with primary infection with tuberculosis.

19-12. **The answer is D** (Chapter 65). Induration of 15 mm should be used as the criteria for a positive PPD test in this patient. The nurse works in a suburban area, which presumably has a low incidence of TB. She does not report a history of immunosuppression, and although she works in a health care facility she is in a lower risk category. It is accepted practice in most health care institutions to mandate PPD screening of employees. Greater than 5 mm of induration is the recommended criterion for a positive PPD in patients with HIV, close contact to a TB patient, abnormal chest radiograph resembling TB, or other form of immunosuppresion. Greater than 7.5 mm is not one of the defined levels of induration to diagnose TB. Greater than 10 mm of induration is considered positive in patients who use intravenous drugs, patients who belong to a group with a high prevalence of TB such as immigrants and nursing home patients, patients from regions with a high prevalence of TB, and patients with predisposing conditions such as silicosis, diabetes, or cancer. In addition, children <4 years old are considered positive with a PPD test >10 mm.

19-13. **The answer is A** (Chapter 66). A period of observation is recommended because of the possibility for progression of the pneu-

mothorax. Catheter aspiration with or without Heimlich valve mechanism followed by a period of observation may be acceptable. Simple observation and clinical reassessment or placement of a small thoracostomy tube are also acceptable alternatives. Availability of the above equipment and practice patterns varies with regard to the management of small pneumothoraces, but simply discharging the patient with analgesics is probably not the best option.

19-14. **The answer is D** (Chapter 63). This chest radiograph demonstrates a cavitary lesion. Patients with community-acquired pneumonia will present with an acute onset of cough and fever. Their typical radiographic patterns include lobar consolidation or a diffuse interstitial process. Pleural effusions may be seen in up to 25% of patients. Intravenous drug abusers are prone to *Staphylococcus* infections. *S. aureus* pneumonia may be associated with pleural effusions and empyemas. Patients with tuberculous reactivation may have a necrotizing pneumonia, which can lead to cavitary lesions on chest radiograph. This patient was diagnosed with cavitary tuberculosis with an air fluid level. The patient was eventually placed on antituberculous medications. Transplant patients due to immunosuppression may develop atypical pneumonias including viral and fungal pneumonias. These patients may develop cavitary lesions on chest radiograph.

19-15. **The answer is D** (Chapter 65). Miliary tuberculosis develops from hematogenous seeding of various organ systems. It is most commonly seen in immunocompromised hosts. The chest radiograph has a characteristic multinodular appearance similar to the millet seed, from which the name was derived. The radiographic appearance of community-acquired pneumonia can present differently depending on the etiology. It is unlikely, however, to find a miliary pattern in pneumococcal, *Chlamydia*, or *Mycoplasma* pneumonia. Viral pneumonias may have seasonal variability, but their radiographic appearance is unlikely to have a miliary pattern. *P. carinii*, now known as *P. jiroveci*, the causative agent of *Pneumocystis* pneumonia, presents with an insidious onset of cough and fever. *Pneumocystis* pneumonia is found in immunosuppressed patients. The chest radiograph varies but classically is described as a bilateral interstitial pattern.

19-16. **The answer is C** (Chapter 67). This patient's description of hemoptysis as bright red and frothy is consistent with true hemoptysis, rather than a gastrointestinal source or a swallowed nasopharyngeal source (dark red). All patients with true hemoptysis require radiographic imaging, starting with a chest radiograph. This patient is at high risk for a neoplastic cause of hemoptysis because he is male, >40 years of age, and has a smoking history. All patients with these risk factors should receive a chest radiograph as part of their ED evaluation for true hemoptysis. An abnormal chest radiograph is present in 80–90% of individuals with a neoplastic source of hemoptysis. A complete blood count, sputum for culture and stain, and coagulation studies are diagnostic studies that should be guided by clinical suspicion. A complete blood count and coagulation studies are appropriate in the evaluation of massive hemoptysis or in unstable patients with airway compromise. A complete blood count and sputum stains and cultures may be appropriate in patients suspected to have an infectious source of hemoptysis, such as patients presenting with a fever, an abrupt onset of cough with purulent blood-tinged sputum, or night sweats.

19-17. **The answer is B** (Chapter 68). Pregnancy leads to a general state of hyperventilation, and pregnant patients will have a higher PaO_2 and a lower $PaCO_2$ than nonpregnant patients. Therefore, a PaO_2 of <70 mmHg in a pregnant patient represents fairly significant hypoxemia. During an asthma exacerbation, the normal alkalosis of pregnancy is exaggerated, leading to a decrease in pla-

cental blood flow and more severe hypoxemia in the fetus than the mother. In addition, a $PaCO_2$ of >35 mmHg represents respiratory failure in the pregnant asthmatic patient. Studies suggest that 11–18% of pregnant asthmatics will have 1 or more visits to the ED for an asthma exacerbation. Appropriate management of acute asthma exacerbations in pregnant patients is similar to that of nonpregnant patients but may include fetal monitoring. This includes using peak expiratory flow rate (PEFR) or forced expiratory volume in 1 second (FEV_1) measurements for assessment, administering repetitive inhaled β_2-agonists, and early administering systemic corticosteroids. Although no asthma medications have been labeled in category A by the Food and Drug Administration (medications for which adequate well-controlled trials in pregnant women have failed to demonstrate risk to the fetus), no problems have been reported as a result of asthma treatment in the ED. In patients with mild persistent or more severe asthma, inhaled corticosteroids should be considered after ED treatment for an exacerbation.

19-18. **The answer is A** (Chapter 68). Current guidelines for patient disposition are based on responsiveness to aggressive treatment in the ED. A good response to treatment includes complete resolution of symptoms and a peak expiratory flow rate (PEFR) or forced expiratory volume in 1 second (FEV_1) of >70% predicted. Patients with persistent symptoms and a PEFR or FEV_1 of <50% predicted after treatment should be hospitalized. The patient with an incomplete response to treatment may need more detailed evaluation before an appropriate disposition decision can be made. The patient with an incomplete response to treatment will have some persistence of symptoms and a PEFR or FEV_1 between 50% and 70% predicted. Most of these patients can be discharged safely to home if they have no risk factors for death from asthma. Patients with significant risk factors for death from asthma should be admitted to an observation unit or the hospital. These risk factors include past history of sudden severe exacerbations, prior intubation for asthma, prior admission to an intensive care unit for asthma, 2 or more hospitalizations for asthma within the last year, hospitalization or emergency care visit for asthma within the last month, 3 or more emergency care visits for asthma within the past month, use of more than 2 canisters of inhaled short-acting β_2-agonist, current use of systemic corticosteroids or recent withdrawal from systemic steroids, comorbidity such as cardiovascular disease or chronic obstructive pulmonary disease, serious psychiatric illness or psychosocial problems, low socioeconomic status in urban residents, or illicit drug use.

19-19. **The answer is C** (Chapters 68, 69). Patients with COPD are generally older than patients with asthma and are more likely to have comorbidities that complicate the accuracy of diagnosis. Decompensation in COPD is usually caused by a worsening of baseline airflow obstruction resulting from superimposed respiratory infection, increased bronchospasm, or other respiratory pathology such as pulmonary embolism, cardiovascular deterioration, medication noncompliance, or smoking. Chest radiography in this group of patients should be strongly considered to help elucidate the underlying cause of the exacerbation. Radiographic abnormalities are common in COPD exacerbations and may guide additional treatments for findings such as pneumonia, pleural effusion, and pulmonary congestive heart failure. Routine chest radiography is not indicated for patients with asthma exacerbation but is clinically indicated if there is concern for pneumothorax, pneumonia, or other medical problems. The goals of treatment for both asthma and COPD include ensuring adequate oxygenation and reversing airflow obstruction. Thus, administration of oxygen and inhaled β_2-agonist medications is appropriate in both conditions. Bedside spirometry utilizing peak expiratory flow volume or forced expiratory volume in 1 second is useful in assessing both severity of the exacerbation and response to treatment in asthma and COPD.

19-20. **The answer is B** (Chapter 69). This patient meets criteria for some method of assisted ventilation, but a rapidly deteriorating mental status would make her a poor candidate for NIPPV. To review, indications for mechanical ventilation (intubation) in the setting of COPD exacerbation include evidence of respiratory muscle fatigue, worsening respiratory acidosis, deteriorating mental status, and clinically significant hypoxemia despite supplemental oxygen therapy. NIPPV can be used instead of intubation in this situation and has been associated with better outcomes in terms of short-term mortality rates, symptomatic improvement, intubation rates, and length of hospitalization in patients. Contraindications to the use of NIPPV include an uncooperative or obtunded patient, inability to clear airway secretions, hemodynamic instability, respiratory arrest, recent facial or gastroesophageal surgery, burns, poor mask fit, or extreme obesity.

19-21. **The answer is A** (Chapter 71). The most common complication in the first 3 months after transplant is bacterial pneumonia. This is due to decreased mucociliary clearance, diminished cough reflex, disrupted lymphatics, reperfusion injury, and immunosuppression. Infectious agents may be present in the donor lung that can generate infection in the immunosuppressed posttransplant patient. Acute rejection is also common and can occur 3 to 6 times in the first year after transplant. Clinically acute rejection may be difficult to distinguish from infection because both complications may cause cough, chest tightness, fever, hypoxemia, and infiltrates on chest radiographs. Airway stenosis is now an uncommon postoperative complication, and bronchiolitis obliterans is a complication that occurs later after transplantation and is thought most commonly to be the result of chronic rejection.

19-22. **The answer is C** (Chapter 72). Inspiratory and expiratory chest radiographs may show hyperinflation on the affected side caused by air trapped behind the foreign body. A ventilation-perfusion scan is used primarily for diagnosing pulmonary embolism. A chest CT scan may demonstrate the presence of a foreign body but requires exposure to intravenous contrast, patient ability to cooperate with the exam, and radiation exposure. In a child with suspected foreign body aspiration, additional pulmonary imaging beyond a chest radiograph is usually unnecessary, and additional investigation with bronchoscopy can be both diagnostic and therapeutic. Thoracic ultrasonography in the ED may be useful in identifying pulmonary effusions and pneumothoraces. In addition it can be used as a guide in aspiration and the placement of drains.

19-23. **The answer is D** (Chapter 72). In the PIOPED study, it was found that patients with a normal ventilation-perfusion scan had a 4% overall prevalence of pulmonary embolism on subsequent pulmonary angiogram. However, none of the patients in this category demonstrated morbidity or mortality. Therefore, a normal or near-normal ventilation-perfusion scan is sufficient to withhold further diagnostic study or treatment. A high-probability ventilation-perfusion scan had a specificity of 98% for diagnosing a pulmonary embolism in the PIOPED study. This result is sufficient to diagnose and treat a patient for pulmonary embolism without further imaging. A patient with a nondiagnostic ventilation-perfusion scan requires further imaging to confirm or eliminate pulmonary embolism from the differential diagnosis. In the PIOPED study, patients with a nondiagnostic ventilation-perfusion scan went on to pulmonary angiography, and 25% were found to have a pulmonary embolism. In many centers, helical CT scan of the chest is used for the initial diagnostic evaluation of pulmonary embolism. Patients with abnormal chest radiographs or underlying pulmonary disease are likely to have nondiagnostic ventilation-perfusion scans and require further diagnostic testing for the evaluation of a possible pulmonary embolism.

19-24. **The answer is B** (Chapter 72). PA and lateral chest radiographs are the best views to examine the lung parenchyma, cardiac and mediastinal size, and bony structures of the chest wall. A portable AP view may be necessary in trauma patients or those who are unstable or can't cooperate with a PA and lateral exam. Lateral decubitus views generally help with the evaluation of pleural effusions or detection of small pneumothoraces. Inspiratory and expiratory views are generally helpful for diagnosing pneumothoraces or possible foreign body aspiration.

Renal and Urologic Emergencies
Questions

20-1. Which of the following findings are consistent with acute prerenal failure?

(A) BUN to creatinine ratio of <10, fractional excretion of sodium (FeNa) <1, red cells in urine sediment.

(B) BUN to creatinine ratio of >20, FeNa >1, normal urinalysis.

(C) Urine osmolality <350, moderate proteinuria, granular casts.

(D) Urine osmolality >500, red cell casts, proteinuria, FeNa <1.

20-2. Which of the following is NOT a cause of postrenal failure?

(A) Bladder tumor.
(B) Phimosis.
(C) Neurogenic bladder.
(D) Urethral prolapse.

20-3. Which of the following is NOT a cause of acute renal failure?

(A) Rhabdomyolysis.
(B) Nonsteroidal anti-inflammatory drugs (NSAIDs).
(C) Iron.
(D) Penicillin.

20-4. A chronic renal dialysis patient is brought to the ED in cardiac arrest. Which of the following is the MOST likely cause?

(A) Pericardial effusion.
(B) Hyperkalemia.
(C) Malignant hypertension.
(D) Postdialysis hypotension.

20-5. Which of the following statements regarding infection in patients with continuous ambulatory peritoneal dialysis (CAPD) is TRUE?

(A) Gram-negative bacteria are responsible for most cases of CAPD peritonitis.

(B) Cell count in cases of peritonitis is >250 leukocytes.

(C) Infection is the most frequent complication of CAPD.

(D) The peritoneal catheter should be changed at the first sign of peritonitis.

20-6. Which of the following is TRUE regarding vascular access in a chronic renal failure patient on hemodialysis?

(A) Vascular graft thrombosis requires immediate surgical thrombectomy.

(B) A nonfunctioning or infected Hickman catheter should be pulled in the ED.

(C) Vascular graft infection often presents with signs of systemic sepsis and few classic signs of local infection.

(D) "Steal syndrome," resulting in shunting of arterial blood away from the extremity distal to the vascular access, is common in patients with AV fistulas.

20-7. Which of the following is NOT a risk factor for urinary tract infection (UTI) in women?

(A) New sexual partner.
(B) Uterine prolapse.
(C) Use of diaphragm and spermicide.
(D) Oral contraceptive use.

20-8. What is the MOST common causative organism for uncomplicated UTI?

(A) *Chlamydia trachomatis.*

(B) *Proteus* species.

(C) *Escherichia coli.*

(D) *Staphylococcus saprophyticus.*

20-9. Which of the following structures needs to be repaired in a fractured penis?

(A) Tunica albuginea.

(B) Corpus spongiosum.

(C) Corpora cavernosum.

(D) Urethra.

20-10. Which of the following is NOT an appropriate treatment for priapism?

(A) Terbutaline 0.25 mg administered subcutaneously in the deltoid.

(B) Sedation.

(C) NeoSynephrine instillation into the corpora cavernosa.

(D) Exchange transfusion.

20-11. A 19-year-old man complains of acute onset of scrotal pain. Which of the following procedures is LEAST indicated?

(A) Treat with ceftriaxone and doxycycline, then discharge.

(B) Obtain a radionuclide scan of the testes.

(C) Attempt manual detorsion.

(D) Obtain a Doppler ultrasound study.

20-12. What is the MOST appropriate test for diagnosing kidney stones?

(A) Ultrasound.

(B) Urine dipstick.

(C) Plain abdominal radiograph.

(D) Noncontrast computed tomography.

20-13. Which of the following patients with nephrolithiasis can be safely discharged home?

(A) A 50-year-old diabetic man with associated urinary tract infection and signs of obstruction.

(B) A 30-year-old man with a single kidney and signs of obstruction.

(C) A 40-year-old man with a 4-mm stone in the distal ureter.

(D) A 25-year-old woman with uncontrolled pain and persistent vomiting.

20-14. Which of the following is NOT a common cause of hematuria?

(A) Rifampin.

(B) Glomerulonephritis.

(C) Cancer.

(D) Schistosomiasis.

20-15. A patient with a history of ureteral stricture presents to the ED 3 days after placement of a ureteral stent. The patient reports urgency, frequency, and dysuria for the last 24 hours. The patient denies flank pain, gross hematuria, fever, nausea, or vomiting. A urinalysis in the ED confirms the presence of microscopic hematuria but is otherwise unremarkable. Which of the following diagnoses is MOST likely in this patient?

(A) Bladder irritation secondary to stent placement.

(B) Stent migration.

(C) Pyelonephritis.

(D) Urinary obstruction.

20-16. What is the MOST common site of infection in a renal transplant patient during the first year posttransplant?

(A) Urinary tract.

(B) Mucocutaneous tissue.

(C) Respiratory tract.

(D) Cerebrospinal fluid.

20-17. Which of the following commonly used immunosuppressive agents can cause nephrotoxicity in a renal transplant patient?

(A) Prednisone.

(B) Mycophenolate mofetil.

(C) Azathioprine.

(D) Cyclosporine.

20-18. Which of the following imaging modalities used in evaluating renal colic is the MOST sensitive and specific for identifying renal calculi or hydronephrosis?

(A) Ultrasonography.

(B) Kidneys, ureters, and bladder (KUB) plain radiograph.

(C) Helical CT without intravenous contrast.

(D) Intravenous pyelography (IVP).

20-19. During the initial trauma evaluation of a 24-year-old male involved in a motor vehicle accident, blood is discovered at the urethral meatus, and there is concern for a pelvic fracture. Which of the following diagnostic modalities should be used to evaluate a possible urethral injury?

(A) Helical abdominal CT scan with intravenous and oral contrast.

(B) Retrograde urethrogram.

(C) Focused assessment with sonography in trauma (FAST) scan.

(D) IVP.

Renal and Urologic Emergencies
Answers, Explanations, and References

20-1. The answer is B (Chapter 92). Prerenal failure is due to volume loss, decreased cardiac output, or renal artery and small vessel disease. When the clinical picture is not clear, chemistry and urinalysis can aid in distinguishing prerenal from intrinsic and postobstructive renal failure. Prerenal failure is associated with a BUN to creatinine ratio of >20, urine osmolality of >500, FeNa of >1, and normal urinalysis. In postrenal failure, urine osmolality is <350. Active urine sediment and FeNa of >1 are associated with intrinsic renal failure.

20-2. The answer is D (Chapter 92). Postrenal failure can be caused by obstruction anywhere along the urinary tract from the kidney and the ureters to the bladder and the urethra. Bladder neck obstruction may result from neurogenic bladder or medications. Prostatic hypertrophy and functional bladder neck obstruction are the most common causes of postrenal failure. Urethral strictures or atresia, but not prolapse, may cause obstruction and lead to postrenal failure.

20-3. The answer is C (Chapter 92). Myoglobinuria from rhabdomyolysis can cause acute tubular necrosis. NSAIDs cause preferential reduction in renal blood flow leading to renal failure from hypoperfusion. Penicillin is a cause of allergic interstitial nephritis. Iron does not usually have direct renal toxicity.

20-4. The answer is B (Chapter 93). Although all of the choices can lead to cardiac arrest in chronic dialysis patients, hyperkalemia is the most common cause. Treatment should start with intravenous calcium, then dextrose and insulin, as well as sodium bicarbonate. Other electrolyte disturbances seen in uremic patients include hypokalemia, hypocalcemia, and hypermagnesemia.

20-5. The answer is C (Chapter 93). Infection is the most common complication of CAPD, and the majority of cases of peritonitis are caused by staphylococcal species. Peritonitis is usually defined as >100 leukocytes with >50% neutrophils. Therapy typically consists of infusion of antibiotics with the dialysate into the peritoneal cavity rather than delivered intravenously. The peritoneal catheter needs to be changed when there have been multiple episodes of peritonitis or evidence of tunnel infection or intra-abdominal abscess.

20-6. The answer is C (Chapter 93). Vascular access thrombosis or stenosis is not an emergency and can be treated by angiographic clot removal, angioplasty, or direct injection of thrombolytics within 24 hours. Hickman and other tunnel catheters used for dialysis should not be removed by pulling because they are cuffed. Steal syndrome is an uncommon complication of vascular access. Graft infection often leads to sepsis and may not present with classic signs of pain, erythema, swelling, and discharge from the site in dialysis patients.

20-7. The answer is D (Chapter 94). A new sexual partner in the last 12 months and use of diaphragm and spermicide are demonstrated risk factors for UTIs. Oral contraceptives, personal hygiene, and postcoital voiding are not. Some spermicides enhance vaginal colonization with *Escherichia coli*. Uterine and bladder prolapse and neurogenic bladder cause incomplete bladder emptying and thus reduce the ability of the bladder to clear bacteria. These conditions are commonly associated with asymptomatic bacteriuria (ABU), and ABU is a strong predictor of subsequent UTI.

20-8. **The answer is C** (Chapter 94). All of the organisms listed may cause uncomplicated UTIs. However, *E. coli* is by far the most common bacterium. Unusual organisms, such as yeast or *Enterococcus* species are often found in complicated UTIs, especially in patients with underlying renal disease, recent hospitalization, or instrumentation of the urinary tract.

20-9. **The answer is A** (Chapter 95). Tear of the penile tunica albuginea, the thick fascial layer around the corpora cavernosum, can occur during sexual intercourse or other sexual activity. The urethra is rarely injured, but a retrograde urethrogram may be necessary for full evaluation. The tunica albuginea should be surgically repaired.

20-10. **The answer is B** (Chapter 95). Priapism is a painful, pathologic erection secondary to engorgement of the corpora cavernosa but not the glans or corpus spongiosum. There are multiple etiologies for priapism including sickle cell anemia, medications, spinal cord injury, leukemic infiltration, and idiopathy. Neither sedation nor ice water enemas are effective in reducing the erection. Corporeal aspiration followed by irrigation with saline or α-adrenergic agonists is performed in persistent cases.

20-11. **The answer is A** (Chapter 95). Testicular torsion is a urologic emergency. It can be difficult to distinguish clinically from torsion of the appendix testis or epididymitis. Urologic consultation for operative exploration should be obtained immediately when testicular torsion is suspected. Radionuclide scans and Doppler ultrasound studies may help confirm the diagnosis but are time consuming and have limited sensitivity and specificity. Manual detorsion should be attempted in the ED if there is any delay in surgical consultation.

20-12. **The answer is D** (Chapter 96). Noncontrast computed tomography (CT) is the diagnostic test of choice for kidney stones, with the advantages of speed, no need for radiocontrast material, and ability to detect alternate diagnoses. Plain films have poor sensitivity and specificity. A urine dipstick can be misleading, especially if hematuria is absent. Ultrasound can miss small stones and those in the middle third of the ureter. Sensitivity and specificity of ultrasound is slightly less than CT but is the study of choice in pregnancy.

20-13. **The answer is C** (Chapter 96). Stones <4 mm and in the distal ureter have a high likelihood of passing spontaneously. Patients with any of the other features should be hospitalized for management and urologic consultation. Patients with renal insufficiency, severe underlying disease, stones >5 mm, or evidence of complete obstruction should also be considered for admission and discussion with a urologist. Uncomplicated patients whose pain can be controlled with oral medications and whose stones are likely to pass may be discharged home with a urine strainer and outpatient follow-up with a urologist.

20-14. **The answer is A** (Chapter 97). Rifampin, phenazopyridine, beets, berries, rhubarb, iodide, and bromide are all causes of discolored urine that may be mistaken for hematuria. All the other choices are included in the broad differential diagnosis for hematuria. Schistosomiasis is the most common cause of hematuria worldwide. The patient's age, history, and urinalysis results help determine etiology. For example, bacteria and white blood cells are seen with infection. Red cell casts are found in rapidly progressive glomerulonephritis (usually associated with acute renal failure). Cancer is more likely in older smokers presenting with painless hematuria.

20-15. The answer is A (Chapter 98). Symptoms of bladder irritation such as mild flank pain, dysuria, urgency, and frequency are common in patients with ureteral stents. All of these patients should be evaluated for possible infection, but a urinalysis that is not suggestive of infection points to the diagnosis of bladder irritation. This may be treated with analgesics, anticholinergic medications, or in severe cases with belladonna alkaloid and opioid suppositories. Stent migration, urinary obstruction, or pyelonephritis is usually accompanied by severe flank pain. Microscopic hematuria in these patients is usually of no clinical significance, but gross hematuria is suggestive of a serious problem such as stent migration, and requires imaging studies to locate the stent position.

20-16. The answer is B (Chapter 99). Renal transplant patients receive aggressive immunosuppression therapy until 3–6 months posttransplant. In the first year after transplant, 40–80% of patients will experience at least one infection. The most common infections are mucocutaneous, commonly oropharyngeal, esophageal, or vaginal candidiasis. Urinary tract infections and respiratory infections are the next most likely sites of infection in the first posttransplant year, with meningitis being less likely.

20-17. The answer is D (Chapter 99). All of the drugs listed are commonly used immunosuppressant agents used to treat renal transplant patients. The initial posttransplant period begins with an induction regimen, followed by a modification after 3–6 months after the period of greatest risk of rejection has passed. Cyclosporine may be directly nephrotoxic and cause renal insufficiency and hypertension in these patients. Common side effects of prednisone include Cushing syndrome, hyperglycemia, adre-

nal suppression, and hyperlipidemia. Azathioprine can cause bone marrow suppression. Mycophenolate mofetil can also cause bone marrow suppression as well as diarrhea and vomiting. Transplant patients who are on cyclosporine should have drug levels and serum creatinine drawn to check for the possibility of drug toxicity and renal failure.

20-18. The answer is C (Chapter 100). Helical CT without intravenous contrast has become increasingly popular for many institutions as the modality of choice in evaluating renal colic. It has been shown to be 95–98% sensitive and 95% specific for detecting either renal calculi or hydronephrosis. In contrast, IVP (intravenous pyelography) has been shown to be 80–85% sensitive and 95% specific for detecting either renal calculi or hydronephrosis. Ultrasonography has a sensitivity of 65–93% and 90–95% specificity for detecting either renal calculi or hydronephrosis. Plain radiography of the kidneys, ureter, and bladder (KUB) can be used to identify renal calculi, but may be difficult to interpret because of the presence of phleboliths and bowel shadows. One study comparing plain radiography to IVP or CT found that KUB had a 45–60% sensitivity for identifying renal calculi.

20-19. The answer is B (Chapter 100). This patient should undergo retrograde urethrogram to evaluate a possible urethral injury prior to placement of a foley catheter. The exam may be performed in the resuscitation bay, and involves the insertion of 50–60 cc of radiocontrast solution into the urethral meatus using either a 60 cc syringe or a foley catheter inserted only 2 to 3 cm into the meatus. Fluoroscopy or plain radiographs of the urethra are then taken and examined for evidence of contrast extravasation. Helical abdominal CT, FAST (focused assessment with sonography in trauma) scan, and IVP (intravenous pyelogram) do not provide information about the integrity of the urethra.

Resuscitative Problems and Shock
Questions

21-1. You witness the sudden collapse of a middle-aged male at a college basketball game. He is pulseless and unresponsive. The emergency medical services (EMS) system is activated and bystander CPR is immediately started with adequate ventilations and compressions. EMS providers arrive after 5 minutes. The patient is still unresponsive and pulseless. The patient is placed on a cardiac monitor. Which finding on the monitor would be associated with the highest chance for survival?

(A) Regular, rate 30, P waves, narrow QRS complex.

(B) Regular, rate 110, P waves, narrow QRS complex.

(C) Irregular, rate 160, narrow QRS complex.

(D) An erratic tracing with variable amplitude and rate, indistinguishable complexes.

21-2. While jogging through the park on a warm summer afternoon you hear a man scream for help. At his side, you see a morbidly obese woman, standing in distress, with both hands grasping her neck. No one else is assisting her, but 911 has been called. She continues to coughing forcefully and is able to speak only 1 word at a time; however, she is not improving. What is the next MOST appropriate step?

(A) Encourage spontaneous efforts.

(B) Perform the Heimlich maneuver.

(C) Perform finger sweep.

(D) Perform chest thrusts.

21-3. Which of the following is NOT an acceptable indication for open-chest cardiac massage?

(A) Arrest after penetrating chest trauma with minimal downtime.

(B) Arrest after blunt trauma with signs of life in the ED.

(C) Arrest with severe hypothermia.

(D) Arrest due to myocardial infarction.

21-4. Which of the following is consistent with guidelines published by the American Heart Association in 2000?

(A) Compression depth in adults: 1–1.5 inches.

(B) Compression rate in adults: 100 per minute.

(C) Compression to ventilation ratio with 2 rescuers and a nonintubated victim: 5:1.

(D) Location of pulse check for lay rescuers: carotid.

21-5. A pregnant 15-year-old who is 28 weeks into the pregnancy arrives at the ED by private car in severe distress. She has ruptured her membranes and is having contractions. During your rapid assessment, the neonatal head is delivered. Thick particulate meconium is noted in the amniotic fluid. The nose, mouth, and pharynx are suctioned with a catheter, the infant is delivered, and the cord is clamped and cut. The neonate is placed under the radiant warmer, staff begin to dry the baby, and free-flow oxygen is administered. The child is blue and pale, has a weak cry, and has decreased muscle tone. Heart rate is estimated at 120. What is the next MOST appropriate step?

(A) Vigorous stimulation, assessment of reflex irritability, and continued bulb suction as necessary.

(B) Pharyngeal suction followed by repeated endotracheal intubation and extubation with suction until secretions clear.

(C) Pharyngeal suction, endotracheal intubation, and bag-valve mask ventilation.

(D) Pharyngeal suction, endotracheal intubation, bag-valve mask ventilation, and chest compressions.

21-6. A multigravida 25-year-old female delivers a term infant en route to the ED. The mother is healthy, had prenatal care without complication, and reports no substance abuse. She describes rupture of membranes that occurred approximately 30 minutes before delivery. The umbilical cord is clamped and cut, and the infant is placed under the radiant warmer and dried. No evidence of meconium is noted. The baby has a strong cry and good muscle tone but has subcostal retractions and is blue and pale. Heart rate is 150 beats per minute. The chest is enlarged, with decreased breath sounds on the left and cardiac impulse displaced to the right. No murmur is auscultated. The abdomen is scaphoid. What is the most likely cause of respiratory distress?

(A) Congenital diaphragmatic hernia.

(B) Tracheoesophageal fistula.

(C) Pneumothorax.

(D) Tetralogy of Fallot.

21-7. A 1-week-old infant presents with a history of poor feeding. The child is afebrile with a heart rate of 160 beats per minute and respirations of 40 breaths per minute. The child is noted to have fine movements of the limbs that respond to stimuli and stop with manual stimulation. There are no accompanying movements of the eyes or tongue. Blood glucose is found to be 21 mg/dL. After IV access is obtained, what is the MOST appropriate dose of IV glucose to administer?

(A) 4 cc/kg of D10W.

(B) 4 cc/kg of D25W.

(C) 2 cc/kg of D25NS.

(D) 1 cc/kg of D50.

21-8. Which of the following statements regarding the pediatric airway is TRUE?

(A) The MacIntosh blade is preferred in children younger than 2–4 years of age.

(B) Using the standard age-based formula for estimating endotracheal tube size, a normal 4-year-old child would require a 4-mm endotracheal tube.

(C) The blind finger sweep is the preferred maneuver to clear a suspected airway obstruction in an unconscious child when advanced airway equipment is unavailable.

(D) A child is more likely than an adult to develop airway obstruction due to positional variation.

21-9. A 2-year-old female is brought to the ED by paramedics in cardiac arrest. Per the paramedic report, the victim was playing with her older brother, then suddenly stopped breathing. The child was previously healthy, and there were no signs of trauma at the scene. The child's father has accompanied the child to the ED. He is in severe emotional distress and is unable to assist with the history. The child is cyanotic, flaccid, and unresponsive. Attempts to ventilate the child are made with a bag-valve mask, but chest rise is not seen and no breath sounds are audible. There is no pulse. Rhythm is sinus at a rate of 88. CPR is in progress. Vascular access was attempted once en route but was unsuccessful. No medications have been given. Total time from onset of event is estimated at 9 minutes. What is the MOST appropriate next step?

(A) Bilateral needle thoracostomy.

(B) Immediate circulatory access.

(C) Direct laryngoscopy.

(D) Terminate efforts.

21-10. A 2-year-old male is rushed in by his parents after being found unconscious near open bottles of his grandfather's medications. The airway is secure, and successful bag-valve ventilations are started. He is pulseless and unresponsive. Intravenous access is being obtained. The cardiac monitor shows a wide complex tachycardia at a rate of 260. What is the next step in management?

(A) Shock the patient with 200 J.

(B) Shock the patient with 0.5 J/kg.

(C) Shock the patient with 2 J/kg.

(D) Administer epinephrine 0.01 mg/kg IV.

21-11. A 6-year-old male is brought in by paramedics because parents noted decreased responsiveness. The child was seen in your facility 2 days prior and discharged with a diagnosis of acute gastroenteritis. Vital signs include a blood pressure of 70/22 mmHg, heart rate of 184 beats per minute, temperature of 39.8°C, respiratory rate of 44 breaths per minute, and O_2 saturation of 90% on room air; child's weight is 20 kg. The patient is lethargic. The airway is patent without secretions, and breathing is spontaneous, shallow, and rapid. Distal pulses are rapid, regular, and weak. Eyes are closed and do not open to command. All extremities are moving spontaneously. Oxygen is administered via nonrebreather face mask, and peripheral venous access is obtained. Aggressive fluid resuscitation is started, without improvement in vitals. Exam is most significant for diffuse abdominal tenderness and peritoneal signs. Extremities are cool with weak peripheral pulses. Cultures are drawn, labs are sent, antibiotics are administered, and consultants are notified. X-rays are pending. However, despite vigorous resuscitation, respiratory status deteriorates. You decide to intubate the patient. Which of the following is the best induction agent for this child?

(A) Ketamine.

(B) Thiopental.

(C) Propofol.

(D) Midazolam.

21-12. A 4-year-old female with trisomy 21 presents with a 1-day history of fever, vomiting, and altered mental status. She is obese but active and was riding her bike yesterday when she began feeling sick. She has a past history of a seizure disorder for which she takes phenobarbital. She is lethargic, and the airway is unprotected. Vital signs are blood pressure of 110/68, heart rate of 148, temperature of 41°C, and respiratory rate of 28. Oxygen saturation cannot be obtained due to a poor waveform. Weight is 24 kg. The patient has a very short neck, small mouth, and large tongue, but bag-valve mask ventilation appears to be working successfully. What combination of medications is MOST appropriate for rapid sequence intubation?

(A) Atropine, ketamine, and rocuronium.

(B) Atropine, etomidate, and succinylcholine.

(C) Versed and vecuronium.

(D) Ketamine and succinylcholine.

21-13. Which of the following is TRUE regarding maternal physiology in normal pregnancy?

(A) Tidal volume increases significantly.

(B) Oxygen consumption decreases.

(C) Cardiac output increases steadily until delivery.

(D) Mean arterial blood pressure increases.

21-14. Which of the following statements is TRUE regarding ACLS in pregnancy?

(A) The method of chest compressions is unchanged prior to 20 weeks of gestation.

(B) During the third trimester, aortocaval compression can be minimized in the supine patient if an assistant displaces the uterus to the right.

(C) Epinephrine is category D in pregnancy and should not be used during resuscitation because it may cause uteroplacental vasoconstriction.

(D) Fetal viability should be evaluated prior to initiating perimortem cesarean section in the term victim presenting in cardiac arrest.

21-15. Which of the following statements best describes current consensus on ethical issues related to resuscitation?

(A) Family members of your patient should be discouraged from observing resuscitative efforts.

(B) Postmortem procedures should not be done on recently deceased patients for teaching purposes.

(C) Physicians may withhold a requested intervention such as CPR if they judge the intervention to have no realistic chance of providing benefit.

(D) There is little downside to performing resuscitative efforts that are judged to be futile.

21-16. Which of the following statements about the laryngeal mask airway (LMA) is TRUE?

(A) The LMA can provide an effective airway if bag-valve mask ventilation is unsuccessful or if endotracheal intubation has failed.

(B) Proper LMA placement requires visualization of the larynx.

(C) LMA placement decreases the risk of aspiration in the conscious patient.

(D) The LMA can stay in placed for an indefinite amount of time.

21-17. A 62-year-old male with a history of coronary artery disease, congestive heart failure, and emphysema on home oxygen comes in complaining of chest pain and shortness of breath. For the past 2 days he has had URI symptoms. He has been intubated twice before, most recently 3 months ago, and required a 2-week stay in the ICU. He has no known drug allergies. He is agitated, is having respiratory difficulty, and cannot list his medications. He is full code. Vital signs are blood pressure of 106/52 mmHg, heart rate of 138 beats per minute, temperature of 38°C, respiratory rate of 34, O_2 saturation of 84% on nonrebreather face mask. He is distressed, agitated, and uncooperative. The airway is patent but with copious secretions. Breath sounds are severely diminished but symmetric bilaterally. Pulse is irregular and rapid. IV access is obtained, and the patient is given aspirin, nitroglycerin, and furosemide, but he is not improving. What is the MOST appropriate step in management of the airway?

(A) Decrease the concentration of oxygen delivery.

(B) Initiate CPAP therapy.

(C) Initiate BIPAP therapy.

(D) Perform rapid sequence intubation (RSI).

21-18. Which of the following statements regarding endotracheal intubation in adults is TRUE?

(A) Preoxygenation in the conscious patient with adequate tidal volume is best accomplished with an oral airway and a properly fitting bag-valve mask.

(B) Observing symmetric chest rise and auscultation is still the quickest and most accurate method of confirming endotracheal intubation.

(C) Nasotracheal intubation is no longer a recommended airway strategy because of associated discomfort, risk of aspiration, significant incidence of profound epistaxis, and risk of significant vagal-induced bradycardia.

(D) Digital intubation does not require visualization of the vocal cords.

21-19. Which of the following nondepolarizing paralytic agents has the shortest onset of action?

(A) Atracurium.

(B) Vecuronium.

(C) Rocuronium.

(D) Pancuronium.

21-20. A 52-year-old obese male presents with new-onset shortness of breath. Despite treatment he appears to be worsening. Because of his body habitus you are concerned about the possibility of a difficult airway. While asking him to extend his tongue you are able to visualize the tongue and hard palate but cannot see the faucial pillars, the soft palate, or the uvula. By Mallampati criteria, what class airway is this?

(A) I.

(B) II.

(C) II.

(D) IV.

21-21. A blunt trauma patient is comatose after significant head injury. There is no visible face or neck injury. He is obese with significant micrognathia and a full beard. He is desaturating despite dual-operator bag-valve mask ventilation and an adjunct oral airway in place. Orotracheal intubation has failed twice. An intubating laryngeal mask airway (ILMA) is inserted, allowing adequate oxygenation and ventilation. What is the next step in establishing definitive airway management?

(A) Orotracheal intubation through the ILMA.

(B) Emergent needle cricothyroidotomy with jet ventilation.

(C) Emergent surgical cricothyroidotomy.

(D) Emergent tracheostomy.

21-22. An adult male trauma patient requires an emergent cricothyroidotomy for airway management after failed rapid sequence intubation due to body habitus. A 5-mm endotracheal tube is advanced 5 cm into the trachea and the tube cuff is inflated. Minimal venous blood is noted at the incision site. An inline capnometer confirms exchange of CO_2. Moderate resistance to ventilation is noted. As the tube is being stabilized, the patient acutely deteriorates, becoming hypoxic and hypotensive. Which of the following is MOST likely to benefit the patient?

(A) Needle thoracostomy.

(B) Exchange of the endotracheal tube with a larger one.

(C) Normal saline bolus.

(D) Suction.

21-23. Which of the following statements regarding central venous access (subclavian, internal jugular, or femoral) is TRUE?

(A) Arterial punctures are most common with internal jugular access.

(B) Infection is most common with internal jugular access.

(C) Thrombosis is most common with subclavian vein access.

(D) Malposition is least common with the femoral approach.

21-24. Which of the following statements regarding vascular access in children is TRUE?

(A) Intraosseous access is contraindicated in children older than 5 years.

(B) Intraosseous access is associated with more infection-related complications than peripheral access.

(C) In neonates, the infection rate from umbilical vein access is equivalent to that from peripheral venous access.

(D) All venous cutdown techniques require sacrificing the vein.

21-25. Which of the following statements is TRUE regarding accessing indwelling catheters?

(A) Arteriovenous shunts should never be accessed in the ED except for dialysis.

(B) An externalized device can be flushed with normal saline.

(C) Coagulation studies drawn from indwelling devices are often unreliable.

(D) An implanted device should be flushed with 100 U/mL heparin solution.

21-26. Which of the following statements regarding arterial cannulation is TRUE?

(A) Ischemic complications of arterial cannulation requiring surgical intervention are common.

(B) Radial artery cannulation is associated with lower infection rates than femoral artery cannulation.

(C) Radial artery cutdown is discouraged because it involves sacrificing the artery.

(D) The umbilical artery is the most accessible artery for arterial cannulation in the neonate.

21-27. Which of the following statements regarding pulmonary artery catheters is TRUE?

(A) Pulmonary artery catheter placement is associated with a decrease in mortality.

(B) Septic, neurogenic, and cardiogenic shock are all associated with decreased systemic vascular resistance.

(C) Cardiogenic shock is the only form of shock associated with an increased pulmonary wedge pressure.

(D) Hypovolemic shock is associated with decreased cardiac output, decreased pulmonary capillary wedge pressure, and decreased systemic vascular resistance.

21-28. A 68-year-old man loses consciousness in the hospital parking lot. CPR is started within seconds of his collapse. A bystander reports the patient jerking several times after collapsing. Total downtime is 2 minutes.

Ventilation is adequate with a bag-valve mask device with symmetric chest rise and equal breath sounds. He remains pulseless and unresponsive. The initial rhythm on the monitor is ventricular tachycardia, but while preparing to defibrillate, the patient's entire body jerks once forcefully, and the person performing chest compressions reports receiving an electrical shock. The rhythm converts to sinus tachycardia. What is the next MOST appropriate course of action?

(A) Place a magnet over the subcutaneous device to prevent further defibrillation during resuscitation.

(B) Instruct all staff to stand clear for 30 seconds before resuming care in order to avoid serious injury.

(C) Hold chest compressions and check for a pulse.

(D) Continue with defibrillation because the device may be malfunctioning.

21-29. Which of the following statements is TRUE regarding clinical management after acute anoxic brain injury?

(A) The most important treatment is reestablishing spontaneous circulation.

(B) Mannitol is helpful in the acute management of ischemic brain injury.

(C) Hyperglycemia is correlated with improved outcomes after ischemic brain injury.

(D) Tissue plasminogen activator is beneficial in anoxic brain injury.

21-30. Which of the following statements is TRUE regarding the use of epinephrine during cardiac arrest?

(A) High-dose epinephrine protocols lead to improved neurologic outcome.

(B) Escalating-dose epinephrine protocols lead to improved neurologic outcome.

(C) Conventional-dose epinephrine (1 mg in adults) is superior to placebo based on large randomized controlled trials in improving neurologic outcome.

(D) Conventional-dose epinephrine recommendations are based on animal models and anecdotal clinical evidence.

21-31. Which of the following assessment techniques is MOST likely to be clinically useful in predicting the likelihood of successful resuscitation after cardiac arrest?

(A) Serial blood gases.

(B) End-tidal CO_2 monitoring.

(C) Ventricular fibrillation waveform analysis.

(D) Invasive hemodynamic pressure monitoring.

21-32. An obtunded patient is found to have an elevated anion gap, indicating the presence of a wide anion gap metabolic acidosis. What information may be gained by calculating the delta gap in a patient with an elevated anion gap acidosis?

(A) The delta gap calculation can diagnose methanol poisoning.

(B) The delta gap calculation can help detect the presence of a concomitant acute respiratory acidosis or alkalosis.

(C) The delta gap calculation can help detect the presence of a concomitant metabolic alkalosis or the presence of a concomitant nonanion gap metabolic acidosis.

(D) The delta gap calculation can distinguish diabetic ketoacidosis from alcoholic ketoacidosis.

21-33. Blood gas analysis for a pregnant patient suspected of having diabetic ketoacidosis reveals a normal pH. On further evaluation, the serum P_{CO_2} and HCO_3^- are both decreased. Which of the following best describes this patient's acid-base disturbance?

(A) Metabolic acidosis and metabolic alkalosis.

(B) Metabolic acidosis and respiratory alkalosis.

(C) Metabolic alkalosis and respiratory acidosis.

(D) Physiologic compensation and no acid-base disturbance.

21-34. Pulse oximetry is used frequently in the ED as a noninvasive measurement of arterial oxygen saturation. In some clinical situations, the pulse oximetry measurement will be falsely elevated and should not be relied upon. In which of the following clinical scenarios would the pulse oximeter reading be expected to be falsely elevated?

(A) Cyanide poisoning.

(B) Chronic obstructive pulmonary disease.

(C) Carbon monoxide poisoning.

(D) Neonate who is producing fetal hemoglobin.

21-35. A patient arrives in the ED via ambulance with cardiopulmonary resuscitation in progress. The patient is intubated, and an end-tidal CO_2 monitor is attached to the endotracheal tube. The monitor reads a value of 8 mmHg. The endotracheal tube is visually verified and is seen passing through the vocal cords. Which of the following clinical conditions could explain this low reading?

(A) The patient is hyperthermic.

(B) The patient is hypoventilatory following aggressive oxygen therapy for a chronic obstructive pulmonary disease exacerbation.

(C) The patient received 2 ampules of $NaHCO_3$ during resuscitation efforts in route to the ED.

(D) The patient has had a massive pulmonary embolism.

21-36. A patient with a 5-day history of severe nausea and vomiting is found to have a serum sodium concentration of 165 mEq/L, and urine osmolality of >1000 mOsm/kg water. Which of the following intravenous fluid choices would be the BEST choice for beginning volume repletion for this patient?

(A) Normal saline.

(B) 0.45% normal saline.

(C) D_5W.

(D) 3% saline.

21-37. What is the MOST common cause of an elevated potassium finding in the ED?

(A) Excess intake of potassium supplements.

(B) Hemolysis during phlebotomy.

(C) Potassium-sparing diuretics.

(D) Renal failure.

21-38. A 57-year-old female is brought to the ED by ambulance complaining of lightheadedness and palpitations beginning 30 minutes prior to arrival. The patient is placed on a monitor, and the rhythm strip shown in Figure 21-1 is obtained. The patient is noted to have an accompanying blood pressure of 90/40 mmHg, a respiratory rate of 20 breaths per minute, and an oxygen saturation of 92% on room air. Which of the following preexisting conditions could make cardioversion of this rhythm contraindicated?

(A) History of previous successful cardioversions for these symptoms.

(B) History of chronic obstructive pulmonary disease.

(C) History of current digoxin therapy with recent increase in dosage.

(D) Failure of vagal maneuvers to induce cardioversion during ambulance transport.

21-39. A 70-year-old male has electrocardiogram changes consistent with an acute inferior myocardial infarction. Shortly after being placed on a monitor, his cardiac rhythm is a second-degree Mobitz type I (Wenckebach) atrioventricular block. His ventricular rate has fallen from 60 to 38 beats per minute and is accompanied by a decrease in blood pressure to 80/40 mmHg and a decreased level of consciousness. Which of the following chemical therapies would be MOST appropriate for treating this symptomatic heart block?

(A) Atropine.

(B) Isoproterenol.

(C) Nitroglycerin.

(D) No therapy.

21-40. Which of the following is the MOST common adverse effect seen in the acute setting in patients who receive intravenous amiodarone?

(A) Change in mental status.

(B) Tachycardia.

(C) Pulmonary edema.

(D) Hypotension.

21-41. For which of the following rhythms would intravenous diltiazem therapy be contraindicated?

(A) Paroxysmal supraventricular tachycardia.

(B) Atrial fibrillation.

(C) Wide-complex tachycardias.

(D) Atrial flutter.

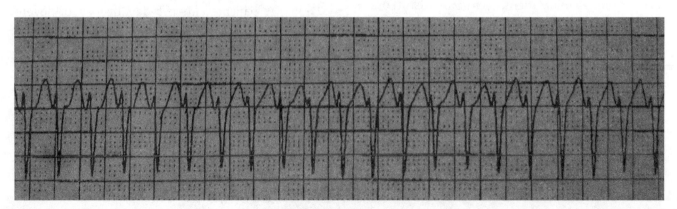

Figure 21-1.

21-42. Which of the following is NOT a concern about stored blood products (packed red blood cells)?

(A) Stored red blood cells have depleted 2,3-diphosphoglycerate, leading to decreased offloading of oxygen at the tissue level.

(B) Stored blood products exacerbate splanchnic hypoperfusion.

(C) The increased pliability of stored red blood cells allows them to seep into the interstitium.

(D) Stored red blood cells are characterized as having decreased deformability.

21-43. A 65-year-old patient from a long-term nursing facility presents with altered mental status. You notice an indwelling Foley catheter with turbid urine. The patient currently has no peripheral intravenous access and is hypotensive. You successfully place a right internal jugular intravenous catheter. Which of the following parameters is LEAST helpful for detecting systemic hypoperfusion?

(A) $ScvO_2$.

(B) Base deficit.

(C) Urine output.

(D) Arterial lactate level.

21-44. Which of the following sets of data constitute the 4 clinical criteria of systemic inflammatory response syndrome (SIRS)?

(A) Temperature (T) >37°C or <36°C, heart rate (HR) >100 bpm, respiratory rate (RR) >20, white blood cell count (WBC) >12,000 × 10⁹/L.

(B) T >38°C or <36°C, HR >90 bpm, $PACO_2$ <35 mmHg, >2% immature bands.

(C) T >38°C or <36°C, HR >90 bpm, $PACO_2$ <32 mmHg, >10% immature bands.

(D) T >38°C or <34°C, HR >90 bpm, $PACO_2$ <32 mmHg, WBC >12,000 × 10⁹/L.

21-45. Larger benefits for the treatment of patients with severe sepsis or septic shock in the ED are seen with which of the following therapies?

(A) Early-goal-directed therapy employing early detection of patients with evidence of tissue hypoperfusion and goal-directed administration of fluids and vasopressors.

(B) Administration of activated protein C for patients with evidence of multiple organ failure in the setting of sepsis.

(C) Administration of corticosteroids in septic patients with evidence of adrenal insufficiency.

(D) Administration of intravenous antitumor necrosis factor antibodies in patients with sepsis.

21-46. What is the most common cause of mortality in patients with acute myocardial infarction?

(A) Stroke.

(B) Pulmonary embolism.

(C) Cardiogenic shock.

(D) Oliguric acute renal failure.

21-47. What is the most common cause of severe allergic reaction in the United States?

(A) *Hymenoptera* stings.

(B) Penicillin or other antibiotics.

(C) Shellfish.

(D) Peanuts.

21-48. Which of the following substances is known to induce an anaphylactoid or non-IgE-mediated hypersensitivity reaction?

(A) Peanuts.

(B) Radiocontrast.

(C) Shellfish.

(D) Antibiotics.

21-49. Spinal cord injury is most commonly caused by which of the following?

(A) Motor vehicle accident.

(B) Gunshot wound.

(C) Knife wound.

(D) Fall from height.

Resuscitative Problems and Shock
Answers, Explanations, and References

21-1. **The answer is D** (Chapter 11). This patient is presenting with sudden cardiac arrest. Sudden cardiac death (SCD) is most commonly associated with ischemic heart disease. Nonischemic cardiomyopathies (dilated, hypertrophic) are less commonly associated with SCD. The remaining cardiovascular abnormalities associated with SCD (valvular, infiltrative, congenital) contribute to relatively few cases. Factors associated with increased likelihood of survival with sudden cardiac arrest include having a witnessed event, early CPR, and early defibrillation of an appropriate rhythm. Sudden cardiac arrest correlates positively with survival if the initial rhythm is a ventricular tachyarrhythmia, especially ventricular tachycardia, although ventricular fibrillation is the most commonly encountered tachyarrhythmia in SCD. Sudden cardiac arrest correlates with poor survival when the initial encountered rhythm is pulseless electrical activity (PEA) or asystole. Combined with an unresponsive and pulseless patient, any organized rhythm such as sinus bradycardia (A), sinus tachycardia (B), or atrial fibrillation (C) would clinically indicate PEA and likely result in a bad outcome. The tracing described in answer (D), however, is ventricular fibrillation and, compared to the other scenarios, would correlate best with survival.

21-2. **The answer is A** (Chapter 12). This patient presents with acute distress and the universal sign for an airway obstruction, both hands grasping the neck. Techniques to clear an obstructed adult airway without the presence of advanced airway equipment include the Heimlich maneuver, chest thrusts, and finger sweep. Choice of technique is based on the patient's level of consciousness and body habitus. In the conscious patient, however, none are indicated if the patient is able to forcefully cough, speak, and visibly or audibly exchange air and is not deteriorating. Therefore, the correct action is to encourage spontaneous efforts to remove the obstruction. Performing a maneuver when not indicated may lead to unnecessary injury and worsening obstruction and may interfere with more effective spontaneous efforts. In the conscious patient who is deteriorating or who presents with inadequate spontaneous efforts (unable to speak, inadequate cough, inadequate air exchange, cyanosis, deteriorating consciousness), the standing Heimlich maneuver is indicated. If the patient becomes unresponsive or is found unresponsive with an airway obstruction, the finger sweep is initially recommended, followed by the prone Heimlich maneuver, repeating this sequence until the rescuer is successful. Chest thrusts are reserved for the late gravid female or the morbidly obese patient.

21-3. **The answer is D** (Chapter 12). ED thoracotomy accompanied by open-chest cardiac compressions should be considered in patients who arrest after penetrating trauma to the chest or abdomen or after blunt trauma, although recommendations vary with regard to downtime. Outcome is better after penetrating trauma, when a reversible cause is identified. Arrest from severe hypothermia is also an acceptable indication for ED thoracotomy, allowing for aggressive mediastinal rewarming and open cardiac massage. ED thoracotomy and open cardiac massage is not recommended after cardiac arrest from most medical conditions, including ischemic heart disease.

21-4. **The answer is B** (Chapter 12). According to the most recent guidelines published by the American Heart Association in 2000, the recommended rate for chest compressions in adults is approximately 100 per minute. The recommended compression depth in adults is 1.5–2 inches. Compression to ventilation ratio for a nonintubated patient with 1 or 2 rescuers is 15:2. With 2 rescuers for an intubated patient, the recommended ratio is 5:1. For health care rescuers, the recommended location for a pulse check is the carotid artery, although the femoral artery may also be used. Since lay rescuers may have technical difficulty with pulse assessment that could lead to incorrect or delayed intervention, they are instead taught to quickly evaluate for alternate signs of perfusion rather than check for a pulse.

21-5. **The answer is B** (Chapter 13). This neonate has multiple risk factors that correlate with the need for neonatal resuscitation including extremes of maternal age, prematurity, precipitous delivery, and thick meconium in the amniotic fluid. Other risk factors can include maternal diabetes or hypertension, sepsis, trauma, shock, inadequate prenatal care, maternal substance abuse, abnormal presentation, multiple gestation, and umbilical cord prolapse. Although maintaining body temperature, suctioning, and stimulation are the mainstay of routine newborn resuscitation, stimulation should be delayed in this case because of the risk of significant meconium aspiration. Recommended management includes pharyngeal suction followed by repeated endotracheal intubation and extubation with suction until secretions clear. Once the airway is clear,

the neonate can be vigorously stimulated. Positive pressure ventilation (PPV) is not indicated if respiratory effort improves with airway clearance and stimulation as long as the heart rate (HR) remains >100. In this case PPV without proper endotracheal suction will increase the risk of meconium aspiration. Neonatal chest compressions at 120 per minute or greater are indicated only if the HR <60. In general, pharmacological therapy with epinephrine is indicated if the HR does not respond after 30 seconds of chest compressions.

21-6. **The answer is A** (Chapter 13). Congenital diaphragmatic hernia presents with respiratory distress soon after birth. Clinical features include dyspnea, cyanosis, retractions, unilateral decreased breath sounds with a displaced cardiac impulse, and a scaphoid abdomen. Careful auscultation may reveal bowel sounds within the chest cavity on the affected side. Pneumothorax in the newborn is usually associated with prematurity or delivery requiring aggressive resuscitation especially after aspiration, intrapartum asphyxia, or any form of positive pressure ventilation (PPV). Decreased breath sounds, mediastinal shift, and distant heart sounds may be present, however, a scaphoid abdomen is not characteristic. Tracheoesophageal (TE) fistulas present with respiratory distress temporally related to feedings. Exam is unremarkable unless associated abnormalities exist (i.e., an imperforate anus). There are 5 types of TE fistula, the most common being upper esophageal atresia with a distal fistula. Tetralogy of Fallot (TOF) is characterized by a ventricular septal defect (VSD), overriding aorta, right ventricular outflow obstruction, and right ventricular hypertrophy. This neonate does not have a VSD murmur, and the other physical findings are inconsistent with TOF.

21-7. **The answer is A** (Chapter 13). Hypoglycemia in neonates is best treated with 2–4 cc/kg of D10W. Higher concentrations of glucose are associated with phlebitis, extravasation, and rebound hypoglycemia. Hypoglycemia in children is treated with 2–4 cc/kg of D25W. Adult hypoglycemia is treated with ampules of D50.

21-8. **The answer is D** (Chapter 14). The MacIntosh (curved) blade is generally not recommended in children younger than 2–4 years because it is often difficult to displace the flaccid epiglottis with indirect upward pressure on the vallecula. The Miller (straight) blade allows direct displacement• of the epiglottis and easier visualization of the cords. Additionally, the straight blade is more forgiving than the curved blade if an incorrect size is used. The standard age-based formula for estimating endotracheal tube size [(16+ years in age)/4] is more accurate than estimating appropriate tube size based on the diameter of the little finger. Using this formula, the correct initial tube size in a 4-year-old is 5 mm. Length-based charts (Breslow) are also accurate in selecting equipment size and provide the advantage of simultaneously selecting medication dosing. Use uncuffed tubes in children younger than 8 years to prevent pressure-related injury to the trachea. Although recommended in unconscious adults, the blind finger sweep is not a recommended maneuver for clearing a suspected foreign body from the pediatric airway. In unconscious children younger than 1 year, back blows and chest thrusts are recommended. As in adults, abdominal thrusts are recommended for unconscious children older than 1 year. Once advanced airway equipment is available, McGill forceps combined with direct laryngoscopy are used to remove a foreign body. Because of multiple anatomical reasons such as flaccid cartilage, disproportionate tongue and epiglottis size, and occipital prominence, the pediatric airway is much more sensitive to obstruction from positional variation. In children, it is important to maintain the head in the sniffing position, use the jaw-thrust technique to prevent posterior displacement of the tongue, consider using an oral airway in the unconscious child, and

meticulously reassess for evidence of obstruction.

21-9. **The answer is C** (Chapter 14). Cardiac arrest in children has extremely poor prognosis since it often results from prolonged hypoxia or from a severe comorbid condition (SIDS, trauma, sepsis, shock), rather than a primary cardiogenic cause. This child had been otherwise healthy with no report of trauma. The sudden onset of cardiopulmonary arrest in this age group and the unsuccessful bag-valve mask ventilation should alert the clinician to an airway obstruction. Direct laryngoscopy is indicated to rule out an obstruction and establish a patent airway. Initiating circulatory access would be time-consuming, delay necessary airway management, and would be unlikely to benefit clinically if hypoxia continues. It would be premature to terminate efforts without ruling out an airway obstruction and a reasonable trial of resuscitation, especially since total downtime has been only 9 minutes. Bilateral needle thoracostomy and subsequent chest tube could be life-saving if a pneumothorax were present, but this diagnosis is unlikely given the clinical picture in the absence of trauma.

21-10. **The answer is C** (Chapter 14). Although ventricular tachycardia and ventricular fibrillation are uncommon in children, they can occur with toxidromes or severe metabolic derangement. This child has pulseless ventricular tachycardia and should be immediately defibrillated. The appropriate initial energy setting for defibrillation in pediatric patients is 2 J/kg, then doubled for subsequent attempts. Cardioversion of unstable tachyarrhythmias with a pulse begins at 0.5 J/kg and if unsuccessful is doubled for subsequent attempts. Epinephrine is indicated for pulseless arrest with ventricular tachycardia in children **after** unsuccessful defibrillation.

21-11. **The answer is A** (Chapter 15). This patient is septic with unstable vital signs not responding to fluid resuscitation. Although all of the agents listed can be used for induction, both thiopental and propofol have a significant propensity to cause hypotension and would not be recommended in this case. Midazolam usually does not cause significant hypotension, except in cases of extreme hypovolemia or critical illness, such as this one. Ketamine is most appropriate, especially since it is likely to cause some cardiovascular stimulation, a side effect that might be helpful in this clinical situation.

21-12. **The answer is B** (Chapter 15). The overwhelming concern in this case is the potential for a difficult airway. Not only is this child obese (24 kg at 4 years of age), but she also has Down syndrome with a characteristic phenotype that may make the airway difficult to secure. In terms of paralytics, succinylcholine is the best choice because it has a short duration of action—an advantage if rapid sequence intubation (RSI) fails. This patient does not have any known contraindication to succinylcholine. It should be administered concurrently with atropine in children younger than 5 years of age. This combination works well with etomidate as an induction agent. Rocuronium and vecuronium are relatively contraindicated because failed RSI will leave the patient without an airway for up to 45 minutes. Ketamine and succinylcholine are a good induction and paralytic combination in this case, but neither should be given without atropine in the child younger than 5 years due to potential vagal side effects (bradycardia and increased secretions). In this patient, it might also be reasonable to attempt endotracheal tube placement without paralysis or to temporarily secure the airway with a laryngeal mask airway if available.

21-13. **The answer is A** (Chapter 16). Despite enlargement of the uterus, tidal volume increases significantly in pregnancy, likely due to progesterone-mediated increases in chest diameter and diaphragm excursion.

Maternal oxygen consumption increases dramatically to accommodate the associated increase in basal metabolic rate. Maternal cardiac output increases steadily for the first two trimesters but then begins to decrease in the third trimester due to decreased stroke volume secondary to uterine obstruction of the vena cava and decreased venous return. However, cardiac output remains elevated from baseline throughout pregnancy. Maternal blood pressure decreases during pregnancy, then returns to normal by the end of gestation. Hypertension with pregnancy is abnormal, and hypertensive disorders of pregnancy are a source of significant pregnancy-related mortality.

21-14. **The answer is A** (Chapter 16). The method of chest compressions is unchanged prior to 20 weeks gestation. After 20 weeks, recommended alterations to assist standard chest compressions include displacing the uterus to the **left** or tilting the patient 15 to 30 degrees if a tilt table or Cardiff wedge is available. Most ACLS medications including epinephrine, vasopressin, adenosine, lidocaine, procainamide, dopamine, and dobutamine are category C in pregnancy, meaning safety is uncertain, but no studies have shown an adverse effect. One notable exception is amiodarone, which is category D, regarded as unsafe. Atropine and magnesium are category B, presumed safe in animal studies. Although recommendations regarding management of maternal arrest and perimortem cesarean section are largely based on case reports, it is generally recommended for delivery of the fetus to be completed within five minutes of maternal arrest for best chance of a meaningful outcome. Prior to perimortem cesarean, the physician should focus on ideal maternal resuscitation and prepare for the upcoming surgery and newborn resuscitation. Time should not be spent attempting to evaluate fetal viability.

21-15. **The answer is C** (Chapter 17). Although the concept of medical futility has proven both difficult to define and difficult to incorporate into practice, consensus sentiment favors the thought that a physician may withhold a medical intervention judged to have no realistic chance of providing benefit. Current opinion favors allowing family members to be present during resuscitation if they so desire. However, to provide the best experience for all involved, family members should be accompanied by a chaperone, and the resuscitation team should be notified in advance of their presence. Although some might have strong opinions about not performing postmortem procedures on patients because of issues of consent, disrespect, or disfigurement, others would argue that postmortem procedures provide a unique learning opportunity without inflicting harm that can provide a potential benefit to future patients. Thus, choice (B) does not reflect an overall consensus sentiment. Potential downsides to performing futile interventions on patients include the cost of the intervention, the cost of prolonging a life that most would not consider meaningful, and the shuttling of resources away from areas that could provide much more benefit.

21-16. **The answer is A** (Chapter 18). The LMA is useful as a temporary airway in situations where bag-valve mask ventilation and orotracheal intubation have both been unsuccessful. The LMA is inserted blindly, requiring no direct visualization of the larynx. Despite having a cuff that inflates over the laryngeal inlet, like most temporary measures, it does not provide adequate protection against aspiration. Additionally, aspiration risk is increased when an LMA is used in a conscious patient.

21-17. **The answer is D** (Chapter 18). Although there is some concern of decreasing respiratory drive in patients with chronic CO_2 retention by administering too much oxygen, oxygen delivery should not be decreased in patients with acute respiratory distress and uncorrectable hypoxia. Noninvasive positive pressure ventilation (NIPPV) in the form of continuous positive airway pressure (CPAP) or bilevel positive airway pressure (BIPAP) may decrease the need for intubation and the associated morbidity in patients with emphysema and congestive heart failure; however, this patient has several contraindications to NIPPV including copious airway secretions, agitation, and the inability to cooperate. Despite the high likelihood of developing a ventilator-associated complication, RSI appears to be unavoidable in this patient. Paralysis and positive pressure ventilation may actually improve his hemodynamic status and decrease the workload on the heart.

21-18. **The answer is D** (Chapter 19). Preoxygenation in the conscious patient with adequate tidal volume is best accomplished with a tight-fitting oxygen mask and reservoir. A bag-valve mask with an oral airway is used for preoxygenation of the **unconscious** patient. Immediate confirmation of tube placement should not depend solely on symmetric chest rise and equal breath sounds. Auscultation should be performed in conjunction with another confirmatory method. Typical confirmatory measures are inline capnometry/capnography or an aspiration device (bulb or syringe). Unexpected deterioration in clinical status such as hypoxia or bradycardia immediately after intubation should raise suspicion of improper tube location despite prior confirmatory measures. Chest x-ray is indicated after intubation to confirm proper tube placement and aid in adjustment of tube depth. Nasotracheal intubation is increasingly becoming a lost art but has specific indications, especially when difficult endotracheal access is anticipated in the conscious patient (habitus, oral trauma, angioedema, Ludwig's angina). If successful, it can prevent the need for a surgical airway. Digital intubation is performed in the unconscious, paralyzed patient and is indicated as an alternative method after failed RSI. Tube placement is guided via tactile recognition of the epiglottis. Laryngeal visualization is not required.

21-19. **The answer is C** (Chapter 19). Onset of action and duration of effect are both important factors in choosing a paralytic for rapid sequence intubation (RSI). Rapid onset allows quicker access to a definitive airway, while short duration allows more rapid return to spontaneous respiration in the event of failed RSI. Succinylcholine is the drug of choice in most cases because it has the shortest onset (45–60 seconds) and duration (5–9 minutes). When paralysis is required and succinylcholine is contraindicated, a nondepolarizing agent must be used. Of the available nondepolarizing agents, rocuronium has the shortest onset of action (as short as 1 minute), while the others take a minimum of 2 minutes to take effect. Duration of action from rocuronium ranges from 30 to 45 minutes. Higher doses allow for more rapid onset at the expense of prolonging the duration of effect.

21-20. **The answer is D** (Chapter 19). The Mallampati classification system is often used to help predict difficulty with intubation. With a Class I airway (rare failure), the faucial pillars, soft palate, and uvula are visualized. With a Class II airway (rare failure), the faucial pillars and soft palate are visualized, but the tongue partially obstructs the uvula. With a Class III airway (moderate chance of failure), only the soft palate and base of the uvula are visualized. With a Class IV airway (high chance of failure), only the hard palate is visualized.

21-21. **The answer is A** (Chapter 20). The airway has been stabilized with an ILMA, however, more definitive airway access is required to ensure the airway is not lost and that there is adequate protection from aspiration. Although two attempts at orotracheal intubation with direct laryngoscopy have been unsuccessful, the next most reasonable step, since the airway has been temporized with the ILMA, would be to attempt blind orotracheal intubation through the ILMA. Fiberoptic-guided intubation via the ILMA would also be a reasonable alternative, but this option is often not immediately available. Needle cricothyroidotomy with jet ventilation would be no better than the ILMA protecting the patient from aspiration and would be inferior in providing adequate ventilation. Surgical cricothyroidotomy should be reserved for cases where (1) rapid sequence intubation has failed and nonsurgical alternatives have failed or are contraindicated; (2) time does not permit for other alternatives (i.e., hypoxia, aspiration); or (3) there is a clear indication for a primary surgical airway (i.e., grossly unstable C-spine, extensive oral trauma). Emergent tracheostomy is indicated following placement of an emergent surgical airway or when nonsurgical approaches have failed and surgical cricothyroidotomy is contraindicated (i.e., tracheal-laryngeal disruption, thyroid hematoma). Only an experienced surgeon should do an emergent tracheostomy.

21-22. **The answer is A** (Chapter 20). This patient developed a tension pneumothorax secondary to hyperinflation of the right lung and requires needle thoracostomy followed by tube thoracostomy. During surgical cricothyroidotomy the endotracheal tube should not be advanced more than 2 to 3 cm past the incision site because of the close proximity to the carina. Even if properly placed initially, it is common for the tube to migrate during affixation to the neck. A tracheostomy tube is shorter and easier to attach to the neck after cricothyroidotomy. It is better to either use one initially or to replace the endotracheal tube with a tracheostomy tube, via the Seldinger technique, as soon as one is available. Although a 6-mm tube is preferred in the typical adult, the increased resistance to ventilation from the smaller tube is less likely to be the cause of the acute deterioration. Unrecognized bleeding from either the initial trauma or from the procedure are also less likely causes of the acute deterioration, so fluid resuscitation and suction are unlikely to help.

21-23. **The answer is D** (Chapter 21). The most common complications with central venous access are pneumothorax, arterial puncture, malpositioning, infection, and thrombosis. Infection and thrombosis are significantly more common with femoral vein access. Arterial puncture is most common with femoral vein access followed by internal jugular access. Malposition is most common in the subclavian approach and least common in the femoral approach.

21-24. **The answer is C** (Chapter 21). Intraosseous access can be used in older children and adults. The recommended intraosseous access site in children younger than 5 years is the flat portion of the proximal-medial tibia, but in adults other sites are suggested, including the medial malleolus, the clavicle, and the ileum. Unique complications are associated with intraosseous and umbilical vein access, however, the overall incidence of infection is similar to other venous access techniques. Although a traditional cutdown requires sacrificing the vein, the "mini cutdown" technique allows for vein preservation by combining surgical exposure of the vessel with catheter-over-needle access to the venous lumen.

21-25. **The answer is C** (Chapter 21). Indwelling catheters, both implanted and externalized, should always be flushed with heparin after use. Even after dead space volume is discarded, coagulation studies drawn from these sites are unreliable. Although improper access of an arteriovenous shunt is associated with infection, thrombosis, and hemorrhage, its use should be considered if alternative access is not available in critical situations. Implanted devices should be flushed with the more concentrated heparin 1000 U/mL solution. The less concentrated heparin 100 U/mL solution is used with externalized devices.

21-26. **The answer is D** (Chapter 22). Although transient decreased flow is common after arterial cannulation, permanent ischemic complications requiring operative repair are uncommon. Infection rates of arterial cannulation at the radial and femoral sites are equivalent. Either umbilical artery can be accessed for blood pressure monitoring or arterial blood gas in the ill neonate. The umbilical artery is the first choice for arterial cannulation in neonates since other sites might require cutdown procedures for access. Unlike a venous cutdown where the vein is transected after exposure, an arterial cutdown combines surgical exposure with catheter-over-wire access to the arterial lumen. The artery is not sacrificed.

21-27. **The answer is C** (Chapter 22). Pulmonary artery catheters have been associated with increased mortality in one large prospective cohort study, although the findings have been controversial. Although septic shock and neurogenic shock are associated with a decrease in systemic vascular resistance, cardiogenic shock is associated with an increase. Hypovolemic shock is associated with a decrease in cardiac output and pulmonary capillary wedge pressure but an increase in systemic vascular resistance. Only cardiogenic shock is associated with an increase in pulmonary capillary wedge pressure.

21-28. **The answer is C** (Chapter 22). This patient has an automatic implantable cardiac defibrillator (AICD). Placing a magnet over the AICD will deactivate the device and is only indicated for device malfunction such as inappropriate defibrillation. In this case, the patient was appropriately defibrillated. The electrical impulse delivered from an AICD can be felt by caregivers but is generally not uncomfortable, and it is not harmful. Standing clear and delaying treatment for any amount of time during the critical resuscitation period in this case is unnecessary and probably would be detrimental. If the device is working properly, it should not fire again unless an unstable tachyarrhythmia recurs. Continuing with defibrillation is contraindicated, even if device malfunction is suspected, because the patient has converted to sinus. Resuscitation should continue normally by checking for evidence of perfusion and ruling out pulseless electrical activity.

21-29. **The answer is A** (Chapter 23). The pathophysiology of anoxic brain injury after cardiac arrest is complex but can be divided into 3 phases: ischemia, early reperfusion, and late reperfusion. Multiple efforts to decrease the extent of injury at the various phases have been met with disappointing results. However, it is clear that early return to spontaneous circulation is important for meaningful neurology outcome. Hyperglycemia in the stroke patient is associated with worse neurologic outcome, so it is reasonable to recommended strict glycemic control after anoxic brain injury, while simultaneously avoiding additional insult by inducing hypoglycemia. Mannitol has not been shown to be helpful in the management of acute stroke. Although controversial, tissue plasminogen activator is indicated in select stroke patients who present within a specified window period, however, it is not indicated for anoxic brain injury after cardiac arrest.

21-30. **The answer is D** (Chapter 24). Conventional dosing recommendations for epinephrine are not based on large clinical trials but instead on animal trials and anecdotal clinical evidence. Escalating-dose and high-dose epinephrine protocols have been correlated with improved response to defibrillation but have not been shown to improve survival or meaningful neurologic recovery.

21-31. **The answer is B** (Chapter 24). In order for a technique to be clinically useful in assessing the likelihood of successful resuscitation, it should be rapid, require few resuscitative resources, be cost effective, and correlate with clinical outcome. So far, no technique has overwhelmingly met these criteria; however, end-tidal CO_2 has shown some promise. One small prospective observational study of 55 adult, nontraumatic, prehospital arrest victims correlated

higher CO_2 levels on arrival with successful return to spontaneous circulation. Although arterial blood gas parameters are often abnormal in critically ill patients, serial blood gases are difficult to obtain in the arrest patient, and results are delayed, so information obtained is unlikely to affect clinical outcome. Ventricular fibrillation waveform analysis is intended to summarize attempts to identify characteristics of the fibrillation waveform that correlate with the likelihood of successful defibrillation. Waveform analysis has been shown in a small retrospective study to possibly correlate with the likelihood of successful defibrillation, but in order to be effective, waveform analysis would need to be done in real time. Invasive hemodynamic pressure monitoring with central venous and aortic catheters provides the most direct measurement of coronary perfusion pressure; however, the procedure is time consuming, requires significant resuscitative resources, and provides data far into the arrest period unlikely to affect clinical outcome.

21-32. **The answer is C** (Chapter 25). The delta gap is calculated by comparing the change in anion gap to the change in HCO_3^-. Normal is considered to be 12 ± 4. Calculating the delta gap provides the clinician with a rapid way to detect the presence of a concomitant metabolic alkalosis if the measured HCO_3^- is lower than expected by the change in anion gap If the measured HCO_3^- is higher than expected by the change in anion gap, there is a concomitant nonanion gap metabolic acidosis. The delta gap is not affected by acute respiratory acid-base disturbances and provides no information about the possible presence of a concomitant respiratory acidosis or alkalosis. Methanol poisoning, diabetic ketoacidosis, and alcoholic ketoacidosis are all conditions that result in a wide anion gap acidosis, and the delta gap provides no additional information about these particular diagnoses.

21-33. **The answer is B** (Chapter 25). Every blood gas that shows normal or minimal pH imbalance should be examined for abnormalities of the P_{CO_2}, the HCO_3^-, and the anion gap. A decreased P_{CO_2} indicates the presence of a respiratory alkalosis, whereas an increase in P_{CO_2} suggests a respiratory acidosis. A decreased HCO_3^- indicates the presence of a metabolic acidosis, whereas an increase in HCO_3^- suggests a metabolic alkalosis. In this patient, the presence of both a metabolic acidosis (diabetic ketoacidosis) and another disorder resulting in a respiratory alkalosis (pregnancy) results in a patient with a mixed acid-base disorder, with a pH measured within the normal range. In patients with a normal pH but an abnormal anion gap, the presence of both a wide anion gap metabolic acidosis and a metabolic alkalosis should be considered.

21-34. **The answer is C** (Chapter 26). Pulse oximetry relies on the difference between absorption of light in deoxygenated (blue) hemoglobin and oxygenated (red) hemoglobin to produce a saturation reading. Pulse oximetry normally has a minimal error (1–2%) at saturations >60%. In the case of carbon monoxide poisoning, the carbon monoxide molecule binds to hemoglobin at the same position oxygen does, and the pulse oximeter falsely reads the carboxyhemoglobin complex as oxyhemoglobin. In contrast, methemoglobinemia causes a falsely decreased pulse oximeter reading and will read at 85% after the treatment for cyanide poisoning has been instituted. Chronic obstructive pulmonary disease and fetal hemoglobin will not affect the pulse oximeter reading.

21-35. **The answer is D** (Chapter 26). Capnography has become a widely used method in many EDs for ensuring tracheal rather than esophageal intubation. However, not all low CO_2 measurements are indicative of esophageal intubation. Capnography provides a means to noninvasively assess ventilation, respiratory gas exchange, and CO_2 production and gives some indication of cardiac output. Conditions that will decrease the end-tidal CO_2 measurement include esophageal intubation, decreased cardiac output, hyperventilation, hypothermia, pulmonary embolism, cardiac arrest, fat or air embolism, disconnection of the ventilation system, accidental extubation, and endotracheal tube obstruction. Conditions that will cause an increase in the end-tidal CO_2 measurement include increased cardiac output, hypoventilation, hyperthermia, bicarbonate administration, and insufflation of CO_2 (laparoscopic surgery).

21-36. **The answer is A** (Chapter 27). The most common cause of hypernatremia encountered in the ED is depletion of total body water. In otherwise healthy patients with severe volume depletion, the kidneys will conserve water, resulting in decreased urinary output with highly concentrated urine (usually >1000 mOsm/kg water). These patients will respond well to normal saline, which can replete total body water while gradually decreasing serum sodium concentrations. Once the patient's tissue perfusion has been restored, the intravenous fluid should be changed to 0.45% normal saline or another hypotonic solution. If hypernatremia persists for several days, brain cells accumulate amino acids known as idiogenic osmoles, which help to restore brain cell water content. If serum sodium concentrations are lowered too rapidly, these idiogenic osmoles attract even more water into brain cells and can result in cerebral edema. For this reason a more gradual approach to rehydration and serum sodium correction by using normal saline or lactated Ringer's solution as the initial rehydration fluid is recommended. D_5W and 0.45% saline are hypotonic solutions and thus not recommended for initial therapy. A solution of 3% saline is hypertonic and will aggravate the patient's hypernatremic state.

21-37. **The answer is B** (Chapter 27). The most common cause of an elevated serum potassium level in patients is hemolysis during phlebotomy. Patients with unexpectedly elevated serum potassium levels should have an electrocardiogram performed to look for changes associated with elevated serum potassium. These changes may include tall peaked T waves, short QT interval, prolonged PR interval, QRS widening, P-wave flattening, or QRS degradation into a sine wave pattern. In addition, rhythm abnormalities such as ventricular fibrillation, complete heart block, or asystole may occur. If there is no evidence of cardiac derangements, the initial step in treating these patients is to confirm the elevated serum potassium level by collecting and sending a new sample for repeat analysis. Other causes of true hyperkalemia include renal failure, excess intake of potassium supplements, and the use of potassium-sparing diuretics.

21-38. **The answer is C** (Chapter 28). This patient is experiencing supraventricular tachycardia (SVT) and has a history concerning for digoxin toxicity. Symptomatic patients presenting to the ED with SVT should be cardioverted, either electrically or chemically. However, patients who are experiencing SVT secondary to digoxin toxicity should not be cardioverted. The presence of digoxin lowers the ventricular fibrillatory threshold, and cardioversion may induce refractory ventricular tachycardias or ventricular fibrillation. In patients with digoxin toxicity, the treatment for SVT includes correction of any hypokalemia present to reduce the likelihood of atrial ectopy. In patients who are hemodynamically unstable or have serious ventricular dysrhythmia, treatment with digoxin-specific antibody fragments should be considered. Finally, patients may receive antiarrhythmic therapy with phenytoin, magnesium, or lidocaine. A history of chronic obstructive pulmonary disease or previous successful cardioversion for these symptoms is not a contraindication to cardioversion. Vagal maneuvers are a simple, noninvasive means of attempting cardioversion, but their failure to achieve cardioversion is not a contraindication to chemical or electrical therapy to induce cardioversion.

21-39. **The answer is A** (Chapter 28). Second-degree Mobitz type I (Wenckebach) atrioventricular block is not generally dangerous, and specific treatment is not necessary unless the ventricular rate is slow enough to induce signs of hypoperfusion. Wenckebach is often a transient rhythm and is usually found in the setting of acute inferior myocardial infarction, digitoxin toxicity, myocarditis, or the postsurgical period after cardiac surgery. If the patient is experiencing symptomatic Wenckebach, the appropriate chemical treatment would be atropine. Transcutaneous or transvenous electrical pacing may be necessary if atropine is unsuccessful in increasing the ventricular rate. Isoproterenol should not be used in the setting of cardiac ischemia or digoxin toxicity. Nitroglycerin is not an antiarrhythmic agent and could worsen this patient's already low blood pressure.

21-40. **The answer is D** (Chapter 29). Intravenous amiodarone is used in the ED to treat ventricular tachycardia, ventricular fibrillation, atrial fibrillation, atrial flutter, and wide-complex tachycardias. In the acute setting, adverse effects of using intravenous amiodarone are usually limited to bradycardia and hypotension, although shock, cardiac arrest, and asystole have also been reported. Patients who undergo long-term amiodarone therapy face several serious adverse effects including pulmonary fibrosis, thyroid dysfunction, hepatotoxicity, and corneal microdeposits.

21-41. **The answer is C** (Chapter 29). Wide-complex tachycardias may be indicative of the presence of an accessory bypass tract, as in Wolff-Parkinson-White syndrome. The use of calcium channel blockers, β-blockers, and adenosine should be avoided in this setting because of the possibility of inducing refractory ventricular fibrillation and/or cardiac arrest in these patients. Indications for the use of intravenous diltiazem include paroxysmal supraventricular tachycardia, atrial fibrillation, and atrial flutter.

21-42. **The answer is C** (Chapter 31). Red blood cells are actually rendered less pliable when they have been stored for a long period of time. Currently employed preservatives allow packed red blood cells to be stored and last approximately 42 days. Despite improvements in blood storage, 2,3-diphosphoglycerate is diminished. The lack of 2,3-diphosphoglycerate shifts the oxygen-hemoglobin dissociation curve to the left, which allows less oxygen to be delivered to tissues. Red blood cells stored over 2 weeks have been associated with mesenteric hypoperfusion. Stored red blood cells are less deformable and consequently can get lodged in capillaries.

21-43. **The answer is C** (Chapter 31). Although urine output generally correlates well with adequate renal perfusion in normal subjects, this may not be the case in all patients, in particular those with impaired renal function. This patient is elderly and has a Foley catheter that could be obstructed with insipissated urine sediment. The Foley catheter should be flushed but preferably changed. A surrogate for mixed venous oxygen saturation (Svo_2) is central mixed venous oxygen saturation ($Scvo_2$) sampled from either the internal jugular or subclavian vein as they approach the right atrium. $Scvo_2$ provides an estimate of the oxygenation of blood returning to the heart after tissues have been perfused. A low value (<50) indicates increased peripheral tissue oxygen demand and signifies peripheral hypoperfusion. $Scvo_2$ can be sampled from a central venous source and sent to a blood gas laboratory for measurement of venous oxygen saturation. Base deficit, a marker of tissue hypoperfusion, indicates bicarbonate stores are becoming depleted. Lactate is another marker of tissue hypoperfusion, indicating a shift toward anaerobic metabolism when tissues are not receiving adequate substrate.

21-44. **The answer is C** (Chapter 30). It includes all 4 variables defining SIRS: temperature >38°C or <36°C, heart rate >90 bpm, respiratory rate >20 breaths per minute or a $Paco_2$ <32 mmHg, and white blood cell count >12,000 × 10^9/L, <4000 × 10^9/L, or >10% immature forms or bands.

21-45. **The answer is A** (Chapter 32). The Early Goal Directed Trial was a randomized trial performed in the ED which demonstrated early identification and goal-directed therapy of patients with severe sepsis improved survival by 16% compared to patients in the control group. Administration of activated protein C demonstrated a reduction in mortality of 6% in patients receiving this recombinant form of protein C, which is depressed in some cases of severe sepsis. Administration of steroids has also shown an 11% improvement in the mortality of patients with severe sepsis with relative adrenal insufficiency. A study utilizing antitumor necrosis factor antibodies did not show a decrease in mortality in patients with severe sepsis.

21-46. **The answer is C** (Chapter 33). Cardiogenic shock affects up to 40% of patients with acute myocardial infarction. This is seen more frequently with ST-elevation myocardial infarction. Stroke is another result of cardiovascular disease that does not necessarily proceed directly from myocardial infarction. However, these conditions share many of the same risk factors. Pulmonary embolism is not directly related to increased mortality in patients undergoing acute myocardial infarction but can be seen in patients with hypercoagulable disorders, immobility, or previous venous thrombus. There is no direct link between myocardial infarction and mortality from oliguric acute renal failure. Patients with preexisting renal insufficiency with or without diabetes may suffer from acute contrast-related renal disease after cardiac catheterization.

21-47. **The answer is B** (Chapter 34). Antibiotics of the β-lactam variety are associated with severe hypersensitivity reactions. The risk of recurrence upon reexposure is not 100% as would be expected. Patients with confirmed anaphylaxis to common agents are encouraged to carry a self-injectable form of epinephrine and wear a medical bracelet indicating their condition. Stings from *Hymenoptera* species are the second most common form of anaphylaxis in the United States. Shellfish is another cause of severe allergic reaction. In children, food allergies are a common cause of anaphylaxis.

21-48. **The answer is B** (Chapter 34). Radiocontrast has been associated with non-IgE-mediated hypersensitivity reactions previously referred to as anaphylactoid. Current classification schemes includes these reactions along with anaphylaxis. Peanuts, shellfish, and antibiotics are characterized by an IgE-mediated mechanism with mast cell degranulation and release of histamines. Serum tryptase, an enzyme specific to mast cells, may be elevated for several hours after an anaphylactic response and is presumptive evidence that an anaphylactic reaction has occurred. This test is not used clinically in the ED.

21-49. **The answer is A** (Chapter 35). Motor vehicle accidents account for the largest number of spinal trauma cases. The cervical region is the most commonly injured area and often leads to permanent paralysis. Gunshot wounds and stabbings can also cause spinal injury. Usually these events are due to episodes of interpersonal violence. The emergency physician must be skilled in assessing patients with severe spinal injury and be cautious when managing the airway of patients with suspected spinal injury. Falls are the other significant form of blunt trauma causing spinal injury. Patients with complete paralysis above the T1 level can have neurogenic shock identified by hypotension and bradycardia. These patients must be aggressively managed and vasopressors instituted to support blood pressure often hampered by decreased sympathetic tone. Steroids must not be forgotten in the acute management of spinal cord injury patients.

Special Situations
Questions

22-1. A 30-year-old man presents to the ED with right upper extremity pain, redness, and swelling after skin-popping black tar heroin 3 days ago. He also notes a fever but denies shortness of breath, diplopia, dysphagia, or weakness. Vital signs are blood pressure 130/90 mmHg, pulse 92 beats per minute, respirations 20 breaths per minute, and temperature 37.6°C. The right upper extremity is swollen and red, with a central blackened eschar. A bulla has ruptured, releasing serous fluid, which does not have an odor. The arm is tender, but crepitus is absent. The rest of the physical examination is normal except for multiple hyperpigmented sites on the extremities. What is the next MOST appropriate series of actions?

(A) Obtain IV access, send blood to the lab, give parenteral antibiotics, obtain radiograph of the upper extremity, and get a surgery consult.

(B) Prescribe cephalexin and have the patient follow up in 2 days.

(C) Give IV antibiotics and admit.

(D) Obtain IV access and send blood to the lab.

22-2. A 20-year-old woman who is an injection drug user presents with a 3-day history of right eye pain with decreased vision. She denies trauma or prior similar events but recalls having a high fever. Vital signs are blood pressure 130/85 mmHg, pulse 80 beats per minute, respirations 20 breaths per minute, and temperature 38°C. Visual acuity is 20/50 in the right eye and 20/20 in the left. Extraocular movements are intact. The right eye is red and chemotic. The pupils are 3 mm each and reactive. Both eyes have intraocular pressures of 18. Slit lamp examination reveals a cloudy anterior chamber without hypopyon or hyphema. There is no corneal fluorescein uptake. The vitreous is hazy. On funduscopy, several fluffy yellow-white lesions are seen on the retina. What is the MOST likely etiologic agent?

(A) *Staphylococcus.*

(B) Cytomegalovirus.

(C) *Toxoplasma.*

(D) *Candida.*

22-3. Which of the following statements regarding the elder patient is correct?

(A) Common diseases present atypically in the elder patient.

(B) Falls are a normal part of aging.

(C) Functional decline is a normal part of aging.

(D) When functional decline develops, feeding is the first activity that needs assistance.

22-4. Which of the following factors is NOT associated with increased bacteremia or focal infection in the elder patient?

(A) Age >70 years.

(B) Diabetes mellitus.

(C) White blood count >15,000/μL.

(D) Erythrocyte sedimentation rate >30 mm/hour.

22-5. A 40-year-old woman with paraplegia at level T6 presents with a sense of apprehension, pounding headache, vague right shoulder pain, and profuse sweating. She denies fever, vomiting, constipation, or changes in the appearance of her urine during self-catheterization. Vital signs are blood pressure 180/100 mmHg, pulse 50 beats per minute, respirations 20 breaths per minute, temperature 37°C, and room air oxygen saturation 99%. She appears anxious and is diaphoretic above the xiphoid. She has piloerection and pallor below the xiphoid. Funduscopic examination is normal. Examination of the heart and lungs is normal. The nondistended abdomen is soft, and bowel sounds are present. There are no palpable masses. There is no asymmetric swelling of the lower extremities. The patient has spastic paralysis and hyperreflexia of the lower extremities. A peripheral IV is started, and blood is sent to the lab. An electrocardiogram shows sinus bradycardia without ST-segment abnormalities or ectopy. The patient states her normal blood pressure is 110/70. What is the next MOST appropriate action?

(A) Place a Foley catheter and evaluate the urine.

(B) Perform a rectal examination.

(C) Perform a fecal disimpaction.

(D) Start a nitroprusside drip at 0.3 μg/kg/min.

22-6. A 37-year-old male with paraplegia at level T6 from a gunshot wound 5 years ago presents with a sense of feeling unwell complaining of right shoulder pain. He denies fever, vomiting, constipation, or changes in the appearance of his catheterized urine. Vital signs are blood pressure 165/90 mmHg, pulse 60 beats per minute, respirations 20 breaths per minute, temperature 37°C, and room air oxygen saturation 99%. He appears anxious and is diaphoretic above the xiphoid. He has piloerection and pallor below the xiphoid. Funduscopic examination is normal. Examination of the heart and lungs is normal. His abdomen is soft, nondistended, and bowel sounds are present. There are no palpable masses. Rectal exam revealed scant guaiac-negative brown stool. The patient has spastic paralysis and hyperreflexia of the lower extremities. Right shoulder examination is normal. A Foley catheter was placed in the ED and 50 cc of urine was obtained. The urine was clear but dips trace positive for leukocytes and nitrites. Microscopy reveals 1–2 leukocytes and scant bacteria. His repeat blood pressure is 125/85 mmHg but his diaphoresis, pallor, and piloerection continue. What is the next MOST appropriate action?

(A) Oral antibiotics.

(B) Intravenous antibiotics.

(C) Right shoulder film.

(D) Abdominal ultrasound.

Special Situations
Answers, Explanations, and References

22-1. **The answer is A** (Chapter 306). This patient has necrotizing fasciitis, a life-and-limb-threatening soft tissue infection often associated with, but not limited to, injection drug use. Diabetes is also a strong comorbidity. The patient requires IV access, laboratory studies, a film to rule out soft tissue gas, a surgical consult, and parenteral antibiotics. Oral antibiotics and discharge are both inappropriate. Admission will be necessary but surgery must be involved early. Commonly associated clinical signs and symptoms such as hypotension, crepitus, bullae, skin necrosis, and gas on radiographs are frequently absent. Pain out of proportion may be an early clue. The emergency physician should maintain a very high index of suspicion. Necrotizing fasciitis is usually a polymicrobial, aerobic, and anaerobic infection but reports of virulent group A streptococci and *Enterobacter* species are increasing. Broad-spectrum antibiotics and timely surgical debridement are required.

22-2. **The answer is D** (Chapter 306). Endophthalmitis due to injection drug use (IDU) is more commonly caused by fungal, rather than bacterial, infection. Onset of symptoms such as pain, decreased vision, or blurred vision may be acute or indolent. Fluffy yellow-white retinal lesions and vitreous haziness are key features. Infection will progress to involve the anterior chamber, and the yellow-white lesions will grow in the vitreous. Endophthalmitis or chorioretinitis due to candidal species is associated with the use of black tar heroin. A pro-

drome of high fever is followed within 3–4 days by ocular symptoms, cutaneous lesions, and costochondral involvement. *Aspergillus* species are the second most common cause of fungal endophthalmitis in IDU, but cutaneous and musculoskeletal features are absent. *Staphylococcus aureus* and *Streptococcus* species are the most common organisms associated with IDU-related bacterial endophthalmitis. *Toxoplasma* and cytomegalovirus are associated with chorioretinitis in HIV-positive injection drug users.

22-3. **The answer is A** (Chapter 307). Many common diseases present atypically in the older patient. Fewer than half of patients with myocardial infarction who are 85 years and older present with chest pain. More typically, the chief complaint is dyspnea, weakness, dizziness, or syncope. Guarding and rebound may be absent in the patient with an acute abdomen. Generalized weakness or functional decline may signal sepsis or subdural hematoma. Falls are multifactoral in etiology and may indicate a sentinel event, but they are not a normal part of aging. The cause of the fall should be evaluated to determine whether electrocardiogram, computed tomography, lab tests, or social services are required. Functional decline involves a change in the ability to perform activities of daily and independent living and is not a normal part of aging. Diminishing function occurs in a set pattern, which first affects bathing, followed sequentially by dressing, toileting, transferring, and feeding. Organic disease should be suspected if an atypical pattern occurs, such as when feeding declines first. Older patients are more susceptible to infection, which can present atypically. Septic patients may be hypothermic, and pyuria may be absent in urinary infection. Close attention must be paid to the febrile older patient because bacteremia and occult infection are common.

22-4. **The answer is A** (Chapter 307). Factors associated with increased bacteremia or focal bacterial infection include age >50 years, diabetes, white blood count >15,000/µL, neutrophil band count >1500/µL, and erythrocyte sedimentation rate >30 mm/hour. A seven- to eightfold relative risk for bacteremia or focal bacterial infection exists for patients with 1 or 2 of the factors.

22-5. **The answer is D** (Chapter 308). The patient has autonomic dysreflexia, which has markedly elevated her blood pressure above baseline. Since the pressure is above 150 mmHg, and she has a headache, an antihypertensive agent with a rapid onset of action and brief duration is indicated. Either nitroprusside or nitrates would be appropriate. Autonomic dysreflexia occurs in patients with spinal cord injuries above T6. Noxious stimuli originating from below T6 are transmitted up the cord via intact sensory neurons in the spinothalamic tract and posterior columns. Interconnections trigger massive sympathetic outflow from levels T6–L2. Normal inhibition of this reflex is mediated by neurons originating above T6, but the injury level blocks the impulses. Patients with autonomic dysreflexia have elevated blood pressure and a vagally mediated reflex bradycardia. Above the level of injury the skin is vasodilated and diaphoretic. Below the level, pallor and pilo-

erection occur. The noxious stimuli that most commonly trigger autonomic dysreflexia include urinary tract infection, bladder distention, and kidney stone. Fecal impaction is the second most common cause. A patient's blood pressure should be managed prior to performing urinary catheterization or fecal disimpaction. Lidocaine jelly should be applied to the urethra and anus prior to the procedures. Patients with spinal cord injuries and an acute abdomen can also present with autonomic dysreflexia but classic findings such as abdominal rigidity, rebound, and tenderness will be absent. The patient in this case will require additional studies such as ultrasound or abdominal CT, and lab studies.

22-6. **The answer is D** (Chapter 308). The patient has minimal bacteriuria and insignificant pyuria. A urinary tract infection remains a possibility, but he is also at risk for an acute abdomen. Given his right scapular pain, a bedside ultrasound of the right upper quadrant is an appropriate test for possible gallstones. A right shoulder film would not be useful, but a chest radiograph or abdominal series in such a patient could be revealing. Significant bacteriuria in male or female patients who use intermittent catheterization would be >100 colony forming units (CFUs)/mL. Any bacteriuria in patients with indwelling or suprapubic catheters is considered significant. Women who can spontaneously void must have >100,000 CFUs. Males who can spontaneously void or use condom catheters must have more than 10,000 CFUs. *Proteus, Klebsiella, Pseudomonas, Serratia, Providencia*, enterococci, and staphylococci are typically involved organisms. Broad-spectrum antibiotics are required.

Toxicologic Emergencies
Questions

23-1. A 60-year-old woman presents to the ED with severe epistaxis. She is on Coumadin for atrial fibrillation and has recently been in the hospital for an unspecified illness. On examination, she has stable vital signs and, other than some dried blood in her nares, has no other signs of a bleeding diathesis. Her INR is 1.0. It was 2.2 at discharge. Which of the following other medications, if given to the patient on discharge, could be responsible for the sudden change in her INR?

(A) Phenytoin.
(B) Bactrim.
(C) Erythromycin.
(D) Amiodarone.

23-2. A 25-year-old male is brought in by ambulance after a tonic-clonic seizure that was witnessed by his roommates. The patient is obtunded with a blood pressure of 70/30 mmHg and a heart rate of 110 beats per minute. Lungs are clear, heart sounds are normal, and bowel sounds are diminished. Pupils are 5–6 mm and equal, although minimally reactive. The patient's skin appears slightly reddened diffusely and is warm and dry to the touch. An electrocardiogram reveals a wide-complex tachycardia with a QRS of 110 ms. The roommates offer an empty prescription bottle and say the patient was "given these by his therapist for depression." The patient is quickly intubated and two intravenous lines with normal saline are started just as the patient has another seizure, which is quickly controlled with 2 mg of IV Ativan. Which of the following options is the next MOST appropriate intervention?

(A) 15–20 mg/kg of intravenous phenytoin.
(B) Gastric lavage followed by activated charcoal administration.
(C) Lidocaine 20–50 μg/kg bolus.
(D) NaHCO$_3$ 1–2 mEq/kg IV bolus.

23-3. Parents of a 35-year-old woman bring their daughter to the ED. She has recently been diagnosed with the flu and has been taking over-the-counter cold medicine for the last 3 days. Last night, according to them, she began behaving differently, acting confused and agitated. Her parents also noticed that she was shaking all the time. She began having diarrhea this morning. Her past medical history is significant only for depression, and her psychiatrist has recently added a low dose of trazodone to her daily Paxil. On examination, the patient is mildly agitated and anxious but consolable. Her vital signs are as follows: pulse 105 beats per minute, blood pressure 160/95 mmHg, respirations 21 per minute, and temperature 40°C rectally. She has a normal heart and lung examination except for tachycardia, and there are no skin rashes. Examination of the oropharynx reveals prominent salivation but no other abnormalities. She does exhibit some mild rigidity of the muscles of the lower extremities along with diffuse shivering; reflexes are 3+ and equal. There are 3–4 beats of clonus present with plantar reflex examination. Based on this history and physical examination, which of the following is the MOST appropriate treatment for this patient?

(A) Dantrolene 0.5–2.5 mg/kg IV q6h.

(B) Ceftriaxone 2 g IV plus rifampin.

(C) IV hydration, followed by Ativan 2 mg IV.

(D) Cyproheptadine 8 mg orally.

23-4. Which statement about monoamine oxidase inhibitor (MAOI) overdose is TRUE?

(A) The tyramine reaction typically starts 8–10 hours after ingestion of foods high in tyramine.

(B) Once an irreversible MAOI has been stopped, a 2-week "washout" period is necessary before MAO activity returns.

(C) Use of epinephrine and norepinephrine are contraindicated in patients with an MAOI overdose.

(D) For severe hypertension, metoprolol is considered first-line therapy and

should be given in 5-mg boluses every 10 minutes until the mean arterial pressure is decreased by 25–30%.

23-5. Which of the following side effects of neuroleptic medications is paired INCORRECTLY with its clinical presentation?

(A) Dystonic reaction—facial grimacing and oculogyric crises.

(B) Akathisia—motor restlessness.

(C) Neuroleptic malignant syndrome—cogwheel rigidity.

(D) Tardive dyskinesia—choreoathetoid movements.

23-6. Which of the following statements about lithium toxicity is TRUE?

(A) Forced diuresis helps improve lithium excretion in overdose.

(B) If seizures occur and are not controlled with benzodiazepines, phenytoin is the preferred second-line agent.

(C) Lithium toxicity is often manifested by the unlikely combination of lethargy and tremor.

(D) Lithium is not adsorbed by activated charcoal, which should never be used in cases of lithium toxicity.

23-7. Which of the following statements about barbiturates and barbiturate overdose is TRUE?

(A) Barbituric acid, the parent compound for all barbiturates, is the strongest sedative of all barbiturates.

(B) Higher lipid solubility allows more rapid transit of barbiturates across the blood-brain barrier.

(C) Longer-acting barbiturates are more lipid soluble but are more protein bound than short-acting barbiturates.

(D) Multidose activated charcoal is recommended for all barbiturate overdoses.

23-8. Which of the following is an accepted indication for the use of flumazenil?

(A) None—should never be used in the ED.

(B) Unresponsive patients with a suspicion of benzodiazepine overdose.

(C) The need to reverse the effects of benzodiazepines given for therapeutic procedures.

(D) Gamma-hydroxybutyrate (GHB) overdose.

23-9. A 21-year-old woman is brought into the ED by her friends, who think "someone may have slipped something into her drink" earlier tonight. They say the patient has no significant past medical history and takes no medications. On examination the patient is responsive only to deep pain and is normothermic, with a heart rate of 125 beats per minute, blood pressure of 80/40 mmHg, and respirations of 10 breaths per minute. There are no skin rashes or track marks noted. The skin is not notably warm or dry. Her pupils are miotic and only minimally reactive. There is a faint smell of pears on the patient's breath. The remainder of the examination reveals no abnormalities, except for her rectal exam being gastroccult positive. Her ethanol level is 136 mg/dL, and her urine drug screen is negative for cannabinoids, cocaine, benzodiazepines, and amphetamines. Electrocardiogram reveals sinus tachycardia at 130 beats per minute, and the patient's heart monitor is showing repeated runs of ventricular tachycardia. Based on this evidence, what agent has the patient MOST likely been exposed to?

(A) Gamma-hydroxybutyrate (GHB).

(B) Methaqualone.

(C) Glutethimide.

(D) Chloral hydrate.

23-10. Which of the following statements about alcohols is TRUE?

(A) When using ethanol to treat methanol poisoning, a blood ethanol level of 50–75 mg/dL should be maintained to keep enough ethanol in the bloodstream to displace methanol from alcohol dehydrogenase.

(B) Isopropyl alcohol ingestion causes neither an osmolar gap nor an elevated anion gap.

(C) Vitamin B_6 should be given to every patient who presents with an ethylene glycol ingestion.

(D) Use of fomepizole has been shown to decrease the need for dialysis in patients who have ingested methanol or ethylene glycol.

23-11. Which of the following statements about cocaine is TRUE?

(A) Cocaine has no antiarrhythmic effect on cardiac conduction.

(B) Cocaine accelerates conduction of nerve impulses via fast sodium channel activation in the cell membrane.

(C) Neuromuscular blocking agents may have a long duration of effect in patients who have ingested cocaine.

(D) Neuroleptics like haloperidol or droperidol are very effective at calming the agitation or psychosis of cocaine intoxication and should be considered second-line therapy after benzodiazepines.

23-12. Which description of the pathophysiology of salicylate toxicity is FALSE?

(A) As systemic pH decreases, salicylate concentrations in the brain will be higher than plasma concentrations.

(B) While salicylates can mobilize glycogen stores, resulting in hyperglycemia, they are also potent inhibitors of gluconeogenesis.

(C) The centrally mediated increased respiratory rate seen in salicylate poisoning is partially offset by a salicylate-induced decrease in carbon dioxide production.

(D) Despite its antiplatelet activity, hemorrhage from acute, massive salicylate poisoning is an uncommon occurrence.

23-13. A 75-year-old woman is brought in by ambulance accompanied by her family, who state she "hasn't been right" for the past 2 days. They say she has been unusually confused and tired. She has been complaining of nausea and mild abdominal discomfort for the last 24 hours. She's normally an active, independent woman with a history of "heart problems," according to the family. She started a new "heart medicine" recently, but they say she has no known allergies. On examination, the patient is obtunded and responsive to mild pain, with a Glasgow Coma Scale score of 11. Her blood pressure is 70/40 mmHg, with a pulse of 35 beats per minute, a respiratory rate of 18 breaths per minute, and an oral temperature of 36.4°C. She weighs approximately 100 kg. On auscultation, rales can be heard in the lower lung field bilaterally. The heart sounds are normal but slow. The abdominal exam is benign with no peritoneal signs and normal bowel sounds. There are no skin rashes, and the neurologic exam reveals no focal or lateralizing signs except for obtundation. The cardiac monitor shows a junctional bradycardia. The electrocardiogram confirms the junctional bradycardia and in addition, large T waves are noted. Her electrolytes are as follows: sodium 139 mEq/L, potassium 5.5 mEq/L, chloride 106 mEq/L, bicarbonate 18 mEq/L, creatinine 1.7 mg/dL, and BUN 55. Arterial blood gas reveals a pH 7.38, CO_2 35, O_2 96, and HCO_3^- 17. Serum digoxin level is elevated at 3.0 ng/mL. Of the choices listed, which is the MOST appropriate management plan?

(A) Atropine 1 mg IV, 3 vials of Digibind IV, calcium chloride 10% 10 cc IV.

(B) External cardiac pacing, 3 vials Digibind IV, Kayexalate 30 g orally.

(C) Atropine 1 mg IV, 3 vials Digibind IV, 10 units regular insulin IV, 50 cc $D_{50}W$ IV.

(D) Atropine 1 mg IV, 10 units regular insulin IV, 50 cc $D_{50}W$ IV, gastric lavage, and 50 g activated charcoal.

23-14. When comparing acute ingestions of digoxin, β-blockers, and calcium channel blockers, which of the following contrasts is INCORRECT?

(A) Calcium channel blocker overdoses often present with mild hyperglycemia, while β-blocker overdoses usually present with euglycemia or hypoglycemia.

(B) Patients suffering a calcium channel blocker overdose often have a normal mental status even when bradycardic, in contrast to patients with digoxin or β-blocker overdoses.

(C) Patients with acute digoxin overdose are generally hyperkalemic, while patients with calcium channel blocker overdose are generally slightly hypokalemic.

(D) Digoxin and calcium channel blocker overdoses can present with tachydysrhythmias, which are exceedingly rare in β-blocker overdoses.

23-15. Which symptom or sign of iron poisoning is NOT seen in the first 24 hours after ingestion of a toxic dose of elemental iron?

(A) Elevated liver transaminases.

(B) Abdominal pain.

(C) Nausea and vomiting.

(D) Gastrointestinal (GI) bleeding.

23-16. With respect to hydrocarbon ingestions, which chemical property of hydrocarbons has the GREATEST effect on the risk of aspiration?

(A) Volatility.

(B) Viscosity.

(C) Flash point.

(D) Surface tension.

23-17. A 30-year-old male is brought to the ED complaining of severe pain to his left hand beginning 20 minutes ago when a chemical at work accidentally spilled on his hand. He works in a glass etching factory, and there is no one available to identify what the agent was. On exam he appears to be in severe pain. His vitals signs are as follows: afebrile with blood pressure 150/95 mmHg, pulse 115 beats per minute, and respirations 17 breaths per minute. His lung, cardiac, and abdominal examination is normal, and his throat is clear. The skin of his left hand has a slight whitish discoloration up to the distal wrist, corresponding to the area splashed earlier; otherwise the examination of the patient's hand is not significant. After initial irrigation of the area with water, what is the next MOST appropriate treatment for this injury?

(A) Apply Tween 80 or De-Solv-It to the entire left hand.

(B) Coat the hand in a gel made with surgical lubricant and calcium gluconate.

(C) Irrigate until the pH of the skin surface is neutral.

(D) Clean the affected area with a dilute Dakin's solution.

23-18. A 38-year-old farm worker presents to the ED with hypersalivation, urinary incontinence, diarrhea, and muscle weakness after being in a recently "sprayed" field. He has prominent wheezing and is producing copious amounts of clear sputum. Which of the following statements is TRUE of the treatment for this condition?

(A) Atropine should be administered as 1 mg IV every 5 minutes until muscle weakness has resolved.

(B) Supportive care is the only appropriate treatment for this condition.

(C) Pralidoxime will regenerate cholinesterase molecules if given any time after exposure.

(D) Atropine and pralidoxime work synergistically to treat this condition.

23-19. A 6-year-old boy is brought to the ED by his father, who says the child has been complaining of headache, fatigue, and abdominal pain for the past week or so. The father thinks he is being "poisoned" by the

chemicals in their house. Their century-old house is undergoing major renovations, and many chemicals and solvents are present in the basement. The father states that the child has been slightly irritable. On examination, the child appears tired but in no distress, and his vitals signs are normal. The head and neck examination is normal. There is no meningismus. The oropharynx is normal. The abdomen is mildly tender throughout, but there are no signs of peritoneal irritation or masses. There are no skin rashes or discolorations. Musculoskeletal examination is also normal. The neurologic exam is notable for weakened wrist extensors on the right hand and diffusely depressed reflexes and a normal sensory examination. Laboratory tests are as follows: hemoglobin 9.8 g/dL,:WBC 8300, and platelets 345. Basophilic stippling is noted. Electrolytes are sodium 137 mmol/L, potassium 4.9 mmol/L, chloride 111 mmol/L, CO_2 17 mmol/L, glucose 120 mg/dL, BUN 35 mg/dL, and creatinine 1.9 mg/dL. Measured serum osmolarity is 295 osm/L. Urinalysis reveals proteinuria and glycosuria. Based on this evidence, which antidote would be MOST effective at treating this patient's condition?

(A) British antilewisite.

(B) Ethanol infusion.

(C) 6-mercaptopurine.

(D) Physostigmine.

23-20. Which of the following vitamins is CORRECTLY paired with the symptoms associated with a large ingestion of that vitamin?

(A) Vitamin B_1: reddening and itching of the face, neck, and chest.

(B) Vitamin B_2: abdominal pain, polyuria, constipation, and lethargy.

(C) Vitamin C: gout and/or nephrolithiasis.

(D) Vitamin D: no significant toxicity.

23-21. Which statement about cyanide poisoning is CORRECT?

(A) Clinically, cyanosis can be seen before frank signs of respiratory failure occur.

(B) Cyanide has a weaker affinity for methemoglobin than normal hemoglobin.

(C) Sodium thoisulfate allows the body to turn cyanide into a less toxic molecule.

(D) Cyanide binds hemoglobin more avidly than oxygen, impairing oxygen delivery to the tissues.

23-22. Which of the following agent is CORRECTLY paired with its antidote?

(A) Monoamine oxidase inhibitors (MAOIs): physostigmine.

(B) Isoniazid: pyridoxine.

(C) Nitrate compounds: cyanide antidote kit.

(D) Methanol: thiamine.

23-23. Which of the following substances is NOT well adsorbed by activated charcoal?

(A) Acetaminophen.

(B) Tricyclic antidepressant.

(C) Iron.

(D) Calcium channel blockers.

23-24. A 26-year-old psychiatric patient attempted suicide by swallowing 20 Clinitest tablets (containing sodium hydroxide) and "chasing" it with drain cleaner (containing potassium hydroxide). Of the following treatment options, which is the MOST appropriate?

(A) Administration of activated charcoal.

(B) Nasogastric (NG) tube placement and dilution with large amounts of water.

(C) Neutralization with a weak acid via NG tube.

(D) Immediate gastrointestinal consultation for endoscopic evaluation.

23-25. Which of the following statements about methemoglobinemia is TRUE?

(A) The blood is classically described as having a "red currant" color.

(B) Medications that can cause methemoglobinemia include lidocaine, acetaminophen, and dapsone.

(C) Inducing mild methemoglobinemia is part of the treatment of cyanide poisoning.

(D) Sulfhemoglobinemia is more common than methemoglobinemia.

23-26. Which of the following characteristics improves a substance's ability to be cleared from the blood stream by hemodialysis?

(A) Small volume of distribution.

(B) Highly protein bound.

(C) Large molecular weight.

(D) Low pKa.

23-27. A child is brought to the ED by her parents, who found the child chewing on a clonidine patch. Which sign or symptom would be most likely in this patient?

(A) Mydriasis.

(B) Tachypnea.

(C) Hypertension.

(D) Bradycardia.

23-28. A patient with tachycardia, hypertension, diaphoresis, agitation, and mydriasis is MOST likely exhibiting which type of toxidrome?

(A) Sympathomimetic toxidrome.

(B) Cholinergic toxidrome.

(C) Opioid toxidrome.

(D) Anticholinergic toxidrome.

23-29. Which of the following statements concerning hallucinogens is TRUE?

(A) Patients with symptomatic phencyclidine (PCP) ingestions should have its excretion enhanced by acidification of the urine.

(B) Jimson weed can be ingested or smoked and can cause include delirium, mydriasis, tachycardia, dry mouth, dry skin, and urinary retention.

(C) Prolonged psychosis following lysergic acid diethylamide (LSD) ingestion occurs in over 40% of people who use the drug.

(D) Urine tests are useful in distinguishing acute marijuana usage from usage in the recent past.

23-30. What is the half-life of naloxone?

(A) 30 minutes.
(B) 30–60 minutes.
(C) 60–90 minutes.
(D) 90–120 minutes.

23-31. Which of the following chemical gas exposures typically results in a delayed onset of symptoms?

(A) Inhalational nerve agents.
(B) Phosgene.
(C) Cyanide.
(D) Ammonia.

23-32. Which of the following statements is MOST correct concerning patients with an isoniazid overdose?

(A) The onset of symptoms is often delayed up to 12 hours.
(B) The anion gap metabolic acidosis associated with isoniazid toxicity should be treated with sodium bicarbonate.
(C) Isoniazid-induced seizures are often refractory to typical therapeutic interventions.
(D) Thiamine is the drug of choice for isoniazid poisoning.

23-33. An 80-year-old female presents following ingestion of a full bottle of quinine. Which of the following potential complications is associated with quinine toxicity?

(A) Pancytopenia.
(B) Noncardiogenic pulmonary edema.

(C) Hyperkalemia.
(D) Sodium channel blockade.

23-34. You are called to the resuscitation room to examine a 34-year-old factory worker rescued from an industrial plant fire. He is profoundly hypotensive and suddenly becomes apneic. Following airway management, empiric therapy with which of the following agents is MOST likely to benefit this patient?

(A) Oxygen, 100%.
(B) Methylene blue and oxygen.
(C) Sodium thiosulfate and oxygen.
(D) Amyl nitrite, sodium nitrite, and oxygen.

23-35. Which of the following is UNLIKELY to be associated with the development of methemoglobinemia?

(A) Phenazopyridine.
(B) Inhalation of paint-stripping solvents that contain methylene chloride.
(C) Severe gastroenteritis in a 3-month-old infant.
(D) Benzocaine.

23-36. Which of the following statements regarding significant methemoglobinemia poisoning is TRUE?

(A) In the absence of underlying pulmonary disease, pulse oximetry readings are normal.
(B) The arterial Pa_{O_2} measurement is abnormal.
(C) Anemic patients exhibit cyanois at lower methemoglobin concentrations.
(D) Venous cooximetry is accurate in determining methemoglobin levels.

23-37. A 14-month-old child presents after swallowing 2 of his grandmother's glyburide pills approximately 3 hours prior to arrival. The patient is currently alert and playful. Which of the following statements is TRUE concerning the management of this patient?

(A) The patient is safe for discharge as symptoms should have developed by 3 hours postingestion.

(B) Prophylactic glucagon is indicated for glyburide ingestion in a patient without diabetes.

(C) Octreotide would not be useful in refractory hypoglycemia secondary to sulfonylurea poisoning.

(D) The patient should be admitted and monitored for up to 24 hours as hypoglycemia may be delayed in onset.

Toxicologic Emergencies
Answers, Explanations, and References

23-1. **The answer is A** (Chapter 157). Drug interactions are both common and commonly missed in the ED; a high index of suspicion should be maintained, and patients should always be asked if their medications are new or if the doses have been changed. Drugs that induce the cytochrome P450 enzyme system of the liver such as phenytoin, griseofulvin, and carbamazepine, among others, accelerate the metabolism of other medications such as warfarin. Amiodarone can cause the formation of idiosyncratic hepatotoxins, which can prolong the metabolism of warfarin. Erythromycin and sulfonamides are inhibitors of the cytochrome P450 system, thereby increasing warfarin levels.

23-2. **The answer is D** (Chapter 158). This patient is presenting with symptoms typical of a tricyclic antidepressant (TCA) overdose, namely, dilated pupils, warm and dry skin, decreased bowel sounds, seizures, and wide-complex dysrhythmias. Indications for bicarbonate therapy in TCA overdose include QRS widening >100 ms, hypotension, ventricular dysrhythmias, and a terminal right axis deviation in aVR of more than 3 mm. Lidocaine is considered second-line therapy after $NaHCO_3$ for wide-complex ventricular dysrhythmias. Gastric lavage is recommended only for very recent ingestion (i.e., less than 1 hour prior to presentation) and should not supercede the need for cardiovascular resuscitation. Phenytoin is not recommended in TCA overdose as it has been shown ineffective in seizure control for these patients and is also potentially proarrhythmic.

23-3. **The answer is C** (Chapter 159). This patient is exhibiting a classic serotonin syndrome, which can occur when a patient on a selective serotonin reuptake inhibitor (SSRI) begins another serotoninergic medication. Such medications include prescription medication (trazodone, meperidine, lithium), over-the-counter medications (dextromethorphan, St. John's Wort), and drugs of abuse (MDMA, LSD). Emergency physicians should be careful with patients on SSRIs lest they precipitate the syndrome themselves. Patients often present with the typical clinical triad of agitation, autonomic instability (diarrhea, diaphoresis, hyperthermia, hypertension), and increased muscular tone (hyperreflexia, muscle rigidity more prominent in the lower extremities). Conditions that can mimic serotonin syndrome include malignant hyperthermia, meningitis, neuroleptic malignant syndrome, and sympathomimetic overdose, to name a few. Treatment is symptomatic, aimed at stabilizing vital signs and decreasing muscular rigidity. Cyproheptadine is recognized anecdotally as a potential serotonin antagonist, but no clear guidelines on its use have been formed.

23-4. **The answer is B** (Chapter 160). MAOIs have mostly been supplanted by newer antidepressants due to MAOI toxicity and the availability of safer alternatives like selective serotonin reuptake inhibitors. Commercially available MAOIs irreversibly block both subtypes of MAO, leading to the accumulation of aminated neurotransmitters in the presynaptic terminals. MAOIs, however, have a minimal role on the effect of circulating catecholamines, which are metabolized by a different enzyme system. The tyramine reaction occurs about 15–90 minutes after the ingestion of foods high in tyramine (aged or pickled foods), causing headache, hypertension, neck stiffness, and palpitations. Hypertension is typically treated with phentolamine or nitroprusside. Beta-blockers are contraindicated in MAOI ingestions due to the resulting unopposed alpha effect, causing worsening hypertension.

23-5.   **The answer is C** (Chapter 161). Neuroleptics can cause numerous side effects. Dystonic reactions are involuntary muscle contractions commonly seen after a first dose. Muscles of the neck and jaw are commonly affected, as are ocular muscle (oculogyric crises). Akathisia is motor restlessness combined with agitation and can often be mistaken for worsening psychosis. Tardive dyskinesia is a result of chronic neuroleptic use, taking months to years to appear. It is characterized by rhythmic choreoathetoid movements of the face and limbs; lip smacking and rhythmic tongue protrusion are classic signs. Neuroleptic malignant syndrome (NMS) is a rare idiosyncratic reaction characterized by muscle rigidity, hyperthermia, autonomic instability, and alterations in mental status. The rigidity of NMS is characterized as a "lead-pipe" rigidity. Parkinsonism (also seen with neuroleptic use) is classically associated with "cogwheel" rigidity.

23-6.   **The answer is C** (Chapter 162). Lithium toxicity can present in many different ways, but among the most common is a unique combination of fine tremor (mostly in the hands) and fatigue or lethargy; few other intoxications present similarly (e.g., baclofen, Quaaludes). Other symptoms include polyuria, nausea and vomiting, ataxia, and a maculopapular rash. Signs and lab abnormalities include long QTc interval, atrioventricular blocks, nephrogenic diabetes insipidus, acne, and leukocytosis,

among others. While lithium is not well adsorbed by activated charcoal, it is not contraindicated until a multidrug ingestion is ruled out. Forced diuresis may actually be harmful, as loop diuretics and thiazides can increase sodium and water loss to which lithium handling by the kidney is closely tied. Fluid repletion is the key to treatment. Phenytoin is often ineffective in controlling lithium-induced seizures, and phenytoin can decrease the renal excretion of lithium. Barbiturates are an effective second-line therapy.

23-7.   **The answer is B** (Chapter 163). Barbiturates, although less popular due to safer sedatives, are still among the most common toxic agents in overdose as reported by national poison control centers. The parent compound, barbituric acid, has no central nervous system depressant activity. While alkalinizing the urine is an effective modality for the treatment of long-acting barbiturate overdose, it is not believed effective in short-acting barbiturate toxicity, as the short-acting agents are primarily hepatically metabolized. The lipid solubility of the barbiturate governs the rapidity of its transit across the blood-brain barrier. Longer-acting barbiturates have less lipid solubility and are less protein bound, which accounts for their smaller volume of distribution and their longer duration of action. While activated charcoal is recommended for barbiturate overdose, multidose activated charcoal should be considered only in cases of overdose with long-acting barbiturates.

23-8.   **The answer is C** (Chapter 164). Flumazenil is a competitive antagonist of the benzodiazepine receptor in the central nervous system. It is considered an antidote for all benzodiazepine overdoses as well as for the nonbenzodiazepine sedative zolpidem. It is ineffective in reversing other sedative hypnotics, including barbiturates and GHB. Flumazenil has limited utility in the ED and is generally reserved for the reversal of procedural sedation. Administration of flumazenil can lower the seizure threshold of the patient and has been known to cause refractory seizures in patient who have coingested other substances, notably tricyclic antidepressants. Flumazenil should never be given to a patient with an unknown ingestion. Supportive care remains the cornerstone of treatment.

23-9. **The answer is D** (Chapter 165). While the patient appears to have been the victim of a sedative/hypnotic ingestion, it is often difficult to ascertain the exact offending agent. Occasionally, subtle clinical clues can lead to the correct diagnosis. In this case, the smell of pears on the breath and the ventricular dysrhythmia point to chloral hydrate as the potential agent. Chloral hydrate has often been used in the past as a so-called "knockout drug" or "rape drug" but has largely been supplanted by GHB and other agents. The combination of ethanol and chloral hydrate is what is commonly referred to as a "Mickey Finn." The chloral hydrate is metabolized by alcohol dehydrogenase to form trichloroethanol, which in turn slows the enzyme's metabolism of ethanol, but alcohol intake creates the NADH needed to metabolize chloral hydrate; the result is a powerful vicious cycle. GHB is possible; however, it does not present with the scent of pears on the breath. Methaqualone (Quaaludes) ingestion often presents with seizures, tremor, and lethargy, while glutethimide is often associated with anticholinergic symptoms, as well as a unique fluctuating and prolonged comatose state.

23-10. **The answer is C** (Chapter 166). Ethanol has 10–20 times the affinity for alcohol dehydrogenase as methanol (the ratio is 100:1 for ethylene glycol); when using IV ethanol, blood levels should be maintained at 100–150 mg/dL. Lower levels are considered much less effective. Using fomepizole also causes displacement of the atypical alcohols from alcohol dehydrogenase but does not alter the indications for dialysis, as significant levels of toxins have likely already accumulated in the bloodstream in the time between ingestion and treatment. Isopropyl alcohol is unique among the common atypical alcohols. It can cause an osmolar gap, but an elevated anion gap is not seen. Treatment of ethylene glycol poisoning should always include 100 mg of pyridoxine (vitamin B_6), the cofactor that aids in the breakdown of the metabolite glycoxylic acid into the nontoxic glycine.

23-11. **The answer is C** (Chapter 168). Cocaine is a sympathomimetic agent with local anaesthetic and central nervous system stimulant properties. Its stimulant activity comes mainly from blockade of presynaptic uptake of dopamine, serotonin, and norepinephrine. Like other local anesthetics, cocaine inhibits conduction of nerve impulses by blocking fast-acting sodium channels in neural tissue. Cocaine has many effects on the heart. Its ability to cause widened QRS complexes and QTc prolongation comes from a type 1A quinidine-like effect on cardiac conduction tissue. Cocaine is metabolized by plasma cholinesterase so neuromuscular blocking agents (both depolarizing and nondepolarizing) should be used with some caution—they may have a prolonged effect as a result of decreased metabolism. Haloperidol and droperidol can cause hyperthermia, dysrhythmia, and lowered seizure threshold in patients who have ingested cocaine, and they should be avoided in the cocaine-intoxicated patient.

23-12. **The answer is C** (Chapter 170). Salicylates have multiple effects on the body, and an understanding of the mechanisms of their toxicity is the key to understanding the treatment principles. Salicylates are mostly ionized at a physiologic pH. However, as acidemia progresses, more of the salicylate molecules will be ionized and will be free to cross the blood-brain barrier, allowing for relatively higher concentrations of salicylates in the brain with larger ingestions. This higher degree of ionization is also the key to the principle of ion trapping in the kidney used to treat the condition. Salicylates have profound effects on glucose homeostasis. While they do cause mobilization of glycogen stores, they can also inhibit gluconeogenesis. Normoglycemia, hyperglycemia, or hypoglycemia can be seen in the salicylate-poisoned patient. Hemorrhage is a surprisingly rare complication of acute massive salicylate poisoning, although it is slightly more common with chronic salicylate poisoning. Although it is true that the respiratory stimulation of salicylates is centrally mediated, salicylates also cause increased metabolism of skeletal muscle, thereby increasing the amount of carbon dioxide in the blood. Once the buffering capacity is overcome and the ventilatory compensation can no longer keep up with carbon dioxide production, a respiratory acidosis superimposes upon the anion gap metabolic acidosis.

23-13.   **The answer is C** (Chapter 174). This patient is suffering from an acute digitalis overdose, as evidenced not only by the elevated serum level but also from the corroborating clinical signs of nausea, abdominal pain, confusion, and, most convincingly, the junctional bradycardia. Oral medications are not appropriate in an obtunded patient. Activated charcoal, while appropriate in most toxic ingestions, and Kayexalate, while appropriate in the context of the patient's hyperkalemia, are best not given orally to an obtunded patient. Activated charcoal should not be administered to an obtunded patient unless the airway is properly protected against aspiration. Even in that case, gastric lavage has been associated with asystole in digitalis-poisoned patients, presumably due to the intense vagal stimulation caused during lavage. When calculated, 3 vials of digoxin-specific Fab fragments (Digibind) is the correct dosage via the equation: serum digoxin level multiplied by the patient's weight in kilograms divided by 100. Choice D the only option not to include Fab fragments, and this patient meets the criteria for Digibind (specifically, hyperkalemia in excess of 5.5 mEq/L associated with a toxic digitalis level).

Treatment for hyperkalemia should proceed as in any other clinical situation with one exception: calcium should never be given to a digoxin-poisoned patient. The blockade of the Na/K pump on the cardiac myocyte cell membrane causes increased use of the Na/Ca antiporter, resulting in increased cytosolic calcium—an effect which accounts for digoxin's inotropic effects. Administration of calcium may exaggerate this effect, creating a hypercontracted "stone heart" that is unable to maintain proper cardiac output.

23-14.   **The answer is D** (Chapters 174–176). The differentiation between digoxin, β-blocker, and calcium channel blocker toxicity is difficult. However, subtle clinical clues can help guide the diagnosis. These are guidelines and should not be used as absolute rules. Hyperglycemia occurs with calcium channel blocker overdoses via antagonism of calcium channels on pancreatic islet cells. β-blocker overdoses can present with hypoglycemia due to blockade of the β2 receptor. Patients with calcium channel blocker overdoses often maintain a normal mental status even in the face of bradycardia and hypotension, much more so than β-blocker- or digoxin-poisoned patients, who manifest confusion and depressed mentation. Hypokalemia is seen in severe calcium channel blocker overdoses, while hyperkalemia is commonly seen in acute digoxin ingestions. Tachydysrhythmias are often seen in digoxin overdoses but are rare in β-blocker overdoses and even rarer in calcium channel blocker overdoses.

23-15.   **The answer is A** (Chapter 179). Iron poisoning is generally divided into 5 stages. The first stage generally consists of abdominal pain, nausea, vomiting, and diarrhea and lasts up to 24 hours. Most toxicologists agree that the absence of GI symptoms within 6 hours of ingestion virtually rules out a significant iron ingestion. The latent stage (stage 2) occurs within 6–24 hours; GI symptoms typically resolve by this time. Stage 3 marks the beginning of systemic toxicity, with iron causing disruption of normal cellular metabolism, giving rise to lactic acidosis and, potentially, a shock state. Stage 4 is the hepatic stage, beginning 2–5 days postingestion. This stage is usually noted by elevated liver transaminases and occasionally by frank hepatic failure. Stage 5 refers to the delayed sequalae of iron poisoning, such as gastric outlet obstruction due to corrosion of the pyloric mucosa, which occurs 4–6 weeks after ingestion.

23-16.   The answer is B (Chapter 180). Viscosity, which is the resistance to flow, is the major determinant for the risk of aspiration for a given ingested hydrocarbon. Substances with viscosities below 60 Saybolt seconds universal (SSU), such as gasoline and turpentine, are at greater risk for aspiration than compounds with viscosities above 100 SSU (e.g., mineral oil, petroleum jelly). Volatility refers to the chemical's ability to vaporize—highly volatile chemical are less likely to be aspirated. Surface tension also plays a role in determining the aspiration risk but is not as significant as viscosity. Flash point has no effect of the risk of aspiration.

23-17.   The answer is B (Chapter 181). Hydrofluoric acid is the agent most likely to have caused this injury. It is used commonly in industry for such purposes as metal cleaning, glass etching, and petroleum processing, and it can also be found in dilute form in some household products (e.g., rust remover). With dermal exposure, the patient usually complains of severe pain to the affected area in the face of fairly benign examination—the skin often has a whitish discoloration to it. Depending on the route and degree of exposure, hydrofluoric acid is associated with significant morbidity and mortality due to hypocalcemia. The fluoride ions readily form complexes with calcium and magnesium, resulting in both cell death and systemic hypocalcemia. Severe injuries can give rise to hypocalcemia, hypomagnesemia, hyperkalemia, and ventric-

ular dysrhythmias. After thorough irrigation, the affected areas should be coated in a calcium gluconate gel. This can be most easily accomplished by combining calcium gluconate powder with surgical lubricant and placing the gel inside a glove that is then placed on the patient's hand. In areas that are not amenable to this kind of coverage, intradermal injection of 5% calcium gluconate can be done. For distal extremities and a worsening clinical picture, intra-arterial calcium gluconate can be used. Oral calcium supplementation in a milliequivalent-for-milliequivalent basis should be given as a calcium or magnesium salt. Continued irrigation is appropriate but does not address the underlying pathophysiologic derangements. Tween 80 and De-Solv-It are used for dermal exposure to tar or asphalt in an attempt to remove the adherent substance. Cleaning with a dilute bleach solution can be used for dermal organophosphate exposures. The patient is not presenting with a cholinergic toxidrome.

23-18.   The answer is D (Chapter 182). This patient is manifesting symptoms of a cholinergic crisis, as evidenced by the hypersalivation, urinary incontinence, muscle weakness, and bronchorrhea, as well as his recent exposure to a "sprayed" field (presumably with insecticide). It is unknown exactly whether the agent involved is an organophosphate or a carbamate. While both agents inhibit cholinesterase, thus causing an accumulation of acetylcholine in neurons of the central and autonomic nervous systems as well as the neuromuscular junction, organophosphates do so irreversibly. Atropine and pralidoxime are the two main antidotes used for these types of patients. Atropine should be given to adults every 5 minutes until muscarinic effects are reversed. Atropine has no effect on muscle weakness. Pralidoxime acts by regenerating phosphorylated acetylcholinesterase and may also directly detoxify free organophosphate molecules. Its use with atropine appears to be synergistic, and pralidoxime does reverse both nicotinic and muscarininc symptoms of cholinergic toxicity. However, pralidoxime will not regenerate cholinesterase molecules once aging of the organophosphate-cholinesterase bond has occurred so it must be given early to reverse muscle paralysis.

23-19.   The answer is A (Chapter 184). The combination of abdominal pain, fatigue, wrist drop, depressed reflexes, anemia, basophilic stippling, and renal failure is highly suggestive of lead poisoning. Symptoms include headache, fatigue, and abdominal pain. Neurologically, the classic finding is wrist drop and depressed reflexes in the face of a normal sensory examination. Mental status changes range from encephalopathy with acute poisoning to irritability and depression due to chronic exposure. A hemolytic anemia is noted as is basophilic stippling, a classic, although nonspecific, finding of lead poisoning. Interstitial nephritis is seen chronically, while acute exposures manifest Fanconi's syndrome of aminoaciduria, glycosuria, and phosphaturia. Treatment for lead poisoning can include British antilewisite (BAL), Ca-EDTA, or succimer (DMSA), depending on the severity. An ethanol infusion is used for atypical alcohol poisoning, a diagnosis supported by neither the complaints nor the laboratory findings (no anion or osmolar gap). 6-mercaptopurine was an antidote for copper poisonings. BAL is used for copper poisoning by many clinicians. Physostigmine is the antidote for severe anticholinergic exposures.

23-20.   The answer is C (Chapter 186). While beneficial, many vitamins, when taken in excess, can have significant adverse effects. Vitamin C, which is important for proper collagen formation, can cause exacerbation of gout and nephrolithiasis when taken in excess. Vitamin B_1 (thiamine) is believed to be nontoxic in overdose. Niacin can cause a reddening and itching of the skin when taken in doses above the recommended 20 mg per day. Vitamin B_2 (riboflavin) is an

antioxidant also believed to be nontoxic in large doses. Hypercalcemia is seen with excess vitamin D ingestion.

23-21.   The answer is C (Chapter 188). Cyanide is a chemical asphyxiant, an agent that interferes with tissue oxygenation by either preventing oxygen delivery to the cells or by interfering with oxygen usage at the cellular level. Cyanide has an avid affinity for metal-containing enzyme complexes, and its key physiologic effect is the inhibition of the iron-dependent reduction of oxygen to water by cytochrome aa_3 (the last step of oxidative phosphorylation). Cyanide has no appreciable effect on hemoglobin molecules. Hence, oxygen saturation often remains normal, and the patient is not hypoxic until after respiratory arrest ensues. Methemoglobin has a high affinity for cyanide, explaining the use of nitrites in the antidote kits for cyanide. However, the formation of methemoglobin by nitrites is relatively contraindicated in cases of cyanide poisoning due to smoke inhalation, where other asphyxiants like carbon monoxide may be contributing to the hypoxia. Creation of methemoglobin in these patients theoretically creates less functional hemoglobin for oxygen delivery. Sodium thiosulfate enhances the activity of rhodanase, an enzyme that catalyzes the transfer of sulfate from sodium thiosulfate to cyanide. The resulting thiocyanate molecule is much less toxic than cyanide and is excreted by the kidneys.

23-22.   The answer is B (Chapter 156). Physostigmine is the antidote for anticholinergic toxicity, not for MAOIs. The cyanide antidote contains nitrate compounds. Thiamine (along with pyridoxine) is used for ethylene glycol toxicity to allow for metabolism of the intermediate molecule glycoxylic acid into nontoxic products. Pyridoxine (vitamin B_6) is used for treatment of isoniazid (INH) toxicity, which presents with seizures refractory to conventional treatment, anion gap metabolic acidosis, nausea, vomiting, tachycardia, and ketonemia.

The active version of pyridoxine is a cofactor in many enzymatic reactions, including the synthesis of gamma-aminobutyric acid (GABA). INH interferes with the normal utilization of pyridoxine in a competitive fashion.

23-23. The answer is C (Chapters 156, 176, 179). Activated charcoal is generally agreed upon as the most appropriate agent to decontaminate the gastrointestinal (GI) tract. It is formed by heating charcoal in an anhydrous environment, making it porous and increasing its surface area, allowing toxic agents in the GI tract to be adsorbed to the charcoal more effectively. Maximal benefit for the use of charcoal is generally agreed upon as being within 2 hours of ingestion, although benefit may still exist beyond that time frame. Reasons not to use charcoal include a risk of aspiration without airway protection, ileus, caustic ingestions (charcoal may accumulate in burned areas), and drugs that do not adsorb to activated charcoal. Substances that do not bind to activated charcoal include metals (like iron and lead), small molecules (such as lithium and borates), hydrocarbons (particularly long-chain molecules), liquids (i.e., alcohols, methylsalicylate), organophosphates and carbamates, quinidine, meprobamate (which forms gastric concretions), DDT, cyanide, and hydroxides of sodium and potassium.

23-24. The answer is D (Chapter 181). Just over 100,000 caustic exposures are reported to poison control centers in the United States annually. Most are unintentional, and many are children under the age of 6 years. While both acids and alkalis can cause significant tissue damage, alkalis like the hydroxides ingested by the patient in question have greater potential for proximal esophageal injury. Alkalis cause a rapidly penetrating liquefactive necrosis, whereas acids tend to cause a coagulative type of necrosis. The resulting eschar from acid burns tends to limit the damage more than is seen in alkali ingestions. Dilution of a strong type of ei-

ther agent can be associated with a powerful exothermic reaction, so dilutional therapy is not recommended, although the exothermic nature of neutralization therapy has recently been questioned. Charcoal should not be given to patients who have ingested caustic agents since caustic agents do not adsorb well to activated charcoal and charcoal can impede visualization during endoscopy. NG tube insertion should be performed by an endoscopist for acid injuries and should not be inserted at all in alkali injuries. Early endoscopic evaluation, ideally performed within 12 hours, is the best way to evaluate the severity and location of tissue injury. There is some debate as to the specific indications for endoscopy, so the hospital's endoscopist should be consulted in all cases of caustic injury.

23-25. The answer is C (Chapters 188, 189). Methemoglobin is a normal product of oxidant stress. The iron moiety in hemoglobin is oxidized to the ferrous (Fe^{3+}) in response to oxygen or any other compound seeking electrons (i.e., an oxidant). An NADH-based enzyme complex normally reduces iron back to its functional ferric (Fe^{2+}). Methemoglobinemia ensues when these normal mechanisms are overwhelmed by an oxidant stress. Many agents can induce methemoglobinemia by this mechanism, including lidocaine, nitrites, and dapsone, but not acetaminophen. Patients usually develop symptoms at a level of 20–30%, when cyanosis anxiety, headache, weakness, and lightheadedness are seen, which may then progress to seizures, dysrhythmias, and acidosis. Classically, patients present with a cyanosis that does not respond to oxygen, and their blood is characteristically described as "chocolate brown." While methemoglobinemia is potentially lethal, formation of methemoglobin is part of the antidote to cyanide poisoning. The use of amyl nitrite or sodium nitrite in the cyanide antidote kit creates methemoglobin, which has a high affinity for cyanide. Sulfhemoglobinemia is much less common than methemoglobinemia but presents similarly.

23-26. **The answer is A** (Chapter 156). Hemodialysis is most effective when the toxic agent to be dialysed has a small volume of distribution and a small molecular weight and is not protein bound. The pKa does not significantly affect the amenability of an agent to dialysis. Dialysis can be used for the following poisonings: lithium, salicylates, methanol, ethylene glycol, and theophylline.

23-27. **The answer is D** (Chapter 177). Clonidine is a centrally acting antihypertensive. It is an α_2 receptor agonist that decreases norepinephrine release in the central nervous system, causing a lowering a heart rate and blood pressure. It also reduces noradrenergic output in locus ceruleus, which is believed to account for the ability of clonidine to mitigate the effects of narcotic withdrawal. Clonidine exposure is not an uncommon occurrence in children. The main symptoms seen are hypotension and bradycardia, an extension of the drug's therapeutic effects. At higher doses, clonidine can have peripheral α-agonist effects, causing a paradoxical increase in heart rate and blood pressure, although the central effects usually predominate. Respiratory depression and apnea can occur and is a common symptom in children. Other symptoms include hypothermia, diarrhea, and miosis.

23-28. **The answer is A** (Chapter 156). Although at first glance both sympathomimetic and anticholenergic toxidromes appear plausible, the presence of diaphoresis in this patient makes a sympathomimetic toxidrome more likely. Cholinergic toxicity is characterized by the SLUDGE syndrome—salivation, lacrimation, urination, defecation, gastric irritation, and emesis. Opioid toxicity manifests as miosis, central nervous system depression, and respiratory depression. Typically the skin of patients suffering from an anticholinergic toxicity is warm, red, and dry, while sympathomimetic toxic patients have moist skin secondary to diaphoresis. This difference is one of the few clues differentiating the two toxidromes.

23-29. **The answer is B** (Chapters 156, 169). Hallucinogenic substances have been used for centuries, but their recreational use has been on the rise since the 1960s and has resurged in the last several years. LSD is the most potent hallucinogenic compound known, believed to exert its effect through the serotoninergic system. The psychedelic effects depend largely on the patient's mood at the time of ingestion and usually last about 8–12 hours. Prolonged psychosis can occur but is relatively uncommon, occurring in about 5% of users. PCP intoxication presents with a sympathomimetic toxidrome that may require a large amount of sedation to achieve control of the patient in the ED. While acidification of the urine does increase the excretion of PCP from the kidneys, acidification has been associated with adverse effects such as rhabdomyolysis and is not recommended as a treatment modality. Marijuana can be detected in the urine for several days after use and up to 2 weeks in chronic users, making it impossible to distinguish between acute and past use. Jimson weed grows naturally in the United States and contains anticholinergic alkaloids. The seeds, and indeed many other parts of the plant, can be ingested, smoked, or even brewed into a tea, producing an anticholinergic toxidrome.

23-30. **The answer is C** (Chapter 167). The half-life of naloxone is 60–90 minutes, and the duration of action is 20–60 minutes. The importance of this point is that the duration of action of naloxone is shorter than the duration of most narcotics, necessitating either repeat doses of naloxone or the administration of a naloxone infusion. The infusion can be calculated by taking the wakeup dose (i.e., that dose that reversed respiratory depression) and administering two-thirds of that dose hourly.

23-31. **The answer is B** (Chapter 185). Inhalation agents that have particle diameters >10 μm or that are water soluble more commonly cause immediate airway-related symptoms. Examples of such agents are ammonia, sulfur dioxide, and acidic gases. Phosgene is not water soluble and thus causes a paucity of symptoms on initial exposure, followed by the delayed onset of noncardiogenic pulmonary edema up to 24 hours later. In fact, the onset of significant pulmonary symptoms within 4 hours of exposure suggests massive exposure and a poor prognosis. Although inhaled nerve agents may have only mild irritant effects, they typically result in a rapid onset of symptoms. Patients suffering from cyanide poisoning are immediately affected but lack any objective evidence of primary pulmonary injury.

23-32.   **The answer is C** (Chapter 187). Isoniazid (INH) is the most commonly cited agent involved in antimicrobial ingestions that result in significant morbidity or mortality. Typical symptoms of INH toxicity include nausea, mental status changes, and ataxia. Severe toxicity is manifested by the triad of seizure, coma, and anion gap metabolic acidosis. INH-related seizures are often refractory to typical therapy and require the use of intravenous pyridoxine. The onset of symptoms postingestion usually occurs within 2 hours, and patients who are asymptomatic at 6 hours can be considered medically stablilized. If present, an anion gap metabolic acidosis is likely due to seizure-induced lactic acidosis, and thus sodium bicarbonate is of little use in this setting.

23-33.   **The answer is D** (Chapter 187). The antimalarial agents are among the potentially most toxic antimicrobial agents. The sodium channel blockade induced by toxic levels of quinine may result in dysrhythmias and cardiovascular collapse. Sodium bicarbonate therapy may be of benefit in this setting. Central nervous system toxicity results in headache, coma, and seizures. Significant ocular toxicity may occur, resulting in blindness. Toxic metabolic disturbances that may occur include hypoglycemia with quinine and hypokalemia due to chloroquine. Hyperkalemia, noncar-

diogenic pulmonary edema, and pancytopenia are not typical findings in quinine overdose.

23-34.   **The answer is C** (Chapter 188). The use of nitrites for the induction of methemoglobinemia as an antidote in the setting of possible cyanide poisoning may potentiate the deleterious effects of a coexisting carboxyhemoglobinemia. Most commonly associated with smoke inhalation exposures involving inhaled hydrogen cyanide, concomitant carbon monoxide poisoning is a relative contraindication to nitrite administration. Induction of a methemoglobinemia in this setting may further reduce an already compromised oxygen-carrying capacity, resulting in worsening cellular ischemia. Thus empiric administration of sodium thiosulfate is recommended. Methylene blue is the antidote for toxicity secondary to methemoglobinemia. Oxygen is beneficial to all patients with apnea who have been exposed to smoke.

23-35.   **The answer is B** (Chapter 189). Acquired infantile methemoglobinemia from gastroenteritis may be due to acidosis-related NADH-methemoglobin reductase impairment. Phenazopyridine (bladder anesthetic agent) and benzocaine (topical anesthetic) are two of the most common causes of methemoglobinemia. Carbon monoxide poisoning can occur after prolonged methylene chloride inhalation (contained in some paint-stripping solvents) through biotransformation via hepatic metabolism.

23-36.   **The answer is D** (Chapter 189). Arterial or venous cooximetry will accurately and definitively identify methemoglobinemia. With significant methemoglobinemia ($\geq 20\%$), cutaneous pulse oximetry will trend toward 85% despite the delivery of increasing oxygen concentrations. Arterial PaO_2 reflects the dissolved (not hemoglobin-bound) oxygen and thus will not reflect the true oxygen delivery to tissues in the setting of significant methemoglobinemia. Anemic patients actually require the presence of a higher percentage of methemoglobin before cyanosis is clinically apparent. The appearance of cyanosis is solely dependent on the absolute concentration of methemoglobin (≥1.5 g/dL).

23-37.   The answer is D (Chapter 190). Children who have ingested even a single oral hypoglycemic agent generally require admission as the onset of hypoglycemia may be delayed for many hours. Glucagon is not indicated in the asymptomatic patient and may lack efficacy due to depleted glycogen stores in certain individuals (children, alcoholics, and the elderly). Octreotide is useful in reversing hypoglycemia secondary to sulfonylurea toxicity by inhibiting insulin release at the pancreatic β-islet cells.

Trauma
Questions

24-1. In which patient is an ED thoracotomy MOST indicated?

(A) A 76-year-old male who was the unrestrained driver in a 70 MPH motor vehicle crash and was found pulseless at the scene.

(B) A 25-year-old female with a gunshot wound to the right chest that upon arrival to the ED is found to have a blood pressure of 40 mmHg by palpation and no breath sounds on the right.

(C) A 40-year-old male with a stab wound to the left chest who lost all vital signs 3 minutes prior to arriving at the ED and has received bilateral needle chest decompressions.

(D) A 27-year-old construction worker with an impaled fence post in his abdomen, a blood pressure of 90/60 mmHg, and fluid in Morison's pouch revealed by ultrasound.

24-2. Which of the following is TRUE regarding imaging of the cervical spine?

(A) A 25-year-old female involved in a 45 MPH motor vehicle crash with a normal neurologic exam, no cervical spine tenderness, and a femur fracture does not need cervical spine radiography.

(B) Once the lateral C-spine radiograph is obtained in a trauma patient, the cervical collar can be safely removed.

(C) As long as a trauma patient is found to be "clinically sober," the cervical collar can be removed if there is no midline cervical spine tenderness.

(D) The final step in clinically clearing the cervical spine is painless rotation of the neck in all four directions.

24-3. An 8-year-old male hit a car door while riding his bicycle. Upon presentation he is crying and complaining of abdominal pain. His physical exam reveals age-appropriate vital signs, an abrasion across his epigastrium, and diffuse tenderness without rebound or guarding. Labs are notable for an amylase level of 220 Iu. A urine sample reveals 2–5 RBCs per high-power field. Which of the following is CORRECT?

(A) Despite a normal abdominal CT, the child could have a pancreatic injury and should be admitted for observation.

(B) An intravenous pyelogram should be performed for evaluation of hematuria.

(C) The bowel is the most commonly injured organ following this mechanism of injury.

(D) Duodenal hematoma is unlikely if a repeat exam reveals no abdominal tenderness.

24-4. A 4-year-old child was struck by a car traveling approximately 30 MPH and was thrown approximately 15 feet. She is complaining of abdominal pain. Physical exam reveals a blood pressure of 68/40 mmHg, a heart rate of 200 beats per minute, and a firm, tender abdomen. She weighs approximately 20 kg. As long as the systolic blood pressure remains below 90 mmHg, what is the most appropriate fluid management?

(A) 800 cc of normal saline followed by 400 cc of blood.

(B) 400 cc of normal saline followed by 200 cc of blood.

(C) 400 cc of normal saline repeated 3 times, then 400 cc of blood.

(D) 400 cc of normal saline repeated 3 times, then 200 cc of blood.

24-5. A 6-year-old male was the rear-seated restrained passenger in a moderate-speed motor vehicle crash. He reported to the EMS providers that his "legs were numb" immediately following the collision, but within 30 minutes these symptoms resolved. His exam is entirely normal, and his plain radiographs are normal. Which of the following is CORRECT?

(A) Regardless of his normal exam and radiographs, he requires urgent magnetic resonance imaging.

(B) He can safely be discharged with close follow-up as long as his exam remains normal during a 4-hour observation period.

(C) Flexion-extension radiographs should be performed to rule out any ligamentous injury.

(D) Computed tomography scan of the cervical spine should be performed to assess for surrounding soft tissue swelling.

24-6. A 15-month-old child fell from a rocking horse while his parents were taking his picture. The parents state the fall was no more than 3 feet, but he did strike his head on the tile floor. The child cried immediately with no apparent loss of consciousness. He

stopped crying within 5 minutes and has otherwise been acting appropriately. Which of the following is TRUE?

(A) Following a 3-hour observation period this child can be safely discharged as long as there is close follow-up within the next 24 hours.

(B) As long as there is no evidence of scalp soft tissue injury and skull radiographs are unremarkable, the child can be safely discharged from the ED with close follow-up.

(C) Due to age alone, this represents a moderate- to high-risk injury, and a computed tomography scan of the head is recommended.

(D) Since there was no loss of consciousness, there is little risk of intracranial bleed, and no further evaluation is required.

24-7. An 82-year-old male slipped in the shower at his assisted living facility. He recalls "slipping" but is not certain if he struck his head. He is currently on a back board and has a cervical collar in place. His only complaint is of mild tenderness in the right shoulder. On exam he has no midline cervical spine tenderness. Which of the following is TRUE?

(A) Epidural hematomas are very common at this age and therefore a computed tomography scan of the head is indicated.

(B) Due to the patient's advanced age, imaging of the cervical spine is warranted even though he has no tenderness.

(C) Cerebral atrophy provides additional protection in this age group, and therefore head injuries are less common.

(D) The most common cervical spine fracture in this age group is a simple wedge compression fracture of C7.

24-8. A 72-year-old female tripped on a rug, striking the edge of a table as she fell to the ground. She complains only of right-sided chest wall pain that is worse with inspiration. She looks extremely uncomfortable. A chest radiograph reveals fractures of the eight, ninth, and tenth ribs without evidence of pneumothorax. Which of the following is TRUE?

(A) The patient can be discharged after her ribs are taped and pain control is provided.

(B) Aortic tear is the most common injury following isolated chest wall trauma.

(C) This patient is likely to develop pneumonia and should be admitted.

(D) If hypoxia is present following this injury, early intubation should be withheld as this can worsen the prognosis.

24-9. A 25-year-old female, currently 34 weeks pregnant, was the restrained driver involved in a 25 MPH motor vehicle crash where she was rear-ended at a stoplight. Her airbag deployed, and the prehospital personnel describe minor damage to the car. There was no loss of consciousness, and the patient complains only of neck pain. She was walking at the scene but was transported in the supine position in full cervical spine precautions on a backboard. Her physical exam is notable for cervical tenderness at the C5–C6 level. Which of the following is CORRECT?

(A) She may be safely discharged following her trauma evaluation as long as the fetal heart rate is >120 beats per minute and fetal activity is noted.

(B) She should not receive radiographs of the cervical spine due to the potential risk of fetal malformations following radiation.

(C) She should not remain supine on the long board and should be immediately removed in order to improve fetal circulation.

(D) Following the appropriate trauma evaluation, the patient should have external fetal monitoring for a minimum of 4 hours prior to discharge.

24-10. Which of the following is TRUE of the full-term pregnant trauma patient?

(A) She should receive the same fluid resuscitation as the nonpregnant patient.

(B) She does not require $Rh_o(D)$ immune globulin (RhoGAM) unless there is evidence of placental abruption.

(C) She requires an open, supraumbilical approach should diagnostic peritoneal lavage be indicated.

(D) She should not have a speculum exam performed due to the risk of placenta previa.

24-11. A 34-week pregnant patient arrives at a level I trauma center following a high-speed motor vehicle crash and within 3 minutes of arrival suddenly becomes pulseless. Which of the following is CORRECT?

(A) If resuscitation attempts are unsuccessful, emergent cesarean section should be performed within 5 minutes of arrest.

(B) If an emergent cesarean section is performed, the horizontal miduterine incision should be used to speed access to the fetus.

(C) Pressors should be withheld from the mother until emergent cesarean section is performed as these agents cause fetal hypoperfusion.

(D) A fetal heart rate should be confirmed prior to the performance of an emergent cesarean section in order to determine fetal viability.

24-12. A 35-year-old male involved in a high-speed motor vehicle crash with obvious head injury is brought to the ED. His vital signs are heart rate 120 beats per minute, blood pressure 110/75 mmHg, and respiratory rate 18 breaths per minute. He opens his eyes with nail bed pressure, is moaning, and appears to flex his upper extremities with noxious stimuli. What is his Glasgow Coma Scale score?

(A) 5.
(B) 7.
(C) 9.
(D) 11.

24-13. A 23-year-old male construction worker presents after a 20-foot fall while at work. According to paramedics he was initially unconsciousness at the scene but has since been acting appropriately. While in the ED the patient begins to become combative and then more somnolent. What is the MOST LIKELY diagnosis?

(A) Subdural hematoma.

(B) Epidural hematoma.

(C) Diffuse axonal injury.

(D) Postconcussive syndrome.

24-14. A 68-year-old female with mental status changes is brought to the ED by her sister, who is her caretaker. According to her sister, the patient fell in the shower 4 days ago. Over the last 24 hours she has become less responsive, and her sister was unable to wake her this afternoon. Her past medical history is significant for atrial fibrillation, for which she takes Coumadin. She is a recovering alcoholic, and according to her sister has not had a drink in 5 years. On exam you note that she has a large contusion over her occiput. What is the MOST likely cause for her change in mental status?

(A) Alcohol intoxication.

(B) Epidural hematoma.

(C) Subdural hematoma.

(D) Concussion.

24-15. A 30-year-old male presents to the ED with a stab wound to the left flank. He has left lower extremity weakness and loss of pain sensation in the right lower extremity. Which type of spinal injury is he suffering from?

(A) Central cord syndrome.

(B) Brown-Séquard's syndrome.

(C) Spinal shock.

(D) Anterior cord syndrome.

24-16. A gunshot victim was brought into the ED with the complaint of weakness in his right arm and leg with preservation of pain sensation on his right shoulder, and loss of pain sensation in his left arm and leg. Where was he most likely shot?

(A) C3 on the left.

(B) T2 on the left.

(C) T4 on the right.

(D) C5 on the right.

24-17. A 60-year-old alcoholic female was brought in by paramedics with the chief complaint of weakness. According to her friends they found her "passed out" at the bottom of the stairs this morning. They put her in bed, but she still complains of weakness. On physical exam she has 4+ reflexes throughout, 3/5 upper extremity muscle strength bilaterally, and 4/5 lower extremity muscle strength. What is this patient's MOST likely injury?

(A) Subdural hematoma.

(B) Anterior cord syndrome.

(C) Central cord syndrome.

(D) Cauda equina.

24-18. Which of the following is the BEST plain film for evaluating orbital fractures?

(A) Caldwell view.

(B) Waters view.

(C) Submental vertex view.

(D) Towne view.

24-19. A 25-year-old motorcyclist is thrown from his bike. He is brought in by paramedics complaining of jaw pain. On physician exam, he has a large intraoral gingival laceration. Panorex film shows bilateral mandibular angle fractures, but the rest of his workup is negative. What is the MOST appropriate disposition for this patient?

(A) Prescribe a soft diet and follow up with oral surgery.

(B) Irrigate and close the wound, prescribe a soft diet, and follow up with oral surgery.

(C) Irrigate and close the wound, prescribe a soft diet and oral antibiotics, and follow up with oral surgery.

(D) Irrigate and close the wound, prescribe a soft diet, give IV antibiotics, and admit with oral surgery consultation.

24-20. A 23-year-old baseball player is brought to the ED after being struck in the right eye by a line drive. On exam, he has tenderness over the inferior orbital rim, periorbital ecchymosis, no subcutaneous emphysema, and mild limitation on upward gaze with the right eye. His pupils are equal and reactive, and his visual acuity is 20/20 in both eyes. Which of the following is the next step in management?

(A) Diagnosis of traumatic iritis based on history and physical exam.

(B) Computed tomography of orbits for suspicion of orbital blowout fracture.

(C) Emergent ear-nose-throat consultation for possible retro-orbital hematoma.

(D) Oral antibiotics for suspected sinus fracture.

24-21. A 20-year-old male presents with a single stab wound to his neck just superior to his clavicle. His vital signs are blood pressure 120/70 mmHg, heart rate 110 beats per minute, respiratory rate 16 breaths per minute, and pulse oxygenation 98%, and he is not in obvious distress. Which of the following describes the BEST management plan for this patient?

(A) Duplex sonography followed by admission for observation.

(B) Duplex sonography, bronchoscopy, laryngoscopy, and esophagoscopy.

(C) Computed tomography of the neck, bronchoscopy, laryngoscopy, and esophagoscopy.

(D) Angiography, esophagoscopy, and esophagram.

24-22. A 40-year-old female presents after a stab wound in the midclavicular line on the left at the third intercostal space. The vital signs are blood pressure 80/70 mmHg, heart rate 100 beats per minute, respiratory rate 22 breaths per minute, and pulse oximetry reading 99%. A left tube thoracostomy is placed, and 2000 cc of blood comes out of the tube initially. Which of the following is the next management step for this patient?

(A) Computed tomography of the chest.

(B) Emergent thoracotomy in the operating room.

(C) ED thoracotomy.

(D) Placement of a second tube thoracostomy on the same side.

24-23. A 50-year-old male presents after a motor vehicle crash with bruising over his sternum. He states that he hit his chest against the stearing wheel. His vital signs are unremarkable, and he is asymptomatic except for anterior chest wall tenderness at the site of the bruising. The initial chest radiograph and sternal view reveal a sternal fracture but are otherwise normal. There are no other associated injuries. The electrocardiogram is unremarkable. Which of the following is the MOST appropriate management plan for this patient?

(A) Admit for 24 hours of telemetry monitoring.

(B) Perform 2 sets of cardiac enzymes and troponin tests, and discharge if negative.

(C) Perform an echocardiogram in the ED, and discharge if negative.

(D) After a repeat electrocardiogram in 6 hours, discharge the patient with pain medication, without any further testing.

24-24. A 45-year-old male presents after a skiing injury in which he fell onto his right chest. He has pleuritic chest pain on the right and is short of breath. His vital signs are blood pressure 120/60 mmHg and heart rate 110 beats per minute. The chest radiograph documents a 35% pneumothorax. Which of the following is the next step in managing this patient?

(A) Place a right-sided 24-French chest tube.

(B) Place a right-sided 32-French chest tube.

(C) Place a 16-gauge angiocatheter in the right fifth intercostal space (midaxillary line), and aspirate air.

(D) Admit for observation, and repeat the chest radiograph in 4 hours.

24-25. A 35-year-old male presents with a single stab wound to the right lateral chest. He has no other injuries. His vital signs are blood pressure 150/80 mmHg and heart rate 100 beats per minute. His breath sounds are clear and equal bilaterally. Which of the following is the BEST management plan for this patient?

(A) Obtain a chest radiograph, and discharge the patient if negative.

(B) Obtain a chest radiograph on presentation, and perform a second one in 6 hours. Discharge the patient if both are negative.

(C) Obtain a chest radiograph on presentation, and perform a second one in 12 hours. Discharge the patient if both are negative.

(D) Discharge home, and instruct the patient to return if he develops shortness of breath.

24-26. Which of the following is the BEST method for diagnosing a diaphragmatic injury in a patient with a stab wound to the left upper quadrant?

(A) Computed tomography.

(B) Diagnostic peritoneal lavage.

(C) Upper gastrointestinal series.

(D) Laparoscopy.

24-27. Which of the following is the BEST screening test for detecting traumatic aortic injury in a stable patient?

(A) Chest radiograph.

(B) Computed tomography.

(C) Transthoracic echocardiography.

(D) Test for unequal blood pressures in the upper extremities.

24-28. Which of the following is the appropriate management for a patient with a right upper quadrant abdominal stab wound?

(A) Diagnostic peritoneal lavage followed by discharge if negative.

(B) Abdominal ultrasound followed by discharge if negative.

(C) Admission for observation and serial physical examinations.

(D) Digital probing of the wound followed by discharge if there is no evidence of violation of the anterior fascia.

24-29. Which of the following BEST describes the role of plain radiographs in abdominal trauma?

(A) Useful for determination of peritoneal penetration in patients with stab wounds to the abdomen.

(B) Useful for determination of free air in patients with blunt abdominal trauma.

(C) Useful for detection of the location of bullets in patients with gunshot wounds to the abdomen.

(D) Useful for detection of free air in patients with penetrating abdominal trauma.

24-30. A 35-year-old female presents 6 hours after a bicycle accident with ecchymosis on her midabdomen from hitting the handlebars. Her abdomen is not tender, and the remainder of her physical exam is unremarkable. She is hemodynamically stable.

Which of the following is the BEST management plan for this patient?

(A) Perform a bedside abdominal ultrasound exam initially and repeat in 4 hours. Discharge if both are negative.

(B) Perform a follow-up physical examination in 4 hours and discharge if negative.

(C) Admit for observation.

(D) Perform abdominal computed tomography and discharge if negative.

24-31. A 27-year-old male presents with a single stab wound to the left flank. He has the following vital signs: blood pressure 110/80 mmHg and heart rate 90 beats per minute. Which of the following is the MOST appropriate next step in management?

(A) Diagnostic peritoneal lavage.

(B) Wound exploration with a cotton swab.

(C) Computed tomography with intravenous contrast.

(D) Computed tomography with oral, rectal, and intravenous contrast.

24-32. A 37-year-old male was the restrained driver in a major motor vehicle crash. His vital signs are blood pressure 90/60 mmHg, heart rate 120 breaths per minute, and respiratory rate 20 breaths per minute. On physical examination, his Glasgow Coma Scale score is 15. He has diffuse abdominal tenderness and an unstable pelvis. His initial radiographs reveal an open book pelvic fracture, and his focused assessment with sonography for trauma (FAST) exam is shown in Figure 24-1. Which of the following is the next step in management?

(A) Exploratory laparotomy.

(B) Pelvic angiography with embolization of the pelvic vessels.

(C) Pericardiocentesis.

(D) Orthopedic surgery consultation.

24-33. A 7-year-old boy is brought to the ED after being hit by a car while walking across the street. The patient has normal vital signs and a Glasgow Coma Scale score of 15. The patient's physical exam is notable only for an obvious deformity of his left femur and an abrasion on his left hip. Plain radiographs confirm a supracondylar femur fracture. The pelvis and chest radiographs are normal. Laboratory evaluation reveals a normal hematocrit and a urinalysis significant only for 70 RBCs/hpf. Which of the following studies would be appropriate to evaluate the microscopic hematuria in this patient?

(A) Intravenous pyelogram.

(B) Repeat urinalysis in 2–3 days.

(C) Renal angiography.

(D) Computed tomography scan.

24-34. What is the MOST commonly injured organ of the genitourinary tract?

(A) Urethra.

(B) Kidney.

(C) Bladder.

(D) Ureter.

24-35. A 25-year-old man arrives in the ED reporting a gunshot wound to the right arm approximately 15 minutes prior to arrival. Which of the following findings on physical exam suggest the presence of an arterial injury requiring expeditious angiography or surgical intervention?

(A) Diminished distal pulses.

(B) Injury to an anatomically related nerve.

(C) Unexplained hypotension.

(D) Proximity of the injury to major vascular structures.

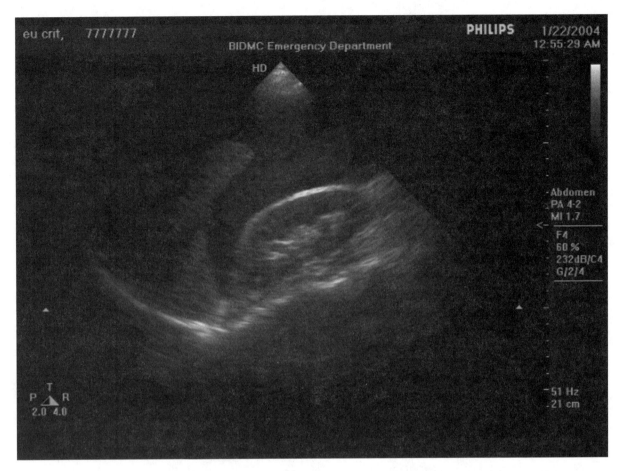

Figure 24-1.

24-36. A 19-year-old male is brought to the ED with a gunshot wound to the right flank. The patient has stable vital signs and an equivocal abdominal exam. No exit wound is found. Which of the following studies would be MOST helpful in locating the bullet and determining possible retroperitoneal and intra-abdominal injury?

(A) Plain radiographs of the abdomen and pelvis taken in planes separated by 90 degrees.

(B) Intravenous pyelogram.

(C) Focused assessment with sonography for trauma (FAST) scan.

(D) Computed tomography scan of the abdomen and pelvis.

24-37. Which of the following details regarding intentional injury is inappropriate for an examining physician without formal training in forensics to document on the medical record?

(A) Description of a bullet wound as the entrance or exit site.

(B) Photographic images of the wounds with a measurement scale in the field.

(C) Anatomic diagrams of the injury size and location.

(D) Description of the distribution of gunpowder residue around a bullet wound.

Trauma

Answers, Explanations, and References

24-1. **The answer is C** (Chapter 251). An ED thoracotomy is beneficial after penetrating chest trauma, especially in patients with stab wounds to the chest. The largest group of salvageable patients are those with vital signs that are lost either en route to the hospital or while in the ED. In this group of patients survival can approach 38%. In a patient with blunt trauma and no vital signs, the likelihood of survival is minimal. When there is hypotension in a patient with penetrating chest trauma, tube thoracostomy should be performed to eliminate tension pneumothorax as a cause of hypotension.

24-2. **The answer is D** (Chapter 251). To clinically clear a patient's cervical spine following trauma, certain criteria must be met. These include: (1) no posterior midline cervical spine tenderness, (2) no evidence of intoxication, (3) normal mental status, (4) no focal neurologic deficits, and (5) no painful distracting injuries. If all of these criteria are met, the patient's neck should be passively moved in all directions to ensure there is no additional pain with movement. At this point the patient is deemed "clinically cleared."

24-3. **The answer is A** (Chapter 252). Trauma is the most common cause of pancreatitis in children and in this child with an elevated amylase level and abdominal pain, admission is required for continued observation, regardless of CT findings. The evaluation of hematuria in the pediatric trauma patient depends on the amount of blood in the urine and vital signs. In this patient with normal vital signs and microscopic hematuria, no further workup is generally indicated as long as the patient is asymptomatic. The spleen, followed by the liver, are the most commonly injured organs, with bowel injuries occurring in <5% of patients with blunt abdominal trauma. Duodenal hematomas can be missed by both physical exam and CT. A contrast-enhanced CT can aid in the diagnosis, but if this injury is suspected based on the mechanism of injury, the child should be admitted for further evaluation and observation.

24-4. **The answer is D** (Chapter 252). In this hypotensive child, 3 20 cc/kg crystalloid fluid boluses should be given consecutively as long as evidence of shock remains. After 3 crystalloid boluses, blood should be used in 10 cc/kg boluses.

24-5. **The answer is A** (Chapter 252). Spinal cord injury without radiographic abnormality (SCIWORA) can present in children with even minor trauma. Increased flexibility of the spine and spinal column in pediatric patients can permit spinal cord injury without fracture or dislocation. Magnetic resonance imaging should be performed and the neurosurgery department should be consulted for any pediatric patient with neurologic complaints following trauma, even if these symptoms are transient. Admission for observation is generally mandated. Flexion-extension radiographs and computed tomography do not exclude the diagnosis of SCIWORA.

24-6. **The answer is C** (Chapter 252). Table 252-5 in the *Study Guide* stratifies the risk groups for pediatric head injury. Based on age alone (<2 years) this child falls within the moderate- to high-risk category. At this age there are no good predictors of intracranial injury. The diagnostic test of choice is computed tomography as skull radiographs may identify a fracture but do not exclude intracranial injury. Further, if there is a fracture identified by skull radiograph, a computed tomography scan is still required. If there is no loss of consciousness in the child older than 2 years, some authors suggest that the otherwise healthy child with a normal exam can forego imaging following a minor closed head injury.

24-7. **The answer is B** (Chapter 253). Clinical clearance of the cervical spine in the patient without cervical tenderness follows clinical decision rules that have been validated in a large series of patients. Although the National Emergency X-Radiography Utilization Study (NEXUS) does not incorporate age as a risk factor for cervical spine injury (see Chapter 251), the Canadian C-Spine Rule does use an age of 65 or older. Further, depending on the amount of shoulder pain present, this likely constitutes a distracting injury and precludes the application of either decision rule. Therefore, this patient cannot have his cervical spine "clinically cleared" and should have radiographs obtained. Epidural hematomas are less common in the elderly due to the dense fibrous bond present between the dura mater and the skull. Cerebral atrophy is present in the elderly, but this leads to increased risk of subdural hematomas—it is not protective. The most common cervical spine fractures in this age group are upper cervical, particularly odontoid fractures, and not lower cervical fractures.

24-8. **The answer is C** (Chapter 253). Chest trauma in the elderly can lead to significant morbidity and mortality. In this patient with multiple rib fractures, respiratory compromise is likely to occur, and admission is warranted. Taping of rib fractures is no longer indicated as this leads to increased complications. In blunt chest trauma, rib fractures are the most common injury, not aortic tear. If hypoxia is present, in addition to adequate pain management noninvasive ventilation can be attempted, but intubation should not be withheld if hypoxia persists.

24-9. **The answer is D** (Chapter 254). Even pregnant patients with seemingly minor trauma warrant at least 4 hours of fetal monitoring when the fetus is beyond 20 weeks gestation. Patients with <3 contractions per hour and normal fetal heart rate can safely be discharged without concern for placental abruption. Assessing fetal heart rate and activity does not completely assess the risk of placental abruption. Diagnostic imaging that is indicated should never be withheld from the pregnant trauma patient. There is little risk to a 34-week fetus. A fetus of <8 weeks gestation is at greatest risk from radiation in excess of 10 rads; a full trauma panel is less than 1 rad. Standard immobilization should be used for the pregnant patient, but the patient should be transported with a wedge under the right pelvis in order to rotate the pelvis 30 degrees to the left and prevent compression of the inferior vena cava.

24-10. **The answer is C** (Chapter 254). The indications for performance of a diagnostic peritoneal lavage in the pregnant trauma patient are the same as those in the nonpregnant patient. However, when a gravid uterus is palpable, the procedure should be performed open, in the supraumbilical location. Although $Rh_o(D)$ immune globulin (RhoGAM) can be given within 72 hours of abdominal trauma, it should generally be given in the ED to pregnant trauma patients who are Rh-negative. Exceptions are rare, and failure to administer $Rh_o(D)$ immune globulin can lead to future pregnancy loss. The dose is 50 μg for gestation 12 weeks or less and 300 μg for those >12 weeks. Alternatively, 300 μg can be given to all patients as additional $Rh_o(D)$ immune globulin is not harmful. Although a *bimanual* exam should not be performed in the pregnant patient with a possible placenta previa, a *speculum* exam is indicated in the pregnant trauma patient with evidence of abdominal or pelvic trauma. Evaluation of fluid in the vaginal vault for pH and "ferning" can indicate rupture of amniotic membranes.

24-11. **The answer is A** (Chapter 254). Fetal survival is greatest if the fetus is delivered within the first 5 minutes of maternal death. There is little chance of survival beyond 20 minutes. Therefore, the emergent cesarean delivery should be started within 4 minutes of maternal death in gestations estimated beyond 23 weeks and be complete within 5 minutes. The procedure involves a vertical midline incision to enter the peritoneum with an additional vertical incision to enter the uterus. This is the fastest method to deliver the fetus. Time should not be spent assessing fetal heart rate or activity as the fetus may not have a heart rate but may still be resuscitated following delivery. If adequate fluid resuscitation has been attempted, pressors should not be withheld from the mother, regardless of potential adverse effects on the fetus.

24-12. **The answer is B** (Chapter 255). The patient receives a 2 for eye opening to pain, a 2 for speech, and a 3 for decorticate (abnormal flexion) motor skills.

24-13. **The answer is B** (Chapter 255). The patient most likely suffered an epidural hematoma due to a laceration of his middle meningeal artery. His story demonstrates a classic presentation of this type of brain injury with an initial loss of consciousness, followed by a lucid interval with subsequent rapid neurological decline. Subdural hematomas occur more often in the elderly or those suffering from brain atrophy and usually have a slower onset of symptoms. Diffuse axonal injury is seen in significant

head trauma, and these patients are usually unresponsive upon presentation to the ED. Postconcussive syndrome is a set of persistent neurological, cognitive, and affective symptoms seen after a traumatic brain injury.

24-14. **The answer is C** (Chapter 255). The patient described has several risk factors for developing a subdural hematoma. She is elderly and has a history of alcoholism. Both of these contribute to brain atrophy and put her at an increased risk for a subdural hematoma. She had a hematoma over the occiput and not the parietal area, which is more commonly associated with epidural hematoma. A concussion is a brief episode of neurological or cognitive change. This patient's symptoms are persistent.

24-15. **The answer is B** (Chapter 256). Brown-Séquard's syndrome is a hemisection injury of the spinal cord, usually due to penetrating trauma that results in loss of ipsilateral motor, position, and vibratory sense, with contralateral loss of pain and temperature sensation below the injury. Central cord syndrome is usually due to hyperextension injuries and results in loss of motor control in both the upper and lower extremities, with the upper extremities being more affected. Anterior cord syndrome results in bilateral motor weakness and is usually due to arterial occlusion. Patients with spinal shock have bilateral flaccid paralysis secondary to acute cord injury.

24-16. **The answer is D** (Chapter 256). C5 on the right is the most likely location of the injury. The patient has suffered a hemisection of the spinal cord at C5 on the right side. He has a Brown-Séquard's syndrome at that level, which explains his loss of ipsilateral motor activity in both the arms and legs and contralateral loss of pain sensation below the lesion. A lesion at C3 on the left would produce left-sided weakness and loss of pain sensation on the right. Lesions in the thoracic location would not result in weakness in the arm.

24-17. The answer is C (Chapter 256). Central cord syndrome is the most likely injury. This is a classic example of a central cord syndrome—a fall with hyperextension injury that results in weaker upper extremities compared with lower extremities. While a subdural hematoma is certainly possible in an elderly alcoholic, it will typically be unilateral in effect. Anterior cord syndrome would produce bilateral paralysis of the arms and legs equally; cauda equina syndrome deals with the distal sacral roots and would have no effect on the arm strength.

24-18. The answer is B (Chapter 257). Multiple studies have found the Waters view to be the most sensitive plain film facial series for evaluating orbital fractures. The Caldwell view or posteroanterior view is best for detailing the upper face and sinus. The submental vertex or jug handle view is useful in evaluating zygoma fractures. The Towne view is part of a mandibular series and evaluates the condyles and ramus of the mandible.

24-19. The answer is D (Chapter 257). The patient has an open fracture as evidenced by gingival lacerations. The appropriate treatment for such a patient involves IV antibiotics, admission to the hospital, and urgent oral surgery consultation.

24-20. The answer is B (Chapter 257). The patient has a history and physical exam consistent with an orbital blowout fracture. Normal pupillary reaction makes traumatic iritis unlikely; normal visual acuity makes retroorbital hematoma unlikely. Some surgeons recommend antibiotics when subcutaneous emphysema is present.

24-21. The answer is D (Chapter 258). The patient described in this scenario has a Zone I injury. After penetrating neck trauma, injuries to Zones I and III should be investigated with angiography since physical examination is not reliable. In addition, Zone I injuries require workup for esophageal injuries, which are also hard to diagnose based on physical examination findings. Angiography remains the gold standard for vascular injuries. Duplex sonography has not been demonstrated to have high enough sensitivity to replace angiography. Esophageal evaluation should be performed with esophagram and esophagoscopy. In combination, the sensitivity is 100% for detecting injury. Significant laryngotracheal injuries are rarely occult. Thus, laryngoscopy and bronchoscopy are reserved for symptomatic patients. Finally, computed tomography may play an important future role in the workup of these patients, but it is technically limited in patients with Zone I injuries and may have a sensitivity of only 90% for detection of major carotid and vertebral arterial injuries.

24-22. The answer is B (Chapter 259). In patients with chest trauma, the volume of blood that comes out of the chest tube is an indication of the severity of bleeding. Patients with massive hemothorax, as defined by >1500 mL of blood from the chest tube or >300 mL per hour for 2 hours, are usually candidates for operative thoracotomy. The management also depends on the stability of the patient. ED thoracotomy is indicated for patients with penetrating chest trauma who lose vital signs en route to or in the ED. A second chest tube may be indicated if the patient remains hypotensive or there is evidence by chest radiograph that the first chest tube is not draining the hemothorax.

24-23. The answer is D (Chapter 259). An isolated sternal fracture is no longer considered an indicator of significant blunt myocardial injury (BMI) and does not mandate a workup for BMI. The incidence of cardiac dysrhythmia requiring treatment is 1.5%. A screening electrocardiogram is indicated. The conservative approach is to repeat the electrocardiogram in 6 hours and then discharge the patient if it is negative. Echocardiography is not useful as a screening test for detecting clinically significant BMI. Cardiac markers are not useful as screening tests for BMI. Creatine kinase lacks specificity. Troponin levels may be elevated in patients with BMI; however, their elevation does not predict clinically significant complications, and they should not be used as screening tests in the ED.

24-24. **The answer is A** (Chapter 259). For a simple pneumothorax, a 24-French or 28-French chest tube should be placed. A larger tube is indicated for hemothorax or hemopneumothorax, since the smaller tube can become obstructed by a blood clot and may not drain the blood adequately. Needle decompression of the chest is warranted if the patient is unstable and a tube thoracostomy set is not readily available. Only small pneumothoraces (<1.0 cm wide and confined to the upper third of the chest) can generally be managed without tube thoracostomy.

24-25. **The answer is B** (Chapter 259). For patients with stab wounds to the chest without a concern for pericardial injury, an initial chest radiograph should be performed with a follow-up chest radiograph in 6 hours. A pneumothorax may be delayed after a stab wound; 12% of patients will require tube thoracostomy for delayed hemothorax or pneumothorax. Most of these will be evident on a chest radiograph performed at 6 hours. Assuming that there are no other associated injuries, the patient can then be discharged.

24-26. **The answer is D** (Chapter 259). With penetrating trauma, the diagnosis of diaphragmatic injury is difficult and may only be made with laparotomy or laparoscopy. Diagnostic peritoneal lavage is not as reliable but can be used. The threshold RBC count for a positive lavage should be lowered since diaphragmatic injury does not result in as much bleeding as with solid organ injury. Computed tomography may miss small diaphragmatic injuries from penetrating trauma. Upper gastrointestinal series

may demonstrate displacement of viscera into the chest after blunt diaphragmatic injury, but this does not occur acutely after penetrating trauma due to the small size of the hole in the diaphragm.

24-27. **The answer is B** (Chapter 259). Up to one-third of cases of traumatic aortic injury (TAI) will not have abnormal chest radiographs on presentation, thus this is not a good screening test. In addition, the specificity is low; an anteroposterior chest radiograph or one in the supine position may demonstrate a widened mediastinum simply due to the technique. Computed tomography has become the preferred initial screening test due to recent improvements in the scanning technique, speed, and radiologist experience with reading the test. Transesophageal echocardiography (TEE) is an alternative in the hemodynamically unstable patient with results that are similar to computed tomography. The disadvantages of TEE as a screening test are that it requires a skilled operator who may not be readily available, and it takes time to perform the procedure. Transthoracic echocardiography is inaccurate for detecting TAI.

24-28. **The answer is C** (Chapter 260). Diagnostic modalities available for patients with anterior abdominal stab wounds now include diagnostic peritoneal lavage with admission to the hospital, local wound exploration, or serial physical exams and observation in the hospital. Patients should be observed in the hospital for 12–24 hours after diagnostic peritoneal lavage. Abdominal ultrasound is not sensitive for detecting bowel injuries or other injuries after penetrating trauma that result in small amounts of bleeding. Thus, the test is helpful if positive, but not if it is negative. Local wound exploration is useful for determining penetration of the anterior fascia. However, it is performed as a surgical procedure with proper lighting, retraction, local anesthesia, and visual inspection. Digital probing does not play a role in the evaluation of penetrating abdominal trauma.

24-29. **The answer is C** (Chapter 260). The only use of plain radiographs in abdominal trauma is for the localization of bullets. They are not sensitive for detecting hemoperitoneum. Patients with hollow viscus injury may have normal radiographs. It is not a cost-effective tool for evaluating stab wounds to the abdomen. In patients with gunshot wounds to the abdomen, pelvis, or chest, plain radiographs are useful for determining the location of bullets in order to plan the operative approach and determine which structures are at risk of injury. A chest radiograph also helps determine the risk of pericardial and lung injury in patients with abdominal gunshot wounds that may have traveled into the chest.

24-30. **The answer is D** (Chapter 260). Pancreatic injury results from a rapid deceleration mechanism or direct trauma to the midabdomen. Bicyclists who hit the handlebars are at risk for pancreatic injury. Even if the patient is hemodynamically stable and has minimal tenderness, computed tomography should be performed to make the diagnosis. Initially, these patients may have limited symptoms and a normal computed tomography scan, but 6–12 hours after injury, the sensitivity of computed tomography increases. Bedside abdominal ultrasound exam is insensitive for small bowel or pancreatic injuries that may be accompanied by minimal intraperitoneal bleeding.

24-31. **The answer is D** (Chapter 261). In a patient who is hemodynamically stable after penetrating flank trauma, diagnostic peritoneal lavage would be helpful for determining intraperitoneal injury but does not sample the retroperitoneal injury. Thus it will miss kidney injuries. Local wound exploration is limited in these patients because it is hard to determine peritoneal penetration with deep wounds, especially when the wound extends into the muscle layer. Computed tomography is the diagnostic modality of choice since it will image the retroperitoneum and peritoneal cavity. Triple contrast should be used (including rectal contrast) to identify rectal or sigmoid injury. Oral contrast may not extend down to these areas. The accuracy of computed tomography for flank stab wounds approaches 98%.

24-32. **The answer is A** (Chapter 260). The ultrasound demonstrates free fluid in Morison's pouch. In a patient who is hemodynamically unstable with pelvic fractures and intraperitoneal bleeding, the FAST exam can be used to help triage to either the operating room for a laparotomy or to the angiography suite for pelvic vessel angiography. In this case, the FAST exam is positive, so the initial management plan should be to perform a laparotomy and then proceed to angiography. There is no evidence of pericardial effusion, thus pericardiocentesis is not indicated. Performing external fixation in the ED would delay operative management of the intraperitoneal bleeding.

24-33. **The answer is D** (Chapter 262). Unlike adult trauma patients, the degree of hematuria found by urinalysis in pediatric patients correlates with the degree of injury. Pediatric patients with a urinalysis result of <50 RBCs/hpf do not have significant genitourinary injury, and further imaging of these patients is not necessary. In stable trauma patients with evidence of hematuria that requires further imaging, a computed tomography scan is the test of choice. In pediatric patients this is especially true because a significant intra-abdominal injury is more likely in these patients than a renal injury.

24-34. **The answer is B** (Chapter 262). The most commonly injured organ of the genitourinary system is the kidney. Contusions account for the majority of renal injuries (92%), followed by renal lacerations, renal pedical injuries, and renal ruptures or shattered kidneys. The second most commonly injured genitourinary organ is the bladder, and bladder injury is usually associated with blunt trauma and pelvic fractures. Urethral injuries occur most frequently in men and are also frequently associated with pelvic fracture. The ureter is the rarest of all genitourinary injuries and is most likely the result of penetrating trauma.

24-35. **The answer is A** (Chapter 263). Classically, exam findings for arterial injury in penetrating extremity trauma have been categorized as "hard" findings, which require expeditious angiography and/or surgical intervention, and "soft" findings, which require inpatient admission for observation and repeat examinations. Hard signs include absent or diminished distal pulses, obvious arterial bleeding, large expanding or pulsatile hematoma, audible bruit, palpable thrill, and distal ischemia. Soft signs include small stable hematoma, injury to an anatomically related nerve, unexplained hypotension, history of hemorrhage, proximity of the injury to major vascular structures, and complex fracture. Patients with penetrating extremity trauma without signs of arterial injury, no bone or nerve injury, no signs of developing compartment syndrome, and minimal soft tissue defect may be safely discharged home with close follow-up after observation in the ED for 3–12 hours.

24-36. **The answer is D** (Chapter 264). The computed tomography scan will provide information about both the intra-abdominal and retroperitoneal organs. In addition, a computed tomography scan can be useful when an injury exclusive to the body wall is suspected. Plain radiographs taken in planes separated by 90 degrees will provide information about the location of the bullet and perhaps demonstrate bony injury or free air but will require further imaging or surgical intervention to determine the extent of any injury. In addition, the trajectory path of a bullet cannot be predicted based on its location on a plain film. Bullets that are not lodged in tissue in the abdominal cavity can migrate to the lower abdomen due to gravity, and the trajectory of the bullet in the body is not always a straight line from the entry wound. An intravenous pyelogram in this patient will reveal information only about his genitourinary system and does not assess the possibility of intra-abdominal injury. A FAST scan provides information about possible renal or intra-abdominal injury but is not useful in locating injuries or missiles confined to the body wall.

24-37. **The answer is A** (Chapter 265). Documentation by an examining physician of an entrance or exit wound is very difficult without forensic training. Although entrance wounds have a characteristic rim of abrasion on the skin caused by friction when contacting the missile, an exit wound may demonstrate a very similar pattern if the skin is resting against a firm surface when the bullet exits. The medical record of an injury victim is a legal document that may be used in future legal action regarding the incident. Thus a careful documentation of the wound itself, along with photographic images that include a measurement scale in the field of view, anatomic diagrams of the location of wounds, and a description of any gunpowder residue found around a bullet wound, can be very helpful for forensic experts and law enforcement in determining actual events surrounding the injury.

ABEM 2004 Continuous Certification Articles
Questions

25-1. Which statement regarding the risks associated with gastrointestinal (GI) decontamination is TRUE?

(A) Syrup of ipecac has a high rate of aspiration even in awake and alert children.

(B) Endotracheal intubation is virtually 100% effective in preventing aspiration.

(C) The risks of aspirating activated charcoal are greater than those of aspirating gastric contents alone.

(D) Mechanical injury to the throat and GI tract is common following gastric lavage.

25-2. According to the NEXUS criteria, which of the following patients can have the cervical spine cleared clinically without radiographs?

(A) A 45-year-old man who trips and falls, striking his head, after several alcoholic drinks at a party.

(B) A 19-year-old boy who complains of neck pain and left arm numbness and tingling after a hard tackle during a football game.

(C) A 26-year-old woman with a distal radius fracture and neck pain after falling while ice skating.

(D) A 55-year-old man with left lateral neck stiffness after a moderate-speed motor vehicle collision the previous day.

25-3. Which of the following statements MOST accurately describes the NEXUS decision instrument for the clinical clearance of the cervical spine following blunt trauma?

(A) It is validated only in Level I trauma centers.

(B) It is designed to be applied only by EM-trained physicians.

(C) It detects all cervical spine injuries.

(D) It is valid in the elderly.

25-4. An 18-year-old boy presents to the ED after injuring his left knee while skiing. He planted his foot abruptly to avoid a collision with another skier, felt his lower leg move forward, and heard an audible "pop." He is having difficulty bearing weight on the knee and has a large joint effusion. Which of the following provocative maneuvers is specific for this injury?

(A) Lachman's test.

(B) Apley's test.

(C) McMurray's test.

(D) Posterior drawer test.

25-5. A 50-year-old man presents to the ED after returning from a trip to Brazil 2 days ago. He has a fever, headache, generalized body aches, and a petechial rash on his ankles. What laboratory abnormality might you expect to see in this patient?

(A) Elevated liver function tests.

(B) Microscopic hematuria.

(C) Leukocytosis.

(D) Thrombocytopenia.

25-6. A 48-year-old woman presents to the ED after returning from vacation in Mexico. She complains of 3 weeks of nonbloody diarrhea and occasional abdominal cramping. Which of the following statements regarding the typical time course of traveler's diarrhea is accurate?

(A) Most patients with diarrhea after international travel have symptoms for at least 2 weeks.

(B) Diarrhea that begins 1 month after travel is still likely to be related to the trip.

(C) The likelihood of a protozoan infection increases if the diarrhea persists >2 weeks.

(D) It is difficult to determine a precise etiology of the diarrhea if the symptoms are present for <2 weeks.

25-7. Which of the following correctly characterizes immune thrombocytopenia purpura in children?

(A) Immune thrombocytopenia purpura in children generally occurs in the setting of underlying disease.

(B) Unlike adults, most children have a palpable spleen tip on examination.

(C) In children, immune thrombocytopenia purpura most commonly resolves with no treatment.

(D) Of children, 50% present with platelet counts <10,000.

25-8. A 36-year-old, previously healthy man presents to the ED following recurrent episodes of epistaxis over the last 3 days. Currently he is not actively bleeding. He has no other symptoms suggestive of a systemic disease. On physical exam he has several large areas of ecchymosis. His platelet count is 10,000. Which of the following is indicated for the initial treatment of this patient?

(A) Platelet transfusion.

(B) Prednisone.

(C) Intravenous immune globulin.

(D) No specific treatment needed.

25-9. Low back pain is one of the most common presenting symptoms to the ED. Which statement CORRECTLY characterizes the emergent management of low back pain?

(A) A thorough history and physical exam typically reveals a precise etiology for the pain.

(B) Most patients who present to the ED with an acutely herniated disc do not require surgery.

(C) If no etiology is found, the patient should be reassured that recurrence of the back pain is unusual.

(D) Pain medication should be prescribed on an as-needed basis only.

25-10. Which of the following statements regarding imaging studies in low back pain is CORRECT?

(A) MRI is preferred over CT scan for the diagnosis of spinal stenosis.

(B) Plain radiographs are a good screening test for early cancers or infectious processes.

(C) Imaging is indicated if a patient fails to improve after a month of conservative therapy.

(D) An MRI of the lumbar spine determines the etiology of the back pain in two-thirds of the patients.

25-11. Which of the following injuries to the physis do not require urgent orthopedic consultation in the ED?

(A) A fracture line that involves the physis and extends into the metaphysis.

(B) An intra-articular fracture of the epiphysis extending into the physis.

(C) An axial compression of the physis.

(D) A fracture line that extends from the epiphysis through the physis and into the metaphysics.

25-12. Which of the following statements regarding changes in the CDC guidelines for the management of occupational exposures to blood or body fluids is accurate?

(A) Because of increasing drug resistance, a 3-drug regimen should be prescribed to prevent HIV transmission following most exposures.

(B) Hepatitis B titers should be routinely obtained in all patients following a blood or body fluid exposure.

(C) Providers exposed to hepatitis C require no specific treatment.

(D) The rapid HIV test is not accurate enough to be used in the setting of occupational exposures in the ED.

25-13. A health care worker in the ED comes to you after he was stuck by a used needle several hours earlier while caring for a patient known to be an intravenous drug user. No additional information is available about the patient, and he is unable to be reached since his discharge from the ED. Which of the following statements is CORRECT regarding the management of this patient?

(A) He should follow up with employee health in 72 hours, and postexposure prophylaxis should be initiated at that time.

(B) He needs follow-up testing for anti-hepatitis C antibodies.

(C) He should be given hepatitis B immune globulin even if he has been previously vaccinated.

(D) He should be reassured that adverse effects from postexposure prophylaxis are rare.

25-14. According to the Harvard Practice Study, adverse events in medicine occur MOST frequently in which of the following scenarios?

(A) Performance of invasive procedures.

(B) Misinterpretation of radiographs.

(C) Ordering and administration of medications.

(D) Inadequate communication between providers at shift change.

25-15. Which of the following is TRUE regarding the interpretation of radiology studies in the ED?

(A) Emergency physicians and radiologists disagree on findings approximately 30% of the time.

(B) The discordance between emergency physicians and radiologists is the same for the interpretation of CT scans and plain radiographs.

(C) Increased radiologist availability for consultation has no effect on the number of subsequent patient callbacks.

(D) Discrepancies between the interpretations by the emergency physician and the radiologist necessitate clinical follow-up approximately half of the time.

25-16. A 45-year-old woman presents to the ED with a severe asthma exacerbation. She has a history of prior intubations and has used her inhaler every 30 minutes for the past few hours with no improvement. Which of the following is TRUE regarding ED management of this patient?

(A) Intravenous magnesium has no role in the management of this patient.

(B) Intravenous administration of steroids would be preferred over the oral route.

(C) Continuous nebulization of β-agonists is likely to be more beneficial for this patient than intermittent treatments.

(D) Levalbuterol is more clinically effective than albuterol for the treatment of severe exacerbations.

25-17. Which of the following CORRECTLY characterizes the use of steroids in the ED for the treatment of acute asthma?

(A) Studies have demonstrated that administration of steroids in the ED reduces admission rates regardless of the severity of the exacerbation.

(B) The dose of steroids should be doubled if the patient is having a severe attack.

(C) Inhaled corticosteroids appear to have no role in the ED treatment of asthma.

(D) In a recent multicenter trial, systemic corticosteroids are used in 70% of ED patients.

25-18. A 55-year-old woman currently on a multiple drug regimen for the treatment of tuberculosis presents to the ED complaining of vision changes. Which drug is the likely culprit?

(A) Ethambutol.

(B) Streptomycin.

(C) Rifampin.

(D) Pyrazinamide.

25-19. Which of the following measurements on the tuberculin test is considered positive in a patient with HIV?

(A) 5 mm.

(B) 10 mm.

(C) 15 mm.

(D) The test is not useful in patients with HIV.

25-20. A 33-year-old man presents to the ED with chest pain and shortness of breath following cocaine use. He has no other cardiac risk factors. Which of the following is TRUE regarding acute myocardial infarction (AMI) following cocaine use?

(A) The incidence of AMI with chest pain following cocaine use is 20%.

(B) Dysrhythmias are a common complication in patients with an AMI following cocaine use.

(C) Most patients with an AMI after cocaine use have underlying coronary disease.

(D) The risk of AMI is highest the first hour after cocaine use.

25-21. Which is the MOST common electrocardiogram finding in patients with acute chest pain following cocaine use?

(A) Premature ventricular contractions.

(B) ST elevation in a distribution consistent with acute myocardial infarction.

(C) Nonspecific changes.

(D) Normal electrocardiogram.

25-22. An 85-year-old woman is found in her apartment by her neighbor. She is confused and appears to be having difficulty breathing. It is mid-August and the apartment is not air-conditioned. Upon arrival to the ED her rectal temperature is 44°C. Her past medical history includes coronary artery disease and type II diabetes mellitus. Which of the following is TRUE regarding the presentation and management of this patient?

(A) Lab studies typically reveal a lactic acidosis.

(B) If properly treated, residual brain dysfunction will not occur.

(C) Antipyretics should be given if the core temperature is >40°C.

(D) The patient's use of β-blockers increases her susceptibility to heat stroke.

25-23. A 30-year-old man develops a dry cough and shortness of breath 24 hours after arriving in Colorado for a skiing trip. He is afebrile. A chest radiograph reveals a normal cardiac silhouette and patchy infiltrates. Which of the following is TRUE regarding the management of this patient?

(A) High-altitude pulmonary edema is unlikely given the rapidity of the symptoms.

(B) He should be started on nifedipine 20 mg orally every 12 hours.

(C) To avoid unnecessary exertion, the patient should not be moved.

(D) He should be observed closely for the development of cerebral edema.

25-24. Regarding acute mountain sickness, which of the following statements is accurate?

(A) Age over 65 years is an important risk factor for the development of acute mountain sickness.

(B) In general, a person must descend 2000–3000 m before acute mountain sickness resolves.

(C) Acetazolamide has been shown to be more efficacious than dexamethasone for the treatment of acute mountain sickness.

(D) High-altitude cerebral edema is the end stage of acute mountain sickness.

25-25. Which of the following statements is accurate regarding acute chest syndrome in sickle cell patients?

(A) Most patients present to the ED complaining of shortness of breath.

(B) Acute chest syndrome is an important risk factor for stroke in sickle cell patients.

(C) A specific etiology for acute chest syndrome is rarely found.

(D) Mechanical ventilation and a prolonged hospital stay are unusual.

25-26. A 34-year-old man with a history of sickle cell disease presents to the ED complaining of chest pain and difficulty breathing. Vital signs include a heart rate of 115 beats per minute, blood pressure of 110/65 mmHg, respiratory rate of 22 breaths per minute, temperature of 36.2°C, and a room air oxygen saturation of 92%. He has no audible wheezing. Which of the following is the CORRECT management of this patient?

(A) Bronchodilators should be initiated early.

(B) Broad-spectrum antibiotics should be given if the patient develops a fever.

(C) Blood transfusions should be avoided to prevent pulmonary edema.

(D) High-dose steroids are beneficial.

25-27. Regarding the use of the D-dimer test in the evaluation of pulmonary embolism, which of the following is TRUE?

(A) Semiquantitative latex assays are very sensitive but impractical because of long laboratory turnaround times.

(B) False negatives are more likely if the patient has had symptoms for more than a week.

(C) The SimpliRED assay is accurate enough to initiate treatment of pulmonary embolism with a positive test.

(D) The patient must have symptoms for at least 6 hours for the D-dimer test to be clinically useful.

25-28. Which of the following statements regarding localized exposure to radiation is TRUE?

(A) The physical signs of a radiation burn are readily apparent an hour after exposure.

(B) Long-term complications following a radiation burn are rare.

(C) All wounds containing potential radioactive substances should be aggressively debrided.

(D) The extent of penetration of the radiation is an important factor in the outcome of local injury.

25-29. Regarding the incidence of the difficult airway in the ED, which of the following is CORRECT?

(A) Because of the unpredictability of ED practice, ED studies suggest that the incidence of difficult airways in the ED is >30%.

(B) According to the National Emergency Airway Registry (NEAR), esophageal intubations occur in 4% of intubations, but only half of these are immediately recognized.

(C) The cricothyroidotomy rate in EDs in the United States has increased as the number of emergency medicine residency programs has increased.

(D) A recent multicenter trial reported that rapid sequence intubation in the ED has a success rate >98%.

25-30. Which of the following statements regarding the lighted stylet in the management of the difficult airway is TRUE?

(A) It is contraindicated in the presence of a suspected cervical injury.

(B) The lighted stylet consistently requires more time to intubate than direct laryngoscopy.

(C) The device has also been adapted for nasotracheal intubation.

(D) The overhead lights in the room must be dimmed for visualization of the light.

25-31. A 6-year-old boy is brought to the ED 2 hours after he ingested his grandfather's diabetes medication, mistaking it for candy. He is currently asymptomatic. It is unclear how many tablets he ingested. Which of the following is TRUE regarding the management of sulfonylurea overdose in children?

(A) Octreotide is an effective treatment for sulfonylurea-induced hypoglycemia in adults but is contraindicated in pediatric patients.

(B) Because of delayed onset hypoglycemia, this patient should be admitted for a minimum of 24 hours for observation.

(C) Intravenous access should be obtained immediately upon arrival.

(D) Some studies have suggested that frequent feedings at home and observation by parents is also a safe option following accidental sulfonylurea ingestion.

25-32. Which of the following CORRECTLY matches the oral diabetes agent with its characteristic adverse effect?

(A) Chlorpropamide and hypernatremia.

(B) Acarbose and elevated hepatic transaminases.

(C) Glipizide and lactic acidosis.

(D) Metformin and prolonged QT syndrome.

ABEM 2004 Continuous Certification Articles
Answers, Explanations, and References

25-1. **The answer is C.** Aspiration of activated charcoal leads to greater complications than aspiration of gastric contents alone. This may be because of its ability to induce a granulomatous reaction and to increase pulmonary microvascular permeability. There is still a 5% incidence of aspiration in intubated patients. Administration of syrup of ipecac in awake, alert children is reasonably safe and not associated with a large risk of aspiration. Esophageal perforation or other mechanical injuries to the throat or GI tract are very unusual following gastric lavage. The main risk of gastric lavage is that associated with the subsequent endotracheal intubation, which may not have been otherwise indicated. **Reference:** Bond GR. The role of activated charcoal and gastric emptying in gastrointestinal decontamination: a state of the art review. *Ann Emerg Med.* March 2002;39:273–286.

25-2. **The answer is D.** According to the NEXUS decision instrument, the patient must satisfy 5 clinical criteria to be considered low risk for cervical spine injury. In order to be clinically cleared following blunt trauma without cervical radiographs, a patient must have no painful distracting injury, no neurological deficit, a normal mental status, no evidence of intoxication, and no posterior midline cervical tenderness. These criteria approach 100% sensitivity for clinically important cervical spine injuries. **Reference:** Hoffman JR, Mower WR, Wolfson AB, et al. Validity of a set of clinical criteria to rule out injury to the cervical spine in patients with blunt trauma. *N Engl J Med.* July 2000;343:94–99.

25-3. **The answer is D.** Elderly patients were not excluded from the multicenter trial that validated the NEXUS decision instrument for the clinical clearance of cervical spine injuries. The decision instrument missed 8 of 818 patients with a cervical spine injury; however, only 2 of these were considered clinically significant by the investigators. The study utilized 21 centers and included both large academic centers as well as private and public community EDs. The specific specialty training of the physicians at the various study sites was not stated. **Reference:** Hoffman JR, Mower WR, Wolfson AB, et al. Validity of a set of clinical criteria to rule out injury to the cervical spine in patients with blunt trauma. *N Engl J Med.* July 2000;343:94–99.

25-4. **The answer is A.** This is a classic presentation for an injury to the anterior cruciate ligament. Lachman's test, the anterior drawer test, and the lateral pivot shift test are the 3 maneuvers specific for anterior cruciate ligament injuries. Lachman's test is performed with the patient in a supine position with the knee flexed at 20–30 degrees. The physician holds the femur above the knee with one hand and the other hand grasps the lower leg at the proximal tibia. The lower leg is pulled forward and a discrete endpoint should be felt. If a discrete endpoint is not felt or there is exaggerated anterior motion of the tibia, then the test is highly suggestive of an injury to the anterior cruciate ligament. The posterior drawer test is specific for injuries to the posterior cruciate ligament, and Apley's compression test and McMurray's test assess for meniscal injuries. **Reference:** Solomon DH, Simel DL, Bates DW, et al. Does this patient have a torn meniscus or ligament of the knee? *JAMA.* October 2001;286:1610–1620.

25-5.   The answer is D. This patient has Dengue fever. Dengue is caused by a mosquito-borne flavivirus and is common in tropical and subtropical areas. After an incubation period of 4–7 days, the patient presents with fever, headache, and myalgias. Approximately 50% of patients will have either a nonspecific maculopapular rash or petechial rash. Leukopenia and thrombocytopenia are characteristic. **Reference:** Ryan ET, Wilson ME, Kain KC. Illness after international travel. *N Engl J Med.* August 2002;347:505–516.

25-6.   The answer is C. The likelihood of diagnosing a protozoan infection increases if the diarrhea has been present for a prolonged period of time. Causative bacterial or viral agents can be identified in 50–70% of travelers with diarrhea <2 weeks in duration. Only 5–10% of travelers have symptoms for >2 weeks. If the diarrhea begins >1 month after travel, it is unlikely to be related to the trip. **Reference:** Ryan ET, Wilson ME, Kain KC. Illness after international travel. *N Engl J Med.* August 2002;347:505–516.

25-7.   The answer is C. Most children with acute immune thrombocytopenia purpura recover completely within a few weeks without treatment. There is no data proving that therapy reduces complications such as intracranial hemorrhage. Only 10% of children have a palpable spleen on physical exam. Unlike children, 50% of adults present with a platelet count <10,000, so most adults will require treatment. **Reference:** Cines DB, Blanchette VS. Immune throm-

bocytopenia purpura. *N Engl J Med.* March 2002;346:995–1008.

25-8.   The answer is B. At platelet counts of <10,000, the patient is at risk for internal bleeding. This patient should be started on prednisone 1.0–1.5 mg/kg/day. Approximately 50–75% of patients respond to treatment typically within 3 weeks. Intravenous immune globulin is indicated in the presence of internal bleeding or if the patient does not respond to a course of steroids. Platelet transfusions are used for bleeding emergencies such as intracranial hemorrhage or gastrointestinal bleeding. Patients with immune thrombocytopenia purpura require 2 to 3 times the usual amount of platelets transfused. **Reference:** Cines DB, Blanchette VS. Immune thrombocytopenia purpura. *N Engl J Med.* March 2002;346: 995–1008.

25-9.   The answer is B. The majority of patients with a herniated disc improve with conservative therapy. Only 10% of patients have sufficient pain at 6 weeks that surgery is considered. Even with a thorough history and physical exam, a precise pathoanatomical diagnosis is not possible in roughly 85% of patients with low back pain. While most patients improve within a few days, recurrences of low back pain are common. Pain medication should be prescribed on a regular schedule for the first few days, as this has been shown to be more effective than an as-needed regimen. **Reference:** Deyo RA, Weinstein JN. Low back pain. *N Engl J Med.* February 2001;344:363–370.

25-10.   The answer is C. The majority of patients who present to the ED with low back pain do not require imaging. However, it is reasonable to obtain radiologic studies if the patient does not improve with conservative therapy after 4–6 weeks as the likelihood of cancer, infection, or another etiology is increased. CT and MRI have a similar accuracy for the diagnosis of spinal stenosis. Plain radiographs are not sensitive for the detection of infection or cancers, particularly in the early stages. Overuse of MRI in patients with low back pain is discouraged as many abnormalities are incidental findings and not necessarily the etiology of the patient's symptoms. MRI should be reserved for patients with neurologic deficits or a strong clinical suspicion for infection or malignancy. **Reference:** Deyo RA, Weinstein JN. Low back pain. *N Engl J Med.* February 2001;344:363–370.

25-11. **The answer is A.** A Salter-Harris Type II fracture is a fracture of the physis extending into the metaphysis. Type II injuries are the most common type of growth plate fracture and have a very favorable prognosis as the blood supply to the physis, which originates from nutrient arteries in the epiphysis, is not disrupted. All the other three fractures listed, Type III, Type V, and Type IV, respectively, involve the epiphysis and therefore the blood supply to the physis may be affected, potentially impacting future growth. Therefore, Type III, IV, and V injuries require urgent orthopedic consultation in the ED. **Reference:** Perron AD, Miller MD, Brady WJ. Orthopedic pitfalls in the ED: pediatric growth plate injuries. *Am J Emerg Med.* January 2002;20:50–54.

25-12. **The answer is C.** The revised CDC guidelines emphasize that 3-drug therapy is being overused after occupational exposures and that the 3-drug regimen should be reserved for employees exposed to blood or fluid from a source known to be HIV-positive. The new guidelines also encourage the use of the rapid HIV test to determine the HIV status of the source patient, therefore eliminating the need for long courses of postexposure prophylaxis if unnecessary. It is now accepted that the hepatitis B vaccine confers life-long immunity and antibody titers are not needed if the person is confident he or she has been vaccinated. There is no recommended treatment for prophylaxis following hepatitis C exposure. **Reference:** Schriger DL, Mikulich VJ. The management of occupational exposures to blood and body fluids: revised guidelines

and new methods of implementation. *Ann Emerg Med.* March 2002;39:319–328.

25-13. **The answer is B.** Postexposure prophylaxis should be initiated as soon as possible in the ED. If the employee has been vaccinated against hepatitis B, hepatitis B immune globulin is not indicated. Hepatitis B immune globulin is reserved for patients who have not been immunized and are exposed to known hepatitis B antigen–positive fluid. Employees should be counseled that half of people on postexposure prophylaxis experience adverse effects. Employees potentially exposed to hepatitis C should have baseline titers drawn as well as follow-up testing in 4–6 months. **Reference:** Schriger DL, Mikulich VJ. The management of occupational exposures to blood and body fluids: revised guidelines and new methods of implementation. *Ann Emerg Med.* March 2002;39:319–328.

25-14. **The answer is C.** While each of the scenarios listed has the potential for medical error, the largest number of adverse events occur during the ordering and administration of medications. Adverse events may be an expected complication of therapy and not necessarily a medical error; however, many are preventable. Interventions such as computerized order entry and standardization of the hospital formulary have been shown to reduce medication errors. **Reference:** Schenkel S. Promoting patient safety and preventing medical error in emergency departments. *Acad Emerg Med.* November 2000;7:1204–1222.

25-15. **The answer is D.** In a large review of over 12,000 radiographs, emergency physicians and radiologists had discordant readings only 1% of the time, and half of these discrepancies required clinical follow-up. The discordance between emergency physicians and radiologists is much higher for the interpretation of CT scans than for plain films. A recent study reported that increased radiologist availability for consultation decreased the number of subsequent patient callbacks by 40%. **Reference:** Schenkel S. Promoting patient safety and preventing medical error in emergency departments. *Acad Emerg Med.* November 2000;7:1204–1222.

25-16. **The answer is C.** Continuous nebulization of β-agonists is likely to be more beneficial than intermittent treatments during severe asthma exacerbations, although there appears to be no difference in the mild to moderate exacerbations. Intravenous steroids have no advantage over the oral route and should be reserved for patients who cannot tolerate oral medications or have impaired gastrointestinal function. Several studies have revealed that magnesium is most beneficial for the treatment of severe exacerbations. Further study is needed to determine if levalbuterol is more effective than albuterol. **Reference:** Gibbs MA, Camargo CA Jr, Rowe BH, et al. State of the art: therapeutic controversies in severe acute asthma. *Acad Emerg Med.* July 2000;7:800–815.

25-17. **The answer is D.** According to a recent multicenter trial, systemic corticosteroids are used in 70% of ED patients. Administration of steroids in the ED reduces the rate of admission following severe exacerbations but has no effect on admission rates following mild to moderate exacerbations. Inhaled steroids have been shown to both improve pulmonary function and reduce admissions to the hospital. There is no additional benefit to doubling the dose of steroids. **Reference:** Gibbs MA, Camargo CA Jr, Rowe BH, et al. State of the art: therapeutic controversies in severe acute asthma. *Acad Emerg Med.* July 2000;7: 800–815.

25-18. **The answer is A.** Ethambutol can cause a decrease in visual acuity and red-green discrimination. Interestingly, these findings can involve only one eye. Streptomycin is ototoxic and can also affect renal function. Common adverse effects of rifampin and pyrazinamide include hepatitis and/or flu-like symptoms. **Reference:** Small PM, Fujiwara PI. Management of tuberculosis in the United States. *N Engl J Med.* July 2001;345: 189–200.

25-19. **The answer is A.** Groups that are at high risk for tuberculosis infection, including HIV patients, should have tuberculin testing routinely. The cutoff value for a positive tuberculin test in patients with HIV or other causes of immune system is 5 mm. The cutoff for low-risk patients is 15 mm, and for everyone else, 10 mm is used. **Reference:** Small PM, Fujiwara PI. Management of tuberculosis in the United States. *N Engl J Med.* July 2001;345:189–200.

25-20. **The answer is D.** The highest risk of AMI is within the first hour after using cocaine. The incidence of AMI in patients with cocaine-associated chest pain is 6%. Most patients with AMI following cocaine use do not have underlying coronary disease. Complications following a cocaine-associated AMI are infrequent. Dysrhythmias occur in less than 3% of patients. **Reference:** Weber JM, Chudnofsky CR, Boczar M, et al. Cocaine-associated chest pain: how common is myocardial infarction? *Acad Emerg Med.* August 2000;7:873–877.

25-21. **The answer is C.** In this retrospective review of 250 patients, only 67 patients (27%) had a normal electrocardiogram. Half of the patients had nonspecific changes, with early repolarization comprising the most common variation. Only 9 patients had changes consistent with an acute myocardial infarction. **Reference:** Weber JM, Chudnofsky CR, Boczar M, et al. Cocaine-associated chest pain: how common is myocardial infarction? *Acad Emerg Med.* August 2000;7:873–877.

25-22. **The answer is D.** This patient is presenting with classic or nonexertional heat stroke. Heat stroke is defined as a core temperature >40°C accompanied by central nervous system dysfunction. Patients at the extremes of age are particularly vulnerable to nonexertional heat stroke. Medications such as β-blockers that interfere with the normal compensatory mechanisms to dissipate heat increase the susceptibility to heat stroke. Patients with nonexertional heat stroke usually have a respiratory alkalosis. In contrast, patients with exertional heat stroke have both a respiratory alkalosis and a lactic acidosis. Residual brain dysfunction occurs in about 20% of patients and is associated with a high mortality. Antipyretics have not been shown to be useful for the treatment of heat stroke. **Reference:** Bouchama A, Knochel JP. Heat stroke. *N Engl J Med.* June 2002;346:1978–1988.

25-23. The answer is D. High-altitude pulmonary edema accounts for most deaths from high-altitude sickness. It commonly develops within the first 2 days after arrival at altitude and rarely occurs after 4 days. Supplemental oxygen and descent to a lower altitude are the mainstays of therapy. Often symptoms can improve dramatically with a descent of only 500 m. Nifedipine is necessary only when supplemental oxygen is unavailable or descent is impossible. High-altitude cerebral edema commonly develops in patients with pulmonary edema, so patients should be observed closely for signs of central nervous system dysfunction. **Reference:** Hackett PH, Roach RC. High-altitude illness. *N Engl J Med.* July 2001;345:107–114.

25-24. The answer is D. Acute mountain sickness is defined as the presence of a headache plus one other symptom such as fatigue, dizziness, or gastrointestinal complaints in a nonacclimatized person who has recently arrived at an altitude of 2500 m. High-altitude cerebral edema is characterized by the onset of ataxia or altered mental status in a patient with acute mountain sickness or high-altitude pulmonary edema and is considered the end stage of acute mountain sickness. Often a descent of as little as 500–1000 m will resolve symptoms of acute mountain sickness. Studies have shown that dexamethasone is as effective or supe-

rior to acetazolamide for the treatment of acute mountain sickness. Both dexamethsone and acetazolamide have also been shown to be effective as prophylaxis to prevent acute mountain sickness as well. While underlying cardiopulmonary disease does increase the risk of acute mountain sickness, advanced age independently is not a risk factor for acute mountain sickness. In fact, persons over the age of 50 years are less susceptible to acute mountain sickness than younger people. **Reference:** Hackett PH, Roach RC. High-altitude illness. *N Engl J Med.* July 2001;345:107–114.

25-25. The answer is B. Acute chest syndrome is the leading cause of death among patients with sickle cell disease. Over half of the patients presenting to the ED were initially admitted with an alternative diagnosis, most commonly pain from a vasoocclusive crisis. Later many of the patients developed fever, chest pain, and shortness of breath and were diagnosed with acute chest syndrome. Therefore, the authors conclude that patients with a pain crisis should be considered at risk for the development of acute chest syndrome. This review found that acute chest syndrome is commonly precipitated by infection or fat embolism. Acute chest syndrome requires aggressive therapy including bronchdilators, antibiotics, transfusions, oxygen, and hydration. The mean hospitalization was 10.5 days in this study, and several patients required mechanical ventilation. Stroke is a common complication of acute chest syndrome in sickle cell patients. **Reference:** Vichinsky EP, Neumayr LD, Earles AN, et al. Causes and outcomes of the acute chest syndrome in sickle cell disease. *N Engl J Med.* June 2000;342:1855–1865.

25-26. The answer is A. Pulmonary infections are the most common cause of acute chest syndrome and therefore antibiotics should be given early in the course even in the absence of fever. Additionally, many patients have improvement with bronchodilators. Routine early transfusions are indicated in patients at risk for complications, such as those with underlying cardiopulmonary disease. High-dose steroids are not used in the treatment of acute chest syndrome. **Reference:** Vichinsky EP, Neumayr LD, Earles AN, et al. Causes and outcomes of the acute chest syndrome in sickle cell disease. *N Engl J Med.* June 2000;342:1855–1865.

25-27.   **The answer is B.** D-dimers are fibrin split products released into the circulation by plasmin during fibrinolyisis. This typically occurs within 1 hour of thrombus formation. The continued fibrinolysis initiated after a thrombus formation will continue to elevate D-dimer levels for a week. A false-negative result is more likely after this time frame. Semiquantitative latex assay tests are performed rapidly but have been criticized for low sensitivity. The SimpliRED assay, the prototypical second-generation test, is highly sensitive, and a negative test can be used to exclude a pulmonary embolism in the low-risk patient. However, the test has a low specificity, and further testing is necessary in the presence of a positive test before the diagnosis of pulmonary embolism can be made. **Reference:** Kline JA, Johns KL, Collucciello SA, et al. New diagnostic tests for pulmonary embolism. *Ann Emerg Med.* July 2001;38: 107–113.

25-28.   **The answer is D.** Localized exposure to radiation is caused by the direct handling of radioactive sources. The extent of penetration of the radiation is an important factor in the outcome of local injury. The physical signs are similar to a thermal burn and include erythema and desquamation of the skin. However, these signs typically develop days later. Long-term complications including ulceration and vascular insufficiency can develop. A wound that contains radioactivity should be rinsed with saline and treated with standard techniques. Excision is reserved for long-lived radionuclides. **Reference:** Mettler FA Jr, Voelz GL. Major radiation exposure—what to expect

and how to respond. *N Engl J Med.* May 2002;346:1554–1561.

25-29.   **The answer is D.** A recent multicenter study revealed that rapid sequence intubation, the predominant technique for emergency department airway management, has a success rate of 98%. The actual incidence of difficult airways ranges from 1 to 30% with some studies suggesting an incidence closer to 5–10%. According to NEAR, esophageal intubations do occur in 4% of ED airways but are almost immediately recognized. Improved intubation techniques and success rates have decreased the cricothyroidotomy rate. **Reference:** Orebaugh SL. Difficult airway management in the emergency department. *J Emerg Med.* January 2002;22:31–48.

25-30.   **The answer is C.** Lighted stylet intubation has been shown in the operating room to be a safe and effective method of airway control and has useful applications in the ED as well. In studies on surgical patients, the lighted stylet was found to have fewer complications and required less time to intubate than direct laryngoscopy. The newer models such as the Trachlite have a powerful light source that does not routinely require dimming of the overhead lights prior to use. The device has been adapted for nasotracheal intubation as well. The lighted stylet intubation technique preserves the immobility of the cervical spine and is a safe option for airway control in the patient at risk for a cervical spine injury. **Reference:** Orebaugh SL. Difficult airway management in the emergency department. *J Emerg Med.* January 2002;22:31–48.

25-31.   **The answer is D.** With the exception of the extended-release formulation of glipizide, sulfonylureas have a time to peak action of <8 hours. A pediatric patient should have a finger stick every 1–2 hours after ingestion of a sulfonylurea for 8 hours. If hypoglycemia develops, then the child should be admitted. If the child remains asymptomatic after 8 hours, he or she can be safely discharged home. Intravenous access is unnecessary if the patient remains asymptomatic. Some advocate that children can be safely observed by educated parents at home with frequent feedings. Octreotide therapy suppresses the release of endogenous insulin. Octreotide is used in cases of refractory hypoglycemia, and while experience is limited, it is well tolerated by pediatric patients. **Reference:** Harrigan RA, Nathan MS, Beattie P. Oral agents for the treatment of type 2 diabetes mellitus: pharmacology, toxicity, and treatment. *Ann Emerg Med.* July 2001;38:68–78.

25-32. **The answer is B.** Acarbose therapy is associated with a risk of hepatic injury. While the incidence is low, it is prudent to consider the potential of hepatic injury in patients taking acarbose and to check hepatic transaminases in patients after overdose. Metformin characteristically causes a lactic acidosis, which is more common in the setting of coexisting renal insufficiency, liver disease, cardiopulmonary disease, infection, and alcohol abuse. Chlorpropamide is associated with hyponatremia. Adverse effects of glipizide include gastrointestinal discomfort and elevated hepatic transaminases. **Reference:** Harrigan RA, Nathan MS, Beattie P. Oral agents for the treatment of type 2 diabetes mellitus: pharmacology, toxicity, and treatment. *Ann Emerg Med.* July 2001;38:68–78.

ABEM 2005 Continuous Certification Articles
Questions

26-1. Which of the following is associated with increased risk of death?

(A) Syncope after sudden unexpected pain, fear, or unpleasant sight, sound, or smell.

(B) Syncope during or immediately after micturition, cough, swallowing, or defecation.

(C) Syncope occurring with exertion.

(D) Syncope occurring with head rotation, shaving, or wearing tight collars.

26-2. Which of the following is the MOST useful diagnostic tool for determining the etiology of syncope in the ED?

(A) History and physical exam.

(B) Computed tomography (CT) scan of the brain.

(C) Electrocardiogram.

(D) Baseline laboratory tests.

26-3. For children younger than 2 years of age with minor head trauma, which of the following is the MOST sensitive clinical predictor of intracranial injury?

(A) Seizure.

(B) Vomiting.

(C) Depressed mental status.

(D) Scalp hematoma.

26-4. A 57-year-old male presents to the ED with acute stroke symptoms that started over 6 hours ago. His blood pressure is consistently 240/120 mmHg. Which of the following interventions is indicated?

(A) Provide supportive care with oxygen by nasal cannula.

(B) Elevate the head of the bed.

(C) Start a nitroprusside drip to lower his blood pressure.

(D) Administer labetalol to lower his blood pressure.

26-5. What is the most sensitive electrocardiographic sign of right ventricular infarction?

(A) ST-segment depression in leads V_1, V_2, and V_3.

(B) ST-segment elevation in leads II, III, and aVF.

(C) ST-segment elevation in V_1.

(D) ST-segment elevation in V_4 using right-sided electrocardiographic leads.

26-6. Which of the following is an indicator of myocardial infarction in the presence of left bundle branch block?

(A) Diffuse ST-segment elevation in all leads.

(B) ST-segment elevation in V_1, V_2, and V_3 with reciprocal changes in the limb leads.

(C) ST-segment deviation of at least 1 mm in the same (concordant) direction as the major QRS vector.

(D) There is no indicator for ischemia in the presence of a left bundle branch block.

26-7. A 12-year-old boy, previously healthy, presents to the ED with 8 days of cough and fever. Vital signs show slight tachypnea but are otherwise normal. Oxygen saturation is 98% on room air. He appears well, and lung exam is significant for coarse rhonchi bilaterally. Chest radiograph reveals a posterior left lower lobe infiltrate. He has no medication allergies. Which of the following is the MOST appropriate antibiotic choice?

(A) Azithromycin.

(B) Ciprofloxacin.

(C) Cefuroxime.

(D) Amoxicillin.

26-8. Which of the following patients with suspected meningitis is safe for lumbar puncture without prior head CT?

(A) A 70-year-old male with no past medical history who has a nonfocal neurologic exam.

(B) A 32-year-old female who is HIV-positive and presents with a seizure.

(C) A 56-year-old male with a serum WBC >15,000 with a nonfocal neurologic exam.

(D) A 48-year-old female with a history of stroke and residual left-sided weakness.

26-9. Which of the following significantly increases the risk of having a febrile seizure?

(A) Group A streptococcal pharyngitis.

(B) Diptheria toxoid, tetanus toxoid, and whole-cell pertussis (DTP) vaccination.

(C) African-American race.

(D) Cystic fibrosis.

26-10. A 4-year-old girl presents to the ED with her first simple febrile seizure. Which of the following is indicated?

(A) Glucose finger stick.

(B) Routine lab studies including electrolytes and CBC.

(C) Noncontrast head CT.

(D) Lumbar puncture.

26-11. Which of the following drugs is first-line therapy for a febrile seizure?

(A) Lorazepam.

(B) Phenytoin.

(C) Fosphenytoin.

(D) Phenobarbital.

26-12. Which of the following drugs is ineffective for treating alcohol withdrawal symptoms?

(A) Clonidine.

(B) Carbamazepine.

(C) Chlordiazepoxide.

(D) Phenytoin.

26-13. Which of the following withdrawal syndromes is described by flulike symptoms (fatigue, diffuse myalgias, headache, vomiting)?

(A) Alcohol.

(B) Amphetamine.

(C) Benzodiazepine.

(D) Opioid.

26-14. Which of the following agents is no longer recommended as an anesthetic for lacerations?

(A) LET.

(B) TAC.

(C) EMLA cream.

(D) Bupivacaine with epinephrine.

26-15. Which of the following is TRUE of tissue adhesives for the repair of lacerations?

(A) They are more time-consuming than sutures.

(B) They are more prone to infections than sutures.

(C) They are more expensive than sutures.

(D) They are more likely to dehisce over high-tension areas.

26-16. A 3-year-old boy is suspected of ingesting 30 tablets of his mother's verapamil perhaps 1 hour ago. Upon discovering the child with the empty bottle, the mother drove immediately to the ED. Vital signs are normal except that the child is hypotensive. The boy is awake, alert, and crying but otherwise appears well. The remainder of the exam is notable only for decreased bowel sounds. Which of the following interventions is MOST appropriate?

(A) Ipecac syrup.

(B) Gastric lavage using an orogastric tube.

(C) Administration of activated charcoal.

(D) Whole-bowel irrigation.

26-17. Which of the following statements regarding ipecac syrup is TRUE?

(A) Its use should be considered only in children who have ingested a potentially toxic substance in the preceding hour.

(B) Ipecac is safe and has not been associated with any complications.

(C) Ipecac can be safely given to a child who is obtunded.

(D) Ipecac has been proven to improve morbidity and mortality in clinical trials.

26-18. A 63-year-old male presents to the ED with an acute ST-segment elevation myocardial infarction. He is hemodynamically stable. Aspirin, a β-blocker, and unfractionated heparin infusion have been administered. There is no catheterization lab at your facility. By transferring him to the nearest catheterization lab for PTCA within 2 hours instead of performing immediate fibrinolytic therapy, which of the following outcomes is TRUE?

(A) Decreased risk of death.

(B) Increased risk of death.

(C) Decreased risk of reinfarction.

(D) Increased risk of reinfarction.

26-19. For a child, which of the following is an indication to obtain a radiograph according to the Ottawa knee rules?

(A) Abrasion at the knee.

(B) Tenderness of the tibial tuberosity.

(C) Tenderness at the head of the fibula.

(D) Severe limping.

26-20. Fomepizole is an antidote for which of the following poisons?

(A) Methanol.

(B) Isopropyl alcohol.

(C) Iron.

(D) Arsenic.

26-21. Which of the following is the vector through which the West Nile virus is passed?

(A) Squirrels.

(B) Birds.

(C) Fleas.

(D) Mosquitoes.

26-22. The majority of patients infected with the West Nile virus develop which of the following clinical symptoms?

(A) None.

(B) Nonspecific viral syndrome with low-grade fever, headache, malaise, and myalgias.

(C) Upper respiratory tract symptoms including rhinorrhea, cough, and sore throat.

(D) Neurologic symptoms consistent with meningitis, encephalitis, or acute flaccid paralysis.

26-23. Nesiritide is a relatively new drug for the treatment of which of the following?

(A) Chronic obstructive pulmonary disease.

(B) Congestive heart failure (CHF).

(C) Asthma.

(D) Acute coronary syndrome.

26-24. Which of the following is the hallmark clinical manifestation for gamma-hydroxybutyric acid (GHB) intoxication?

(A) Bradycardia.

(B) Hypotension.

(C) CNS depression.

(D) Anticholinergic effects.

26-25. Meperidine has been associated with fatalities when given to patients taking which of the following medications?

(A) Monoamine oxidase inhibitor.

(B) Tricyclic antidepressant.

(C) Warfarin.

(D) Sulfonamide.

26-26. Which of the following opioids has the least adverse hemodynamic effects and causes the least amount of respiratory depression?

(A) Hydromorphone.

(B) Morphine.

(C) Meperidine.

(D) Fentanyl.

26-27. Which of the following is a TRUE statement regarding nonsteroidal anti-inflammatory drugs (NSAIDs)?

(A) Ketorolac when given parenterally is more potent than oral ibuprofen.

(B) NSAID-induced gastrointestinal (GI) bleeding is responsible for 16,500 deaths annually.

(C) Cyclooxygenase 2 (COX-2) inhibitors have the same rate of GI bleeding as other NSAIDs.

(D) NSAIDs do not affect platelet function.

26-28. Which of the following features is characteristic of central vertigo?

(A) Sudden onset.

(B) Severe spinning.

(C) Constant.

(D) Frequent nausea and diaphoresis.

26-29. Which of the following is a cause of peripheral vertigo?

(A) Cerebellar hemorrhage.

(B) Multiple sclerosis.

(C) Wallenberg's syndrome.

(D) Meniere's disease.

26-30. Which of the following can cause permanent ototoxicity and vestibulotoxicity?

(A) Aminoglycosides.

(B) Quinolones.

(C) Erythromycin.

(D) Antimalarials.

26-31. Which of the following is a primary indication to perform bedside ED ultrasound?

(A) A 72-year-old male who presents with hypotension and severe low back pain.

(B) A 32-year-old female with recently diagnosed cervical cancer who presents for left leg pain and swelling.

(C) A 25-year-old male complaining of severe testicular pain for 8 hours.

(D) An 80-year-old female with new onset vaginal bleeding and pelvic pain.

26-32. Which of the following is a TRUE statement regarding indications for a bedside pelvic ultrasound performed by an emergency physician?

(A) Exam is indicated for any patient with first-trimester vaginal bleeding or pelvic pain with quantitative β-hCG <2000 MIU/mL.

(B) Exam is indicated for any patient with first-trimester vaginal bleeding or pelvic pain with quantitative β-hCG >2000 MIU/mL.

(C) Exam is indicated for any patient with first-trimester vaginal bleeding or pelvic pain regardless of the quantitative β-hCG.

(D) Exam is indicated for any patient with vaginal bleeding or pelvic pain regardless of pregnancy status.

ABEM 2005 Continuous Certification Articles
Answers, Explanations, and References

26-1. **The answer is C.** In the evaluation of syncope, the presence of structural heart disease (coronary artery disease, congestive heart failure, valvular heart disease, or congenital heart disease) has emerged as the most important factor for predicting the risk of death, as well as the likelihood of arrhythmias. Syncope with exertion is associated with aortic stenosis, mitral stenosis, hypertrophic cardiomyopathy, and coronary artery disease. The other choices are all examples of neurally mediated syncope (vasovagal, situational, and carotid sinus syncope). **Reference:** Kapoor WN. Syncope. *N Engl J Med.* December 2000;343: 1856–1862.

26-2. **The answer is A.** The history and physical examination lead to the identification of a cause of syncope in 45% of patients. CT of the brain provides new diagnostic information in 4% of cases. Electrocardiograms reveal the diagnosis in <5% of patients; however, frequently they provide invaluable clues to underlying structural disease (bundle branch block or previous myocardial infarction). Baseline laboratory tests for electrolytes, renal function, blood sugar, and hemoglobin lead to an assignment of cause in only 2–3% of patients. **Reference:** Kapoor WN. Syncope. *N Engl J Med.* December 2000;343:1856–1862.

26-3. **The answer is B.** Most studies report that skull radiographs are 94–99% sensitive for detecting linear or depressed skull fractures. CT imaging has a lower sensitivity, ranging from 47% to 94%. Skull radiographs may be a useful screen for skull fractures for alert, asymptomatic infants with scalp hematomas, who would not otherwise undergo CT imaging. In these well-appearing young infants, skull radiographs offer the advantage of requiring no sedation. If a fracture is detected, CT imaging is indicated to assess for associated intracranial injury. **Reference:** Schutzman SA, Greenes DS. Pediatric minor head trauma. *Ann of Emerg Med.* January 2001;37:65–74.

26-4. **The answer is B.** Hypertension is common in acute stroke and should be treated cautiously if at all. The blood pressure should not be aggressively treated to bring it into the normal range, but mild forms of drug therapy are acceptable. Simple maneuvers such as elevation of the head of the bed may help control hypertension by increasing the cerebral venous drainage. The American Heart Association recommends treating hypertension in the acute states of stroke if the systolic blood pressure is more than 220 mmHg, or if the mean arterial pressure is more than 130 mmHg. Hypotension can dramatically decrease the cerebral perfusion pressure and cerebral blood flow, extending the area of infarction, and is to be avoided. **Reference:** Lewandowski C, Barsan W. Treatment of acute ischemic stroke. *Ann Emerg Med.* February 2001;37:202–216.

26-5. **The answer is D.** Right ventricular infarction is always associated with occlusion of the proximal segment of the right coronary artery. The most sensitive electrocardiographic sign of right ventricular infarction is ST-segment elevation of more than 1 mm in lead V_4R with an upright T wave in that lead. According to the American College of Cardiology, right ventricular infarction accompanying inferior myocardial infarctions is associated with a significantly higher mortality (25–30% vs. 6%) and thus identifies a high-risk subgroup of patients with inferior myocardial infarctions who should be considered high-priority candidates for reperfusion. **Reference:** Zimetbaum PJ, Josephson ME. Use of the electrocardiogram in acute myocardial infarction. *N Engl J Med.* March 2003;348:933–940.

26-6. **The answer is C.** Spontaneous or pacing-induced left bundle branch block can obscure the electrocardiographic diagnosis of acute myocardial infarction. In the presence of left bundle branch block, right ventricular activation precedes left ventricular activation; this activation of the infarcted left ventricle occurs later and is obscured within the QRS complex. Thus, Q waves cannot be used to diagnose infarction. An indicator of myocardial infarction in the presence of left bundle branch block is primary ST change—that is, ST deviation in

the same (concordant) direction as the major QRS vector. Extremely discordant ST deviation (>5 mm) is also suggestive of myocardial infarction in the presence of left bundle branch block. **Reference:** Zimetbaum PJ, Josephson ME. Use of the electrocardiogram in acute myocardial infarction. *N Engl J Med.* March 2003;348:933–940.

26-7. **The answer is A.** The vignette describes a 12-year-old boy with uncomplicated community-acquired pneumonia that can be treated on an outpatient basis. Antibiotic choice is determined by the age-associated microbial etiologies. Table 26-1 gives a breakdown of age, microbial cause, and empiric outpatient treatment. **Reference:** McIntosh K. Community-acquired pneumonia in children. *N Engl J Med.* February 2002;346:429–436.

26-8. **The answer is C.** In adults with suspected meningitis, clinical features can be used to identify those who are unlikely to have abnormal findings on CT of the head. The clinical features at baseline that were associated with an abnormal finding on CT of the head were an age of at least 60 years, immunocompromise, a history of central nervous system disease, a history of seizure within 1 week before presentation, altered

TABLE 26-1. ETIOLOGIES OF PNEUMONIA BASED ON AGE OF CHILD WITH TREATMENT RECOMMENDATIONS

Age	Cause (in order of frequency)	Treatment
Birth–20 days	Group B streptococci Gram-negative enteric bacteria Cytomegalovirus	Admission
3 weeks–3 months	Respiratory syncytial virus (RSV) Parainfluenza virus 3 *Streptococcus pneumoniae* *Bordetella pertussis* *Staphylococcus aureus*	Macrolide
4 months–4 years	RSV, parainfluenza, influenza, adenovirus, and rhinovirus *S. pneumoniae* *Haemophilus influenzae* *Mycoplasma pneumoniae*	Amoxicillin
5–15 years	*M. pneumoniae* *Chlamydia pneumoniae* *S. pneumoniae* *Mycobacterium tuberculosis*	Macrolide

mental status, and focal neurologic abnormality (specifically an inability to answer 2 consecutive questions correctly or to follow 2 consecutive commands, gaze palsy, abnormal visual fields, facial palsy, arm drift, leg drift, and abnormal language). **Reference:** Hasbun R, Abrahams J, Jekel J, et al. Computed tomography of the head before lumbar puncture in adults with suspected meningitis. *N Engl J Med.* December 2001;345:1727–1733.

26-9. **The answer is B.** Febrile seizures occur at some point in 2–4% of children worldwide. There are no geographic, racial, or ethnic differences in incidence. There is a family history of febrile seizures in 25–40% of cases. Viral infections are frequently associated with febrile seizures (humanherpes virus 6, which causes roseola; human herpesvirus 7; and influenzaviruses A and B). There is also significant increased risk on the day of vaccination with DTP and in 8–14 days after a measles, mumps, and rubella vaccination, but these are not associated with any long-term adverse consequences. Of note, the rates of serious bacterial infections in patients with febrile seizures are equivalent to those in age-matched febrile control patients. **Reference:** Warden CR, Zibulewsky J, Mace S, et al. Evaluation and management of febrile seizures in the out-of-hospital and emergency department settings. *Ann Emerg Med.* February 2003;41:215–222.

26-10. **The answer is A.** Routine lab studies are usually not indicated for patients who have had simple febrile seizures, with the exception of a whole-blood or serum glucose test. The American Academy of Pediatrics recommends that neuroimaging not be routine for a first-time simple febrile seizure. A lumbar puncture should be strongly considered in a child younger than 18 months having a febrile seizure with (1) a history of irritability, decreased feeding, or lethargy; (2) an abnormal appearance or mental status findings on initial observation of the child (after the postictal period); (3) any physical signs of meningitis, such as a

bulging fontanelle, Kernig's or Brudzinski's signs, photophobia, or severe headache; (4) any complex features; (5) any slow postictal clearing of mentation; or (6) pretreatment with antibiotics. Children older than 18 months have more reliable signs or symptoms of a central nervous system infection, and a lumbar puncture can be deferred if these are absent. **Reference:** Warden CR, Zibulewsky J, Mace S, et al. Evaluation and management of febrile seizures in the out-of-hospital and emergency department settings. *Ann Emerg Med.* February 2003;41: 215–222.

26-11. **The answer is A.** A febrile seizure lasting longer than 5 minutes should be treated, usually with a benzodiazepine as first-line therapy. Patients with typical febrile seizures will rarely need more than 1 dose of a benzodiazepine to terminate the seizure. For refractory seizures, fosphenytoin is indicated. Phenobarbital and valproate are effective prophylactic regimens for febrile seizure, but these regimens do not prevent the eventual development of epilepsy, and often the adverse side effects of the medications outweigh any short-term benefit in preventing febrile seizures. **Reference:** Warden CR, Zibulewsky J, Mace S, et al. Evaluation and management of febrile seizures in the out-of-hospital and emergency department settings. *Ann Emerg Med.* February 2003;41: 215–222.

26-12. **The answer is D.** The anticonvulsant medication phenytoin is not an effective treatment for alcohol withdrawal. Clonidine ameliorates symptoms in patients with mild to moderate withdrawal but probably does not reduce delirium or seizures. Carbamazepine is superior to placebo and equal in efficacy to oxazepam for patients with mild to moderate withdrawal symptoms; furthermore, it reduces emotional stress better and permits a faster return to work than does oxazepam. Two major literature reviews of pharmacotherapy for alcohol withdrawal concluded that benzodiazepines are the treatment of choice on the basis of several outcomes, including the severity of the alcohol withdrawal syndrome, occurrence of delirium and seizures, adverse effects of the medication, and completion of withdrawal, as well as subsequent entry into rehabilitation. **Reference:** Kosten TR, O'Connor PG. Management of drug and alcohol withdrawal. *N Engl J Med.* May 2003;348:1786–1794.

26-13.   The answer is D. Opioid withdrawal syndrome resembles a severe case of influenza. In addition, the symptoms include pupillary dilatation, lacrimation, rhinorrhea, piloerection ("gooseflesh"), yawning, sneezing, anorexia, nausea, vomiting, and diarrhea. Seizures and delirium tremens seen with alcohol and benzodiazepine withdrawal do not occur with opioid withdrawal. **Reference**: Kosten TR, O'Connor PG. Management of drug and alcohol withdrawal. *N Engl J Med.* May 2003;348: 1786–1794.

26-14.   The answer is B. A combination of tetracaine, adrenaline, and cocaine (TAC) has been shown to be an effective topical anesthetic before repair of lacerations, particularly in children and on the face and scalp. However, improper use of TAC has been associated with serious adverse events such as seizures and death. This has led to alternative regimens such as LET (lidocaine, epinephrine, and tetracaine) that do not have the associated risks and administrative complications of cocaine. EMLA is commonly used as a topical anesthetic. Its use is commonplace with children. **Reference:** Hollander JE, Singer AJ. Laceration management. *Ann Emerg Med.* September 1999;34:356–367.

26-15.   The answer is D. Advantages of tissue adhesives include rapid application, patient comfort, decreased risk of wound infections, low cost, no need for removal, and no risk of needle stick. Disadvantages of tissue adhesives include a lower tensile strength than sutures with subsequent dehiscence over high-tension areas (joints), the inability to use them on the hands, and

the need to avoid bathing or swimming. **Reference:** Hollander JE, Singer AJ. Laceration management. *Ann Emerg Med.* September 1999;34:356–367.

26-16.   The answer is C. In general, activated charcoal is the sole intervention needed to treat serious poisonings. A slurry consisting of activated charcoal and a flavoring agent should be given to the child. If it has not been swallowed within 20 minutes after ingestion of the toxin, activated charcoal should be administered through a nasogastric tube. Rigorously performed studies have not found any substantial value associated with gastric emptying in the ED; therefore, administration of ipecac syrup and gastric lavage are not routinely recommended. The place of whole-bowel irrigation in the treatment of poisoning in children has not been well established. Data suggest that the most important role of whole-bowel irrigation is as an intervention for the removal of substances that are poorly adsorbed to activated charcoal—for example, iron and lithium. **Reference:** Shannon M. Ingestion of toxic substances by children. *N Engl J Med.* January 2000;342:186–191.

26-17.   The answer is A. The use of ipecac should be considered only when a toxin has been ingested in the preceding hour. When administered 90 minutes or more after a toxic substance has been ingested, ipecac syrup has no identifiable benefit. Increasingly, both the safety and the efficacy of ipecac syrup have been questioned. There have been reports of prolonged vomiting, sedation, Mallory-Weiss syndrome, gastric rupture, and fatal aspiration. Contraindications to ipecac use are specific ingested toxins (e.g., hydrocarbons and corrosives), depressed gag reflex, obtundation, coagulopathy or bleeding diathesis, and age younger than 6 months. Overall, the efficacy of ipecac syrup, even when given appropriately, has not been proved. **Reference:** Shannon M. Ingestion of toxic substances by children. *N Engl J Med.* January 2000;342:186–191.

26-18. The answer is C. For the treatment of ST-segment elevation myocardial infarctions, primary angioplasty is considered superior to fibrinolysis for patients admitted to hospitals with angioplasty facilities. This benefit appears to be maintained for patients who require transportation from a community hospital to a center where invasive treatment is available. By transferring the patient for angioplasty rather than onsite fibrinolysis, there is no difference in death or subsequent stroke; however, there is a significant decrease in reinfarction rates (1.6% vs. 6.3%, *P* < .001). **Reference:** Andersen HR, Nielsen TT, Rasmussen K, et al. A comparison of coronary angioplasty with fibrinolytic therapy in acute myocardial infarction. *N Engl J Med.* August 2003;349:733–742.

26-19. The answer is C. The Ottawa knee rules state that knee roentgenography is required only for patients who have acute knee injury (past 7 days) and at least 1 of the following findings: age 55 years or older, isolated tenderness of the patella, tenderness at the head of the fibula, inability to flex to 90 degrees, or inability to bear weight both immediately and in the ED (4 steps, regardless of severe limping). The Ottawa knee rules were validated for pediatrics in a multicenter study with 750 children and found to be 100% sensitive and 43% specific. **Reference:** Bulloch B, Neto G, Plint A, et al. Validation of the Ottawa knee rules in children: a multicenter study. *Ann Emerg Med.* July 2003;42:48–55.

26-20. The answer is A. Fomepizole appears to be safe and effective in the treatment of methanol poisoning. Although methanol itself is not highly toxic, it is metabolized by alcohol dehydrogenase to formaldehyde and formic acid. These metabolites cause the metabolic acidosis, blindness, cardiovascular instability, and death attributed to methanol toxicity. Intravenous fomepizole inhibits alcohol dehydrogenase and subsequently inhibits the production of the toxic metabolites. There is no antidote for iso-

propyl alcohol; treatment is supportive. The antidote for iron is deferoxamine. The antidote for arsenic is dimercaprol (BAL, British antilewisite). **Reference:** Brent J, McMartin K, Phillips S, et al. Fomepizole for the treatment of methanol poisoning. *N Engl J Med.* February 2001;344:424–429.

26-21. The answer is D. Mosquitoes from the genus *Culex* are the principal maintenance and amplifying vectors. The virus is maintained in a bird-mosquito-bird cycle, with passerine birds serving as the primary amplifying hosts. **Reference:** Petersen LR, Marfin AA, Gubler DJ. West Nile virus. *JAMA.* July 2003;290:524–528.

26-22. The answer is A. Most individuals infected with West Nile virus (WNV) remain asymptomatic. When clinical illness occurs, the incubation period generally ranges from 2–14 days. West Nile fever is a mild illness, typically lasting 3–6 days. Symptoms are of sudden onset and often include malaise, anorexia, nausea, vomiting, eye pain, headache, myalgia, and rash. Approximately 20% of infected individuals develop West Nile fever. Despite the increased clinical severity during recent outbreaks, less than 1% of individuals infected with WNV developed severe neurologic disease (e.g., encephalitis, meningitis, or acute flaccid paralysis). During the outbreak in the United States in 2002, patients with meningoencephalitis had a case-fatality rate of 9%. Advanced age is the most important risk factor for death. **Reference:** Petersen LR, Marfin AA, Gubler DJ. West Nile virus. *JAMA.* July 2003;290:524–528.

26-23. The answer is B. Nesiritide is a recombinant human brain, or B-type, natriuretic peptide that is identical to the endogenous hormone produced by the ventricle in response to increased wall stress, hypertrophy, and volume overload. Nesiritide has venous, arterial, and coronary vasodilatory properties that reduce preload and afterload, increase cardiac output without direct inotropic effects, improve echocardiographic indices of diastolic function, and improve symptoms in patients with acutely decompensated CHF, without increasing heart rate or proarrhythmia. In one large, randomized, double-blind study, the hemodynamic and clinical effects of nesiritide added to standard care for CHF was compared to (1) placebo added to standard care and (2) IV nitroglycerin added to standard care. When compared to placebo after 3 hours of treatment, nesiritide decreased capillary wedge pressure ($P < .001$) and improved dyspnea ($P = .03$). When compared to IV nitroglycerin after 3 hours of treatment, nesiritide improved pulmonary capillary wedge pressures ($P = .03$) but not dyspnea or global clinical status ($P = .09$). **Reference:** Young JB, Publication Committee for the VMAC Investigators. Intravenous nesiritide vs. nitroglycerin for treatment of decompensated congestive heart failure: a randomized controlled trial. *JAMA.* March 2002;287:1531–1540.

26-24.   **The answer is C.** GHB is a naturally occurring analog of gamma-aminobutyric acid (GABA) that has been used in research and clinical medicine for many years. In the past decade it has become very popular as a dietary supplement and recreational drug. The cardinal manifestation of GHB intoxication prompting presentation to the ED is CNS depression, often to the point of coma. Several case series of GHB intoxication report that approximately 25% of patients present with a Glasgow Coma Scale (GCS) score of 3, and 60% with a GCS score of <9. Resolution of CNS depression occurs abruptly, with patients going from unresponsive to agitated and combative over very short periods of time. **Reference:** Mason PE, Kerns WP II. Gamma hydroxybutyric acid (GHB) intoxication. *Acad Emerg Med.* July 2002;9:730–739.

26-25.   **The answer is A.** Meperidine is a synthetic narcotic analgesic that can be administered orally or parenterally. Meperidine is metabolized to normeperidine. Normeperidine can cause dysphoria, irritability, tremors, myoclonus, and seizures. Patients given meperidine who are concomitantly taking monoamine oxidase (MAO) inhibitors or medications with MAO properties can develop severe encephalopathy that can be fatal. Therefore, meperidine should be used only for short-term treatment of acute pain and should not be prescribed in high or repeated doses. **Reference:** Blackburn P, Vissers R. Pharmacology of emergency department pain management and conscious sedation. *Emerg Med Clin N Am.* November 2000;18:803–826.

26-26.   **The answer is D.** Fentanyl is a synthetic opioid most commonly used to provide analgesia during procedural sedation in the ED. When given parenterally, onset of analgesia is rapid (90 seconds). Fentanyl's clinical effects in the acute setting are approximately 30 minutes. In equivalent doses, fentanyl is approximately 100 times as potent as morphine and 1000 times more potent than meperidine. The respiratory depression seen with fentanyl is less than that with either morphine or meperidine. Fentanyl produces minimal hemodynamic effects and because of this is a popular agent during cardiac anesthesia. **Reference:** Blackburn P, Vissers R. Pharmacology of emergency department pain management and conscious sedation. *Emerg Med Clin N Am.* November 2000;18:803–826.

26-27.   **The answer is B.** It is estimated that NSAID GI effects account for 107,000 hospitalizations and 16,500 deaths annually in the United States. Particularly at risk are those on higher dosages, with prolonged use, previous peptic ulcer disease, excessive alcohol intake, and advanced age. Three studies have shown that ketorolac 60 mg IM has equal efficacy to ibuprofen 800 mg PO. Two of the studies noted that speed of onset was also similar. COX-2 inhibitors preferentially inhibit prostaglandin synthesis at sites of inflammation throughout the body rather than in the GI tract. A combined analysis of 8 trials of patients (N = 5435) with osteoarthritis treated with rofecoxib was associated with a significantly lower incidence of GI tract bleeding than treatment with other NSAIDs. NSAIDs do inhibit platelet function; however, unlike aspirin, which inhibits function for the 8–10 day lifetime of the platelet, elimination of the NSAID leads to return of platelet function. **Reference:** Blackburn P, Vissers R. Pharmacology of emergency department pain management and conscious sedation. *Emerg Med Clin N Am.* November 2000;18: 803–826.

26-28. The answer is C. Characteristics distinguishing peripheral and central vertigo are found in Table 26-2 of the reference cited below. **Reference:** Goldman B. Vertigo and dizziness. Tintinalli JE et al (eds): *Emergency Medicine, A Comprehensive Study Guide,* ed. 5, 2000, pp. 1452–1463.

26-29. The answer is D. Peripheral vertigo is caused by disorders affecting the vestibular apparatus and the eighth cranial nerve, while central vertigo is caused by disorders of the cerebellum and brainstem. Meniere's disease is a disorder associated with an increased volume of endolymph within the cochlea and labyrinth. Onset of vertigo is sudden but lasts typically 2–8 hours. It is associated with nausea, vomiting, and diaphoresis. Frequency of attacks varies from several times per week to several times per month. Hallmarks of diagnosis include the triad of vertigo, tinnitus, and decreased hearing. Cerebellar hemorrhage results in acute onset, constant vertigo, and ataxia that may or may not be associated with headache, nausea, or vomiting. Wallenberg's syndrome is a lateral medullary infarction of the brainstem. Multiple sclerosis may cause isolated areas of demyelination in the brainstem, causing vertigo. **Reference:** Goldman B. Vertigo and dizziness. Tintinalli JE et al (eds): *Emergency Medicine, A Comprehensive Study Guide,* ed. 5, 2000, pp. 1452–1463.

26-30. The answer is A. Aminoglycoside antibiotics produce hearing loss and peripheral vestibular dysfunction by accumulating inside the endolymph, where they cause the death of cochlear and vestibular hair cells. However, since both inner ears are affected, vertigo is uncommon. Typical clinical manifestations include ataxia and oscillopsia, which is defined as an inability to maintain visual fixation while moving. The damage is irreversible, although the degree of toxicity depends on the dose and duration of treatment with antibiotics. Quinolones, erythromycin, and antimalarials all cause ototoxicity or vestibulotoxicity that is reversible. **Reference:** Goldman B. Vertigo and dizziness. Tintinalli JE et al (eds): *Emergency Medicine, A Comprehensive Study Guide,* ed. 5, 2000, pp. 1452–1463.

26-31. The answer is A. The 6 primary indications to perform bedside ED ultrasound and their associated key sonographic findings are:

1. Trauma ultrasound: hemoperitoneum, hemothorax, and pericardial tamponade.
2. Abdominal aortic aneurysm: aortic diameter >3 cm.
3. First-trimester pregnancy: intrauterine pregnancy.
4. Cardiac evaluation: cardiac activity, pericardial fluid.
5. Obstructive uropathy: hydronephrosis.
6. Gallbladder disease: gallstones, sonographic Murphy's sign.

TABLE 26-2. DISTINGUISHING CHARACTERISTICS OF PERIPHERAL AND CENTRAL VERTIGO

	Peripheral	Central
Onset	Sudden	Slow
Severity of vertigo	Intense spinning	Less intense
Pattern	Paroxysmal, intermittent	Constant
Aggravated by position	Yes	No
Nausea/diaphoresis	Frequent	Infrequent
Nystagmus	Rotatory-vertical, horizontal	Vertical
Fatigue of symptoms/ signs	Yes	No
Hearing loss/tinnitus	May occur	No
Abnormal tympanic membrane	May occur	No
CNS symptoms/signs	No	Usually present

The elderly patient with hypotension and severe low back pain most likely has a ruptured abdominal aortic aneurysm, which is a primary indication for bedside ED ultrasound. **Reference:** Melanson SW, Heller MB. Principles of emergency department sonography. Tintinalli JE et al (eds): *Emergency Medicine, A Comprehensive Study Guide,* ed. 5, 2000, pp. 1972–1982.

26-32.   The answer is C. Ultrasound evaluation of *all* first-trimester pregnant patients presenting to the ED with any abdominal or pelvic pain and vaginal bleeding has been recommended. Such an approach has been found to markedly decrease the frequency of delayed diagnoses and rupture of ectopic pregnancies at the time of diagnosis. The quantitative beta human chorionic gonadotropin (β-hCG) level is extremely helpful in evaluating pregnant patients with an empty uterus on ultrasound. A number of authors have suggested "discriminatory zones," β-hCG levels above which an intrauterine pregnancy (IUP) should be visualized if present. Based on the work of several authors, it is expected that an IUP is detectable on endovaginal scanning if the β-hCG level is >2000 MIU/mL. Patients with β-hCG levels greater than this (the discriminatory zone) who do not have evidence of an IUP are at very high risk for an ectopic pregnancy. However, it is still recognized that ectopic pregnancies present to the ED with β-hCG levels below the discriminatory zone and have been reported even below 100 MIU/mL. For this reason all first-trimester patients who present with the symptoms previously mentioned should receive a pelvic ultrasound to evaluate for possible ectopic pregnancy. **Reference:** Melanson SW, Heller MB. Principles of emergency department sonography. Tintinalli JE et al (eds): *Emergency Medicine, A Comprehensive Study Guide,* ed. 5, 2000, pp. 1972–1982.

Post Test
Questions

27-1. Which of the following is TRUE for plain radiographs of the skull in the evaluation of pediatric minor head trauma?

(A) There are no indications for skull radiographs.

(B) Skull radiographs have higher sensitivity than CT scans for detecting skull fractures.

(C) Skull radiographs are sensitive for diagnosing basilar skull fractures.

(D) Skull radiographs provide detailed information of intracranial injuries.

27-2. Which of the following agents does not cause photosensitivity eruptions?

(A) Furosemide.

(B) Nickel.

(C) Psoralens.

(D) Thiazides.

27-3. You receive a patient from a warehouse explosion who you suspect has a primary blast injury of the lung. The patient complains of mild chest pain with inspiration and shortness of breath. His vital signs are blood pressure 180/60 mmHg, pulse 90 beats per minute, respirations 14 breaths per minute, and a pulse oximetry of 95% on room air. He has mildly decreased breath sounds on the right, and his physical exam is otherwise normal except for mild abrasions and contusions. Chest x-ray shows mild patchy infiltrates in the right lower lobe. What should your initial management include?

(A) High-flow oxygen.

(B) Immediate endotracheal intubation.

(C) Placing the patient upright in a sitting position.

(D) Rapid infusion of crystalloid fluids.

27-4. In which of the following patients with a toxic ingestion is the use of gastric lavage MOST appropriate?

(A) A 30-year-old male who swallowed 50 pills of acetaminophen 3 hours ago.

(B) A 5-year-old girl who possibly swallowed some household bleach.

(C) A 25-year-old woman who took half a bottle of amitryptiline 30 minutes ago in front of her friends.

(D) A 16-year-old male who accidentally swallowed a glass full of turpentine 15 minutes ago.

27-5. Which of the following infective agents is known to mimic appendicitis?

(A) *Yersinia* species.

(B) *Clostridium botulinum.*

(C) *Vibrio cholerae.*

(D) *Staphylococcus aureus.*

27-6. A 45-year-old male with a history of hypertrophic cardiomyopathy presents with severe dyspnea and bilateral inspiratory rales. What is the appropriate pharmacologic management?

(A) Nitroglycerin.

(B) Nesiritide.

(C) Morphine.

(D) β-adrenergic blocker.

27-7. A 30-year-old woman presents to the ED at 29 weeks gestation in preterm labor secondary to recent cocaine use. You successfully deliver a premature infant and stabilize the mother. The premature infant is found to have progressively worsening retractions, tachypnea, and increasing oxygen requirements. A stat chest x-ray reveals ground glass opacities in the lung parenchyma and prominent air bronchograms. An ABG reveals a Po_2 of 50 mmHg on 100% oxygen by nonrebreather mask. What is the next immediate step you should take in the management of this infant?

(A) Contact the closest tertiary pediatric referral center and immediately make plans for transfer.

(B) Immediately apply continuous positive airway pressure (CPAP) through nasal cannula specially designed for neonates.

(C) Immediately intubate the patient and apply positive end-expiratory pressure (PEEP).

(D) Immediately intubate the patient and apply the appropriate weight-based dose of Surfactant down the endotracheal tube.

27-8. Which of the following electrocardiogram findings, occurring shortly after the onset of acute myocardial infarction, is associated with an increased mortality?

(A) Second-degree Mobitz type I atrioventricular block.

(B) First-degree atrioventricular block.

(C) New right bundle branch block.

(D) Sinus bradycardia.

27-9. Which of the following statements regarding sexual assault is NOT correct?

(A) Lack of genital injuries does not imply consensual intercourse.

(B) Colposcopy and staining techniques enhance documentation of genital injury.

(C) General body trauma is frequently documented.

(D) Forensic evidence is gathered even if the assault occurred more than 72 hours ago.

27-10. An industrial painter presents with a small puncture wound on the volar pad of his dominant index finger. The injury occurred upon accidental contact with a high-pressure spray gun. On examination of the wound, he has mild soft tissue tenderness distal to the proximal interphalangeal joint. He has normal two-point discrimination, capillary refill, and flexor tendon function. He states he is mainly here due to his employer's insistence in documenting this "trivial" on-the-job injury. What statement BEST describes the optimal management of this patient's injury?

(A) Digital nerve block is a useful technique to attain pain control in this condition.

(B) Local cleansing, topical antibiotic application, and dressing placement followed by wound reexamination in 48 hours are adequate treatments.

(C) Prophylactic antibiotics are contraindicated in this type of injury.

(D) Immediate hand specialist consultation is indicated.

27-11. A 4-year-old boy tripped and fell against a table edge. His mother brings in 1 front tooth suspended in milk. His physical exam is normal except for ecchymotic gingiva over his anterior alveolar ridge, which is stable. His one incisor is completely avulsed. His other incisor is extremely loose but still in the socket. What is the MOST appropriate treatment?

(A) Push the avulsed tooth firmly into the tooth socket, securing it to the surrounding teeth with periodontal dressing, and recommend follow-up with a dentist within 24 hours.

(B) Leave the avulsed tooth out, secure the loose incisor to surrounding teeth with periodontal dressing, and recommend follow-up with a dentist within 24 hours.

(C) Extract the loose tooth, soak both teeth in Hank's balanced salt solution for 30 minutes, then push the teeth firmly into the tooth sockets, securing them to the surrounding teeth with periodontal dressing. Recommend follow-up with a dentist within 24 hours.

(D) Extract the loose tooth, and recommend follow-up with a dentist within 24 hours.

27-12. Which of the following injuries is well visualized when performing a focused assessment with sonography for trauma (FAST) exam?

(A) Pancreas injury.

(B) Hollow viscus injury.

(C) Hemothorax.

(D) Retroperitoneal hematoma.

27-13. When is the greatest risk of rejection present in the post–cardiac transplant patient?

(A) First 6 weeks.

(B) First 6 months.

(C) First year.

(D) First 5 years.

27-14. A 10-year-old boy falls out of his tree house, landing on his right arm. His parents bring him to the ED. He is complaining of right wrist pain. Physical exam reveals tenderness at the distal radius but no gross deformity. Which of the following is TRUE regarding the potential for a growth plate injury?

(A) This is unlikely to represent a physeal injury, as growth plate fractures of the distal radius are very rare.

(B) A negative radiograph effectively rules out a growth plate injury.

(C) His age is protective from an injury to the physis, as most occur in toddlers and preschool-age children.

(D) Because of relative skeletal immaturity, injuries to the physis occur more frequently in boys than girls.

27-15. Which of the following diagnoses is MOST consistent with the feeling of intense intermittent spinning and nystagmus in the horizontal plane that fatigues?

(A) Meniere's disease.

(B) Multiple sclerosis.

(C) Vertebral artery dissection.

(D) Brainstem transient ischemic attack.

27-16. Which of the following statements is MOST accurate about peritonsillar abscesses?

(A) Needle aspiration effectively treats only 55% of patients, and often incision and drainage are required.

(B) A physical exam suggestive of peritonsillar abscess with negative needle aspiration requires computed tomography to rule out abscess.

(C) The proper technique of needle aspiration is application of topical anesthesia followed by introduction of an 18-gauge needle halfway between the base of the uvula and the maxillary alveolar ridge, penetrating no more than 2 cm.

(D) Peritonsillar abscess is the third most frequent deep space infection on the head and neck.

27-17. The MOST common site of esophageal obstruction in children occurs at which of the following locations?

(A) Distal esophagus.

(B) Thoracic inlet (T1).

(C) Cricopharyngeal narrowing (C6).

(D) Tracheal bifurcation (T6).

27-18. Which of the following types of anemia is NOT associated with an elevated red cell distribution width (RDW)?

(A) Iron deficiency.

(B) Vitamin B_{12} deficiency.

(C) Thalassemia.

(D) Folate deficiency.

27-19. What is the leading cause of death in patients with infective endocarditis?

(A) Congestive heart failure.

(B) Sepsis.

(C) Meningitis.

(D) Pneumonia.

27-20. Which one of the following statements is TRUE regarding neonatal intubation?

(A) The glottis is more posterior in infants than in older children, making it more difficult to visualize.

(B) A common mistake made during neonatal intubation is to insert the blade into the esophagus and then fail to withdraw it far enough to visualize the glottis.

(C) Placing a rolled-up blanket under the shoulders of an infant helps to hyperextend the neonate neck and increase the likelihood of a successful intubation.

(D) Studies show that physicians are often too cautious during the intubation of a neonate and fail to advance the endotracheal tube to the appropriate depth.

27-21. A 62-year-old man with hypertension, diabetes mellitus, and severe asthma, requiring intubation twice, presents with gradually worsening shortness of breath over the last several hours. On presentation to the ED, he is in respiratory distress and appears to be fatiguing. Vital signs are as follows: blood pressure 174/98 mmHg, heart rate 128 beats per minute, respirations 38 breaths per minute, and O_2 saturation 92% on nonrebreather face mask. Exam shows distended neck veins, poor but symmetric air flow bilaterally, tachycardia, and moderate edema. Which is the BEST choice for induction of anesthesia for rapid sequence intubation?

(A) Etomidate.

(B) Fentanyl.

(C) Ketamine.

(D) Versed.

27-22. Which of the following statements regarding scabies is TRUE?

(A) The mite makes a burrow in the outermost, horny layer of the skin.

(B) Hyperkeratotic areas are least affected.

(C) Lesions may involve the face and scalp of infants and young children.

(D) Crusted scabies produces hyperkeratotic crusting limited to the hands and feet.

27-23. Which of the following does NOT cause galactorrhea?

(A) Prolactinoma.

(B) Fibrocystic breast changes.

(C) Pituitary adenoma.

(D) Drugs.

27-24. Which of the following types of electrical injury is CORRECTLY paired with its resultant complications?

(A) Low-voltage alternating current (AC) and Lichtenburg figures.

(B) Lightning and deep tissue destruction.

(C) High-voltage AC and compartment syndrome.

(D) Lightning and tetanic contraction.

27-25. You are seeing a 7-day-old term infant who was discharged from the normal newborn nursery 5 days ago. Parents brought in the baby because she has been vomiting for the past 24 hours. She fed well initially but now is sleeping more and refusing to nurse. The emesis is nonbloody, nonprojectile but green in appearance. Which of the following conditions MUST be evaluated emergently?

(A) Gastroenteritis.

(B) Gastroesophageal reflux.

(C) Pyloric stenosis.

(D) Malrotation with volvulus.

27-26. A 40-year-old man is brought in by paramedics with a chief complaint of abdominal pain after a 15-foot fall from his roof. He did not lose consciousness and denies neck pain. Past medical history is significant for a deep vein thrombosis 4 months ago. The patient takes Coumadin. He denies allergies. The patient has 2 large-bore IVs and received 1000 cc crystalloid in the field. On arrival, vital signs are blood pressure 130/85 mmHg, pulse 120 beats per minute, respirations 24 per minute, temperature 37°C, and oxygen saturation 100% on 15 L/min face mask. The physical examination is normal except for a tense abdomen with tenderness in the right upper quadrant. A screening ultrasound reveals fluid in Morison's pouch. A Foley catheter is placed, and the urine appears normal. Preliminary cervical spine, chest, and pelvis films are normal. Labs reveal a hemoglobin of 10 g/dL, a hematocrit of 37, and INR of 2. Two units of type-specific packed red blood cells are started. What is the next appropriate step in this patient's care?

(A) Fresh frozen plasma 10–15 mL/kg.
(B) Oral vitamin K 1–2 mg.
(C) Cryoprecipitate 10 units.
(D) Intravenous vitamin K 5–10 mg slowly.

27-27. What is the leading cause of death for Americans between the ages of 1 and 44 years?

(A) Infection.
(B) Cancer.
(C) Injury.
(D) Heart disease.

27-28. Which of the following is a main component of offline medical control?

(A) Development of research projects.
(B) Development of treatment protocols.
(C) Development of mentoring programs.
(D) Development of career advancement tracks.

27-29. A 42-year-old G_1P_0 female presents to the ED complaining of a severe headache with upper abdominal pain and nausea. She is 35 weeks gestation by dates and has had no difficulty with this pregnancy. Her blood pressure on arrival is 135/85 mmHg, and her heart rate is 110 beats per minute. What is the MOST appropriate management option?

(A) Control the headache and nausea with prochlorperazine, and discharge to home with follow-up as scheduled by her obstetrician.
(B) Give a GI cocktail and acetaminophen, and discharge to home with follow-up as scheduled by her obstetrician.
(C) Obtain IV access, control the headache and nausea with promethazine, and discharge to home with follow-up as scheduled by her obstetrician.
(D) Obtain IV access and a urinalysis, and give an IV antiemetic as needed.

27-30. A 55-year-old female with no prior medical or surgical history presents to the ED with 4 days of progressively worsening left lower quadrant abdominal pain, fever to 39°C, and nonbloody diarrhea. She reports no recent travel. Diverticulitis is considered in this patient. Which of the following is the BEST diagnostic plan for this patient?

(A) Obtain a barium enema.
(B) Perform a pelvic exam.
(C) Obtain an abdominal CT scan.
(D) Obtain a nasogastric aspirate.

27-31. Which of the following is TRUE of the prevalence of panic attacks?

(A) Peaks in adolescence and then declines.
(B) Has a bimodal distribution in the early 20s and during middle age.
(C) Has a bimodal distribution in late adolescence and the mid-30s.
(D) Peaks at age 30 and declines.

27-32. A high school football player presents complaining of left third finger pain after injuring his hand during practice. You note the distal phalanx of the third digit is held in 40 degrees of flexion, and the patient is unable to extend it. Which of the following is TRUE regarding this injury?

(A) It is only known to occur after blunt trauma.

(B) It is rarely associated with avulsion fractures of the phalanx.

(C) If untreated, it may develop into a swan-neck deformity.

(D) Appropriate treatment includes immobilization in slight flexion.

27-33. A 60-year-old male smoker with a history of COPD, 30 packs/year history of tobacco use, and alcohol dependency presents with fever, cough, and anorexia. On chest x-ray, the patient has a pulmonary abscess. Which of the following is the most likely organism?

(A) *Klebsiella pneumoniae.*

(B) Pneumococci.

(C) *Staphylococcus aureus.*

(D) *Haemophilus influenzae.*

27-34. A 72-year-old male is brought to the ED by paramedics complaining of an acute onset of lower extremity weakness and numbness for several hours. He has a history of diabetes, peripheral vascular disease, and hypertension. On exam it is noted that the patient has no motor strength in his legs, has lost temperature sensation below his nipples, but has maintained vibratory sensation in his lower extremities. What is the most likely diagnosis?

(A) Cauda equina syndrome.

(B) Central cord syndrome.

(C) Anterior cord syndrome.

(D) Sciatica.

27-35. Which of the following conditions is LEAST likely to be associated with a coagulation factor deficiency?

(A) Intra-articular bleeding.

(B) Delayed bleeding.

(C) Retroperitoneal bleeding.

(D) Gingival bleeding.

27-36. Which of the following is a characteristic of primary hypothyroidism?

(A) Absence of pubic hair.

(B) Soft skin.

(C) Amenorrhea.

(D) Cardiomegaly.

27-37. Which of the following statements regarding the pneumonia severity score system is TRUE?

(A) The pneumonia severity index excludes nursing home patients.

(B) It incorporates medical and psychosocial barriers to accessing health care.

(C) Patients with a Class V pneumonia severity score have a 26% mortality rate.

(D) Immunosuppression is an important predictor in the model and, therefore, is heavily weighted in the scoring system.

27-38. Which of the following is NOT true of aortic dissection?

(A) Commonly presents with pulse discrepancies in the upper extremeties.

(B) May produce tamponade.

(C) May produce cerebrovascular symptoms.

(D) Commonly presents with a tearing pain.

27-39. Which of the following statements is TRUE regarding persistent pulmonary hypertension of the neonate (PPHN)?

(A) The cause of PPHN is usually genetic and should be foreseen prior to delivery.

(B) Placing a pulse oximetry probe on the right and left hands of the infant and comparing the readings can usually detect PPHN.

(C) Maintenance of high-normal blood pressure through the use of fluids and pressors slows ductal shunting.

(D) Heliox has revolutionized the management of PPHN and is considered first-line therapy.

27-40. Which of the following commonly prescribed medications DECREASES serum phenytoin levels?

(A) Warfarin.

(B) Azithromycin.

(C) Folic acid.

(D) Cimetidine.

27-41. What is the MOST sensitive test for carpal tunnel syndrome?

(A) Positive Finkelstein's test.

(B) Positive Phalen's sign.

(C) Positive Tinel's sign.

(D) Nocturnal hand tingling.

27-42. A patient taking clozapine (Clozaril) should have which of the following checked at regular intervals?

(A) Thyroid function tests.

(B) White blood cell count.

(C) Serum cortisol.

(D) Platelet count.

27-43. Which of the following medications should be considered as a first-line agent in a 68-year-old male presenting with a blood pressure of 70/45 mmHg after an ST-elevation myocardial infarction?

(A) Dopamine.

(B) Dobutamine.

(C) Norepinephrine.

(D) Milrinone.

27-44. Which of the following diagnostic tests is the MOST helpful in differentiating acute from chronic pancreatitis?

(A) Elevated amylase and lipase levels.

(B) Elevated bilirubin level.

(C) Pancreatic calcifications on abdominal plain radiographs.

(D) Pseudocyst on ultrasound.

27-45. Which of the following is NOT an appropriate treatment for acute mountain sickness?

(A) Acetazolamide 250 mg PO q8h.

(B) Dexamethasone 4 mg PO q6h.

(C) Oxygen 2–4 L/min.

(D) Nifedipine 20 mg q12h of extended release formulation.

27-46. A patient is being treated in the ED for hypercalcemia. Despite forced saline diuresis and brisk urine output over 2 hours, the patient's repeat serum calcium is 12 mg/dL. What is the next MOST appropriate action?

(A) Decrease the rate of saline infusion, and recheck calcium.

(B) Increase the rate of saline infusion, and recheck calcium.

(C) Correct hypokalemia or hypomagnesemia.

(D) Repeat the dose of furosemide.

27-47. A 30-year-old previously healthy man presents complaining of 2 hours of severe left flank pain and vomiting. What is the MOST appropriate course of action?

(A) Urine culture and broad-spectrum antibiotics for presumed pyelonephritis.

(B) No treatment until the diagnosis is confirmed by computed tomography.

(C) Urine dip and combination analgesia with opiates and nonsteroidal anti-inflammatory drugs (NSAIDs) for pain.

(D) Urine dip and antiemetics only.

27-48. What is the MOST common cause of a unilateral neck mass in patients older than 40 years?

(A) Reactive lymphadenopathy.

(B) Hodgkin's disease.

(C) Squamous cell carcinoma.

(D) Salivary gland infection.

27-49. Which of the following conditions does NOT cause cyanosis?

(A) Acquired deficiency of NADH methyl reductase.

(B) Methemoglobinemia.

(C) Sulfhemoglobinemia.

(D) Carboxyhemoglobinemia.

27-50. Which of the following can cause delirium as well as dementia?

(A) Brief episode of hypoglycemia.

(B) Urinary tract infection.

(C) Alcohol.

(D) Withdrawal from benzodiazepines.

27-51. A 70-year-old man with metastatic prostate cancer and a history of midthoracic back pain presents with 2 hours of bilateral lower extremity proximal weakness, which has acutely impaired his ability to ambulate. Strength testing reveals his lower extremities are able to overcome gravity but not direct resistance. Lower extremity and sacral reflexes (anal wink and bulbocavernosus reflex) are diminished. He has a band of hyperesthesia at the level of the umbilicus. The patient receives IV morphine sulfate and gets partial relief. Plain films reveal a compression fracture at T10. What is the next MOST appropriate action?

(A) Dexamethasone 10 mg IV and magnetic resonance imaging of the spine.

(B) Dexamethasone 4 mg IV and computed tomography without myelography.

(C) Dexamethasone 4 mg IV and computed tomography with myelography.

(D) Dexamethasone 4 mg IV and emergent radiation therapy.

27-52. An 85-year-old man from a nursing home presents to the ED with 1 day of fever and a productive cough. He is somewhat lethargic. Vital signs reveal a heart rate of 130 beats per minute, a blood pressure of 90/56 mmHg, and an oxygen saturation of 93% on room air. Chest radiograph reveals a left lower lobe infiltrate. Which of the follow-

ing is TRUE regarding the ED management of this patient?

(A) Sputum cultures should be obtained if *Legionella* species is suspected.

(B) Obtaining blood cultures in this patient has no demonstrated mortality benefit.

(C) According to the pneumonia severity index, this patient is Class III and therefore should be admitted only if vomiting.

(D) Early administration of antibiotics to elderly patients has been shown to reduce mortality.

27-53. Which of the following statements is TRUE regarding bedside ED ultrasound examination for an abdominal aortic aneurysm (AAA)?

(A) The minimum diameter for AAA is 5 cm.

(B) Ultrasound is not useful in detecting AAA rupture.

(C) Ultrasound is less accurate than CT in detecting AAA.

(D) Up to 90% of AAAs are superior to the renal arteries.

27-54. A 35-year-old male presents with a gunshot wound to his right chest. He has hemoptysis on presentation. Just after endotracheal intubation, he goes into cardiac arrest. What is the MOST likely diagnosis?

(A) Air embolism.

(B) Pericardial tamponade.

(C) Esophageal intubation.

(D) Massive hemothorax.

27-55. A 69-year-old male presents with an acute anteroseptal myocardial infarction, a systolic blood pressure of 130 mmHg, and a pulse rate of 90 beats per minute. His physical examination is significant for extreme tachypnea and inspiratory rales throughout all lung fields. What is this patient's approximate mortality?

(A) 5%.

(B) 10%.

(C) 40%.

(D) 80%.

27-56. Which of the following is the MOST accurate statement about salivary gland enlargement?

(A) Up to 80% of sialoliths occur in the parotid gland (Stensen's duct) because of its more viscous secretions.

(B) Mumps is most commonly caused by paramyxovirus and is more severe in children than adults.

(C) Suppurative parotitis is a potentially fatal bacterial infection.

(D) Suppurative parotitis should be treated by minimal stimulus to the gland.

27-57. Use of which of the following opioids has been associated with both seizures and cardiac disturbances such as interventricular conduction delays, heart block, and long QT interval?

(A) Tramadol.

(B) Meperidine.

(C) Hydromorphone.

(D) Propoxyphene.

27-58. A 25-year-old male sustained an amputation of his left forearm while using a table saw. Paramedics reported significant blood loss at the scene. He has a heart rate of 130 beats per minute and a systolic blood pressure of 90/40 mmHg. What class of hemorrhage is this patient in?

(A) Class I.

(B) Class II.

(C) Class III.

(D) Class IV.

27-59. A patient in the ED reports that she was beaten with fists by her husband 6 hours before presentation but denies any previ-ous injury or abuse. The patient has multiple ecchymoses and contusions on her face, arms, and back. Some of these wounds appear dark red or purple and have well-defined margins. Other wounds appear yellow or brown with margins that are fading. Is her exam consistent with her report of the injuries?

(A) No. Some of the wounds appear to be more than 48 hours old.

(B) Yes. The wounds look different because bruising patterns age differently on different areas of the body.

(C) Yes. The appearance of all the wounds is consistent with an assault within the last 24 hours.

(D) Maybe. It is not possible to determine the age of a contusion or ecchymosis by physical examination.

27-60. A 23-year-old female was found down by a family member. Her mother called 911 and initiated CPR. Per paramedic report, the patient was found unresponsive and pulse-less. The patient was successfully intu-bated, and peripheral access was obtained. The paramedics noted equal breath sounds with ventilation, but no heart sounds or pulses were present. The patient had multiple healing linear lacerations over both wrists consistent with self-inflicted injury. Cardiac monitor shows sinus tachycardia with a rate of 120 beats per minute, wide QRS complexes, and a prolonged QT inter-val. The patient received oxygenation by bag-valve mask, chest compressions, 2 L of normal saline, and 1 mg of intravenous epi-nephrine. What therapy is indicated next?

(A) Atropine.

(B) Calcium gluconate.

(C) Sodium bicarbonate.

(D) Amiodarone.

Post Test
Answers, Explanations, and References

27-1. **The answer is D.** Children younger than 2 years of age are a difficult population to evaluate for minor head injury and must be treated differently. They are more apt to have asymptomatic intracranial injury (especially when younger than 6 months). Skull fractures are a known risk factor for intracranial injury and increase their risk by 20-fold. Most skull fractures are also associated with a scalp hematoma, which turns out to be the most sensitive predictor of intracranial injury compared with other clinical signs. A large hematoma and a hematoma on the parietal scalp are especially high risk. Seizure and vomiting have both poor sensitivity and specificity. Depressed mental status is specific but not sensitive. **Reference:** Schutzman SA, Greenes DS. Pediatric minor head trauma. *Ann Emerg Med.* January 2001;37:65–74.

27-2. **The answer is B** (Chapter 247). Psoralens, such as 5-methoxypsoralen, are furocoumarins, as are compounds found in limes, figs, celery, and parsnips. Topical psoralens have been used to treat vitiligo. Ultraviolet light initiates the eruption, only at sites where the topical photosensitizer contacted the skin. Generally, the eruption resembles a localized sunburn. Furosemide (a sulfonamide diuretic), chlorpromazine, thiazides, tetracyclines, and sulfonamides all cause generalized photosensitivity eruptions in sun-exposed surfaces. Areas of the body less exposed to sunlight are spared, including the eyelid creases and submental anterior neck. Treatment involves topical corticosteroids, sun avoidance, and discon-

tinuation of the agent. Nickel exposure can cause a contact dermatitis but not a photosensitivity reaction.

27-3. **The answer is A** (Chapter 9). The risk of pneumothorax and air embolism is very high in patients with pulmonary primary blast injury. Air embolism from positive pressure ventilation is the most common cause of early death among immediate survivors. The risks and benefits of intubation of the blast patient need to be carefully considered. The risk of arterial air embolism may be lower with the patient placed on the left side slightly forward prone. Rapid infusion of crystalloid fluids may be harmful due to the risk of pulmonary contusion.

27-4. **The answer is C** (Chapter 156). Although there is controversy surrounding the use of orogastric lavage for toxic ingestions, it is still a useful tool for potentially life-threatening ingestions that present within 60 minutes. Liquids have more rapid absorption in the gastrointestinal (GI) tract and are thus more likely to have been fully absorbed by the time the patient arrives. Contraindications to orogastric lavage include nontoxic ingestions, caustic ingestions, ingestion of fragments too large to be removed via the lavage tube, lack of airway protection or control, and toxic ingestions that are more damaging to the lungs than the GI tract. Turpentine is a low-viscosity hydrocarbon that has potentially fatal pulmonary complications but relatively mild GI symptoms.

27-5. **The answer is A** (Chapter 150). *Yersinia* species is known to mimic acute appendicitis. *C. botulinum* can cause vomiting, diarrhea, diplopia, dysphagia, and descending muscle weakness. *V. cholerae* can cause severe watery diarrhea and vomiting. *S. aureus* causes sudden severe nausea, vomiting, and diarrhea.

27-6. **The answer is D** (Chapter 53). Hypertrophic cardiomyopathy is characterized by asymmetric left ventricular hypertophy resulting in impaired relaxation and left ventricular outflow tract (LVOT) obstruction. Maneuvers or pharmacologic agents that decrease preload (or increase chronotropy) will increase LVOT obstruction, thus worsening pulmonary congestion. The cornerstone of therapy is decreased chronotropy to allow for increased diastolic filling time of the noncompliant left ventricle. The end result is a decrease in both LVOT obstruction and pulmonary venous congestion. Nitroglycerin, nesiritide, and morphine will cause a reduction in preload and thus likely worsen the patient's clinical status.

27-7. **The answer is C** (Chapter 4). This preterm infant presents with all of the classical findings of respiratory distress syndrome (RDS). Premature infants with RDS present with progressively worsening retractions, tachypnea, and increasing oxygen requirements because their lungs are too immature to synthesize surfactant. This disease is characterized by ground glass opacities in the lung fields and prominent air bronchograms on chest x-ray. The infant's airway and breathing status needs to be immediately stabilized prior to making transport arrangements. CPAP reduces the collapse of the alveoli in patients with RDS and can be attempted through specialized nasal cannula in patients with mild respiratory distress. This infant is in severe respiratory distress, and thus this approach would be inappropriate. This premature infant should be immediately intubated and provided a PEEP of 4–5 cm H_2O, assuring that there is never a period of negative

pressure during passive exhalation. Surfactant should be administered only by specialists familiar with its complications; generally, this is not in the prevue of the emergency physician.

27-8. **The answer is C** (Chapter 50). New-onset right bundle branch block is most commonly seen in the setting of an anteroseptal myocardial infarction. It portends an increase in mortality as it often leads to complete heart block. First-degree atrioventricular block is usually benign. Sinus bradycardia is not associated with an increased mortality in the absence of hemodynamic instability and may be protective by reducing myocardial oxygen demand. Second-degree Mobitz type I (Wenckebach) is the most common form of second-degree atrioventricular block occurring in the setting of acute myocardial infarction. It rarely progresses to complete heart block.

27-9. **The answer is D** (Chapter 298). Forensic evidence collection should be obtained within 72 hours of the assault and is not performed if this time frame has elapsed. However, even if more than 72 hours have passed, the patient still requires a full history and physical examination, formal documentation of injuries, and prophylaxis for pregnancy and sexually transmitted disease. Documented genital injury rates due to sexual assault range from 9% to 45%. Colposcopy and toluidine blue staining techniques increase the rate of findings. Genital injury may be absent despite a sexual assault. A lack of findings does not imply consensual intercourse. General body trauma is documented in 45–67% of sexual assault cases.

27-10. **The answer is D** (Chapter 47). Acutely, such high-pressure injuries appear relatively innocuous but can rapidly evolve, producing significant morbidity. Aggressive management despite a paucity of early symptoms includes careful neurovascular and tendon function assessment, analgesia, antibiotics suitable for skin flora, tetanus prophylaxis, and Early hand surgeon consultation. Digital nerve blocks are contraindicated as they may contribute or potentiate increased intracompartmental pressures, resulting in worsening ischemic tissue injury.

27-11. **The answer is D** (Chapter 242). Avulsed primary teeth are never reimplanted. Severe luxations generally require extraction as they are a risk for aspiration and damage to the underlying teeth. Posttraumatic sequelae are variable and require close dental follow-up.

27-12. **The answer is C** (Chapter 303). The hallmark finding of a FAST exam is hemoperitoneum. However, both upper abdominal views of the FAST exam are capable of identifying hemothorax, where the anechoic fluid collection appears above the diaphragm. Studies have found ultrasound to be at least as sensitive as chest radiograph in identifying hemothorax. Ultrasound is poor at visualizing injuries to the retroperitoneum, pancreas, bowel, and diaphragm.

27-13. **The answer is A** (Chapter 60). Acute rejection is the most common form of rejection and occurs most commonly within the first 6 weeks after transplantation. Rejection often occurs as the immunosuppressive medications are weaned to maintenance levels. Hyperacute rejection from anti-HLA typing is very rare and occurs almost immediately after transplantation.

27-14. **The answer is D.** Physeal injuries are more common in boys largely because of relative skeletal immaturity as compared to girls, as well as an increased incidence of orthopedic injuries overall. Approximately 80% of physeal injuries will occur between the ages of 10 and 16 years. The distal radius is the most common site of injury. Both a Salter-Harris type I and type V injury may have an initial negative radiograph. **Reference:** Perron AD, Miller MD, Brady WJ. Orthopedic pitfalls in the ED: pediatric growth plate injuries. *Am J Emerg Med.* January 2002;20:50–54.

27-15. **The answer is A** (Chapter 231). The symptoms of intermittent, intense spinning, horizontal nystagmus, and fatigability suggest a peripheral rather than a central vertigo. Meniere's disease is the only choice caused by a peripheral rather than central etiology (due to increased endolymph production within the cochlea and labyrinth).

27-16. **The answer is B** (Chapter 243). A physical exam suggestive of peritonsillar abscess with negative needle aspiration requires computed tomography to rule out abscess despite the fact that the most common mimic is peritonsillar cellulitis. Needle aspiration will effectively treat 85% of abscesses, though incision and drainage are the cornerstone of treatment. The proper technique of needle aspiration is application of topical anesthesia followed by introduction of an 18-gauge needle halfway between the base of the uvula and the maxillary alveolar ridge, penetrating **no more than 1 cm** because the internal carotid artery lies just lateral and posterior to the tonsil. Peritonsillar abscess is the most frequently occurring deep space infection of the head and neck.

27-17. **The answer is C** (Chapter 76). Whereas the majority of foreign body ingestions pass spontaneously without any deleterious effects, when obstruction does occur, predictable and distinct anatomic regions are the more common sites. The pediatric population accounts for approximately 80% of all ingestions. The most common site is the cricopharyngeal narrowing corresponding to the cervical vertebral level C6. There are 4 other anatomic narrow esophageal regions: the thoracic inlet (T1), the aortic arch (T4), the tracheal bifurcation (T6), and the hiatal narrowing (T10–T11). In contrast, esophageal obstructions in adults tend to occur predominately in the distal esophagus.

27-18. **The answer is C** (Chapter 218). Thalassemia is associated with a normal RDW. The RDW is high in iron, vitamin B_{12}, and folate deficiency anemias.

27-19. **The answer is A** (Chapter 145). Acute or progressive congestive heart failure (CHF) occurs in up to 70% of patients with infective endocarditis (IE). The extracardiac manifestations of IE are usually the result of arterial embolization of fragments of the friable vegetation and are second to CHF as the leading cause of complications of IE.

27-20. **The answer is B** (Chapter 4). The glottis is in a more ventral position in infants than in older children; therefore, it is more difficult to visualize. This problem can be minimized by avoiding overextension of the neck and by applying gentle pressure to the cricoid. Because the distance between the thoracic inlet and the carina is extremely short in small children, the position of the endotracheal tube needs to be confirmed radiographically as soon as possible. The endotracheal tube is frequently inserted too deep.

27-21. **The answer is A** (Chapter 19). Etomidate is the induction agent of choice in adults for a wide range of clinical scenarios. It has extremely rapid onset and short duration, decreases intracranial pressure, and has a neutral cardiovascular profile. Although ketamine is recommended for status asthmaticus, this patient also has evidence of congestive heart failure on exam. Ischemic heart disease, a contraindication to the use of ketamine, may also be contributing significantly to this patient's clinical status. Additionally, ketamine often increases blood pressure, and this patient is already significantly hypertensive. The general drawbacks of midazolam (Versed) and fentanyl for induction include relatively poor reliability (especially fentanyl) and relatively longer duration of action compared to other agents. Etomidate is the best choice.

27-22. **The answer is C** (Chapter 249). Scabetic infestations in infants and young children tend to be more generalized and involve the scalp and face. Older children and adults usually have lesions in the finger web spaces and flexor creases of the wrists, axillae, breasts, buttocks, penis, and scrotum. The mite burrows in the stratum corneum, which is in the transition zone between the outer, horny layer and the basal layer of the epidermis. Hyperkeratotic areas are most affected. Crusted scabies produces hyperkeratotic crusting of the hands, feet, and scalp. Debilitated or immunocompromised patients are most susceptible and are at increased risk of secondary bacterial infection. Crusted scabies is highly contagious due to a high mite burden.

27-23. **The answer is B** (Chapter 110). Fibrocystic breast disease is a constellation of breast symptoms with the pathognomonic finding of breast cysts. Fibrocystic changes occur as a response of breast tissue to hormonal cycling. There is no galactorrhea with fibrocystic disease. A milky discharge can occur with pituitary adenoma, prolactinoma, and drugs.

27-24. **The answer is C** (Chapter 202). Low-voltage AC causes tetanic contraction of muscle and may cause victims to pull themselves closer to the source secondary to flexor muscle contraction. High-voltage AC is usually a single blast that throws the victim from the source. Lightning can cause a blast effect also and may result in blunt trauma. Lightning causes superficial burns and minor tissue damage, whereas high-voltage AC results in deep tissue destruction and may result in compartment syndrome, requiring fasciotomy. Lichtenburg figures are a fernlike pattern that is pathognomonic for a lightning strike.

27-25. **The answer is D** (Chapter 127). This infant is having bilious vomiting. Bilious vomiting in infants indicates small bowel obstruction (SBO) until proven otherwise and requires immediate surgical consultation. Malrotation with volvulus is the most common cause of SBO and bilious emesis in the newborn period and is a surgical emergency. If untreated, it can progress to infarction and gangrene of the entire small intestine. Vomiting in gastroenteritis is rarely bilious in infants and young children. Gastroesophageal reflux typically causes effortless, nonbilious regurgitation. Infants with pyloric stenosis present with progressive forceful ("projectile") emesis that is nonbilious.

27-26. **The answer is A** (Chapter 224). Fresh frozen plasma (FFP) is considered a safe method of reversing overcoagulation. A dose of FFP 10–15 mL/kg will raise the coagulation factor levels by about 30% in most adults. Alternatively in this case, coagulation factor concentrates would be ideal for reliable reversal; however, FFP is an excellent temporizing measure, since it is readily available. Cryoprecipitate has high levels of factors VIII, vWF, and fibrinogen but not the full spectrum of coagulation factors contained in FFP. Vitamin K should be given to this patient in intravenous form given his life-threatening intra-abdominal hemorrhage, but his most immediate need is FFP.

27-27. **The answer is C** (Chapter 266). Injury is the leading cause of death for Americans between the ages of 1 and 44 years and accounts for 25% of ED visits nationwide. Because they generally affect the young, injuries are responsible for more years of life lost before the age of 65 than all causes of cancer and heart disease combined. The emergency physician has a unique opportunity to provide information and education about preventing injuries because those injured frequently receive care in an ED.

27-28. **The answer is B** (Chapter 1). Offline medical control is the responsibility of the ambulance medical director. Three main components of offline medical control are (1) development of protocols, (2) development of medical accountability, and (3) development of ongoing education. Online medical control is the provision of direct medical communication to personnel in the field either by radio or phone communication.

27-29. **The answer is D** (Chapter 106). Hypertension during pregnancy is defined as a blood pressure of 140/90 mmHg or a 20 mmHg rise in systolic pressure or a 10 mmHg rise in diastolic pressure. A normal-appearing blood pressure may in fact be in the preeclamptic range for any given patient. This patient has preeclampsia with a normal-appearing blood pressure which progresses to eclampsia. Preeclampsia is the combination of hypertension and proteinuria with or without pathologic edema that develops in the second half of pregnancy. Eclampsia is the superimposition of seizures on preeclampsia. Management of eclampsia includes administration of magnesium sulfate and antihypertensive drugs as needed and delivery of the infant.

27-30. **The answer is C** (Chapter 81). Diverticulitis is a disease that is rare in the young, and its incidence increases steadily after age 40. Patients characteristically complain of left lower quadrant pain. However, the differential diagnosis of abdominal pain is vast and no sign, symptom, or physical exam finding is sensitive enough to make a diagnosis. A pelvic exam is recommended to help guide subsequent testing and imaging but is insufficient to diagnose diverticular disease. Abdominal CT is the diagnostic study of choice and allows the surrounding anatomy to be examined for alternative explanations. Barium enemas are useful to demonstrate colonic diverticula, but the inflammatory changes of diverticulitis are not well demonstrated. Vomiting can be part of the symptom complex in patients with diverticulitis; however, nasogastric tube placement is not necessary in the absence of vomiting.

27-31. **The answer is C** (Chapter 292). Panic disorder appears to have a bimodal distribution in late adolescence and the mid-30s.

27-32. **The answer is C** (Chapter 268). This patient has sustained an injury to zone I of the extensor tendon of the affected finger. This injury after blunt trauma is often referred to as "mallet finger" and is the most common tendon injury in athletes. This injury can also occur after sharp or penetrating trauma. If there is tendon-only rupture or only a small associated avulsion fracture of the distal phalanx, the joint can be splinted in slight hyperextension for 6–10 weeks with follow-up by a hand surgeon. Associated avulsion fractures of >25% of the articular surface of the phalanx may require operative repair and require prompt referral to a hand surgeon. Chronic untreated mallet finger may develop a swan-neck deformity. This deformity is caused when the lateral bands are displaced proximally and dorsally, resulting in increased extension forces on the PIP joint.

27-33. **The answer is A** (Chapter 63). *K. pneumoniae* can cause pulmonary abscesses and pneumonia which come on suddenly. This patient is an alcoholic with poor baseline pulmonary function and is at increased risk of aspiration and abscess formation. Pneumococci are a common etiology in community-acquired pneumonia, and although abscesses can develop with this type of infection, the relationship is not as strong as with *Klebsiella* species. *Staphylococcus* species is also associated with abscesses, but this patient's history of alcoholism makes *Klebsiella* more likely. *H. influenzae* is associated with pneumonia in elderly and debilitated populations, but abscesses are less commonly associated with this type of infection.

27-34. **The answer is C** (Chapter 256). This patient likely has anterior cord syndrome as a result of occlusion of the anterior spinal artery. It produces an injury to the cortical spinal tract and spinal thalamic tract while sparing the posterior columns. This injury results in bilateral loss of motor activity, pain, and temperature sensation at the level of the injury with preservation of vibration and position sense. Cauda equina syndrome involves the nerves below L1 and would not produce a loss of sensation at the nipple line. Central cord syndrome is

often a result of a hyperextension injury and typically affects the upper extremities more than the lower extremities. Sciatica is a peripheral nerve phenomenon and does not cause sensory symptoms in the chest.

27-35. **The answer is D** (Chapter 218). Gingival bleeding is characteristic of platelet disorders. Coagulation factor deficiencies are often associated with intra-articular, delayed, or retroperitoneal bleeding.

27-36. **The answer is D** (Chapter 216). The most common etiologies of hypothyroidism are primary thyroid failure due to autoimmune diseases, idiopathic causes, ablative therapy, and iodine deficiency. Features of primary hypothyroidism include previous thyroid operation, obesity, hypothermia, coarse voice, pubic hair unchanged, dry coarse skin, increased heart size, normal menses and lactation, normal sella turcica, increased thyroid-stimulating hormone (TSH), normal plasma cortisol, no response to TSH, and good response to levothyroxine without steroids.

27-37. **The answer is C.** Patients classified as Class V in the pneumonia severity index have a mortality rate of 26%. A characteristic patient in this category is the elderly patient with hypoxia and abnormal vital signs. These patients typically require admission to the intensive care unit. The pneumonia severity index does include nursing home patients. While clinically useful for risk-stratifying patients in the ED with pneumonia, the pneumonia severity index does have some limitations. For example, the model does not account for potential barriers the patient may have accessing health care or underlying immunosupression, 2 factors that are considered when discharging a patient with pneumonia from the ED. **Reference:** American College of Emergency Physicians. Clinical policy for the management and risk stratification of community acquired pneumonia in adults in the emergency department. *Ann Emerg Med.* July 2001;38:107–113.

27-38. **The answer is A** (Chapter 58). While pulse discrepancies can occur in aortic dissection, they are present in <20% of patients. Pulse discrepancies do not exist with abdominal aortic aneurysms. Tamponade and cerebrovascular symptoms are well-known complications of dissection. The pain of aortic dissection is a tearing or ripping type of pain that is abrupt in onset.

27-39. **The answer is C** (Chapter 4). The rapid transition from fetal to newborn circulation includes a precipitous drop in pulmonary vascular resistance concomitant with lung expansion, followed by increased pulmonary blood flow in the first few minutes of life and then a gradual closing of the ductus over the next 48 hours. Several common conditions can disrupt this progression, including infection, meconium aspiration, and asphyxiation. Genetic predisposition is not a factor. Infants with PPHN demonstrate labile oxygenation despite adequate ventilation due to right-to-left shunting of blood through the ductus arteriosus. This usually can be detected by placing a pulse oximetry probe on the right hand (preductal) and a second probe on a foot (postductal). If the preductal oximeter exceeds the postductal oximeter by more than 5% in a newborn, right-to-left shunting is present. Initial management of PPHN includes intubation, administration of 100% oxygen, and optimization of ventilation, sedation, and maintenance of high-normal blood pressures to slow ductal shunting. Nitric oxide, not Heliox, is a potent pulmonary vasodilator that has revolutionized the management of PPHN.

27-40. **The answer is C** (Chapters 157, 178). Any medication that either inhibits or enhances hepatic microsomal activity can increase or decrease (respectively) serum phenytoin levels. Drug interactions are a common scenario when a known seizure patient, who has been compliant on phenytoin, presents with a seizure and a decreased phenytoin level. Folic acid enhances phenytoin metabolism in the liver and thus can cause de-

creased serum phenytoin levels. Wafarin and cimetidine inhibit the cytochrome P450 system in the liver and thus cause increased levels of phenytoin. Azithromycin does not affect phenytoin metabolism significantly. Some other medications displace phenytoin from protein binding sites, resulting in a decreased serum level but an *increased* free phenytoin fraction. This group includes sulfonamides, valproic acid, and salicylates.

27-41. **The answer is B** (Chapter 285). Phalen's sign, flexing the wrist and holding for at least 1 minute, is the most sensitive (50%) and specific (75%). Finkelstein's test is ulnar deviation, used to detect de Quervain's tenosynovitis. Tinel's sign involves paresthesias when tapping over the median nerve.

27-42. **The answer is B** (Chapter 290). Patients taking clozapine risk agranulocytosis, and those presenting to the ED with fever or other infectious complaints should have a white blood cell count.

27-43. **The answer is A** (Chapter 33). Dopamine is a vasopressor for which dose-dependent response is expected. Patients in acute cardiogenic shock have decreased perfusion and, depending on the extent of myocardial dysfunction, may not respond adequately to fluid boluses. Hemodynamic monitoring in these patients is recommended. Dobutamine is a positive inotrope that can decrease blood pressure. The use of dobutamine should be carefully titrated. It is not prudent to use dobutamine in patients with hypotension (systolic <90 mmHg). Norepinephrine is a potent vasopressor with primarily α_1 agonist properties and can be used if the patient's hemodynamics are not responding to dopamine. Milrinone, a phosphodiesterase inhibitor, has been used for its inotropic properties, but because it can also lower blood pressure through its effects on systemic vascular resistance it should be used in concert with a vasopressor.

27-44. **The answer is C** (Chapter 87). Pancreatic calcifications on radiographs can be seen in up to 30% of patients with chronic pancreatitis and is considered pathognomonic for the disease. Amylase and lipase levels may be elevated or normal in chronic pancreatitis and thus are not useful in differentiating acute versus chronic disease. Compression of biliary ducts may lead to elevations of bilirubin and alkaline phosphatase in a small number of patients with chronic pancreatitis. Pseudocysts are complications of both acute and chronic pancreatitis.

27-45. **The answer is D** (Chapter 207). Acute mountain sickness (AMS) may be treated by descent to a lower altitude or acclimatization to the same altitude if the illness is mild. Oxygen promptly relieves most symptoms of AMS. Acetazolamide and dexamethasone are pharmacologic agents that may be used as an alternative to descent in mild to moderate cases and as adjunctive treatment to descent in severe AMS or high altitude cerebral edema (HACE). Nifedipine may be useful in treatment of high altitude pulmonary edema but is not effective for AMS or HACE.

27-46. **The answer is C** (Chapters 27, 225). Hypokalemia occurs in 50% of hypercalcemic cancer patients and may worsen with the use of furosemide during forced diuresis. Add potassium chloride (20–40 mEq) to each liter of normal saline to prevent or correct hypokalemia; recheck levels every 4 hours. Hypomagnesemia can also make hypercalcemia refractory to therapy. If renal failure is absent, give magnesium sulfate 1–2 g IV over 1–2 hours. Evaluate the hypercalcemic patient for hypokalemia and hypomagnesemia before adjusting the saline infusion rate. Monitor patients carefully to avoid fluid overload or congestive heart failure. Hemodialysis may be required for patients unable to tolerate a saline load or those with renal failure or severe mental status changes. Furosemide may be given every 2 hours.

27-47. **The answer is C** (Chapter 96). This patient has the classic presentation of renal colic. Pain medicine should not be withheld pending test results or definitive diagnosis. Effective analgesia for renal colic includes opiates in combination with NSAIDs. Antiemetics may also be given for nausea and vomiting but should not substitute for adequate analgesia. Urine culture and antibiotics targeted against gram-negative organisms are appropriate when there is evidence of infection such as fever or pyuria.

27-48. **The answer is C** (Chapter 243). In patients older than 40 years, 75% of neck masses are neoplastic. The most common cause of a unilateral neck mass is squamous cell carcinoma. Masses can be initially mobile and then fixed as the cancer invades surrounding tissue. Other tumors presenting unilaterally are neoplasms of the salivary gland and thyroid and lymphomas. They can become superinfected and present as abscesses.

27-49. **The answer is D** (Chapter 62). Carboxyhemoglobin represents hemoglobin tightly bound to carbon monoxide (CO) because of CO's 240-fold higher affinity for hemoglobin than oxygen. Clinically it does not appear as cyanosis, but cutaneously at high levels it may have a cherry-red appearance. Acquired deficiency of NADH methyl reductase is a genetic deficiency associated with methemoglobinemia whereby the iron molecule in heme is in the Fe^{3+} (ferric) state. Methemoglobinemia is a known cause of cyanosis that may manifest as low oxygen saturation (~85%) on pulse oximetry. Blood with high levels of methemoglobin has a brownish hue. Sulfhemoglobinemia can produce deep cyanosis at a very low level.

27-50. **The answer is C** (Chapters 229, 295). Alcohol can cause a transient delirium during the acute intoxication phase as well as in withdrawal. Prolonged use also can lead to dementia via a variety of mechanisms. Infection is frequently a cause of delirium in the elderly. Hypoglycemia not severe or prolonged enough to cause permanent brain injury can cause symptoms of delirium as can drug withdrawal.

27-51. **The answer is A** (Chapter 225). The patient has acute spinal cord compression. Magnetic resonance imaging (MRI) is the study of choice for visualization of the spinal cord and the vertebral fractures. If MRI is unavailable, or if the patient has an implanted ferromagnetic device (or intraocular foreign body), use computed tomography, with or without myelography. Patients with acute spinal cord compression require narcotic analgesia and a timely dose of corticosteroids, e.g., dexamethasone 10 mg IV. Emergent radiation therapy, surgical decompression, or both may preserve ambulatory function if the patient presented with paresis but not paraplegia.

27-52. **The answer is D.** Studies have revealed that the early administration of antibiotics does reduce the mortality of elderly patients. Obtaining blood cultures in elderly patients with pneumonia has also demonstrated a reduction in mortality. *Legionella* species is not detectable on a routine sputum culture. Based on his age and vital signs, this patient has a very risk of mortality and, according to the pneumonia severity scoring system, should be admitted, potentially to the intensive care unit, for intravenous antibiotics **Reference:** American College of Emergency Physicians. Clinical policy for the management and risk stratification of community acquired pneumonia in adults in the emergency department. *Ann Emerg Med.* July 2001;38:107–113.

27-53. **The answer is B.** While ultrasound is very accurate in measuring AAA size, it is often impossible to determine sonographically whether the AAA has ruptured, since rupture most often occurs into the retroperitoneal space. Ultrasound is not a good imaging tool to detect retroperitoneal pathology. The aorta normally tapers as it progresses distally, and any diameter >3 cm is abnormal. Approximately 90% of AAAs are located inferior to the renal arteries. Imaging this portion of the abdominal aorta can be difficult due to underlying small bowel gas. Although pressure on the transducer usually displaces intervening bowel gas, complete visualization is sometimes impossible. Such examinations are considered indeterminate. **Reference:** Melanson SW, Heller MB. Principles of emergency department sonography. Tintinalli JE et al (eds).: *Emergency Medicine, A Comprehensive Study Guide,* ed. 5, 2000, pp. 1972–1982.

27-54. **The answer is A** (Chapter 259). In patients with lung injury, systemic air embolism is a cause of cardiac arrest after endotracheal intubation. The diagnosis should be suspected in patients with penetrating chest wounds who have hemoptysis. Positive pressure ventilation can result in air being forced from an injured bronchus into an adjacent injured vessel, producing a venous air embolism. These patients develop hemodynamic compromise and dysrhythmias with intubation and ventilation. Pericardial tamponade is possible but less likely with a right-sided injury. Massive hemothorax may cause hemodynamic instability but would not necessarily be related to intubation. Esophageal intubation would result in hypoxia and bradycardia before cardiac arrest.

27-55. **The answer is C** (Chapter 50). The Killip Clinical Classification is useful in approximating subsequent mortality in patients with acute myocardial infarction. Patients are classified into 4 subsets based on clinical signs and symptoms, as shown in Table 27-1.

27-56. **The answer is C** (Chapter 240). Suppurative parotitis is a potentially fatal bacterial infection. In contrast to mumps, the onset is rapid and without prodrome. Erythema and warmth are present. It occurs in patients with compromised salivary flow and

TABLE 27-1. KILLIP CLINICAL CLASSIFICATION

Class	Symptoms	Mortality
I	No congestive heart failure	5%
II	Bibasilar rales and an S$_3$	15–20%
III	Frank pulmonary edema	40%
IV	Cardiogenic shock	80%

retrograde migration of bacteria into the duct. The treatment is antibiotics that work against staphylococci and anaerobic bacteria. Maneuvers that stimulate salivary flow, such as hydration, massage, applied heat, and stimulatory sialogues (e.g., lemon drops), are also recommended. Obstructive sialoliths require emergent head and neck surgical referral. Viral parotitis is usually benign in children but can be severe in adults. Treatment is supportive. Up to 80% of sialoliths occur in the submandibular gland (Wharton's duct) because of its more viscous secretions and uphill course.

27-57. **The answer is D** (Chapter 167). Propoxyphene (Darvon) has type 1A antiarrhythmic activity. Both propoxyphene and its metabolite, norpropoxyphene, block fast sodium channels in myocardial tissue, which can lead to conduction delays and ventricular dysrhythmias (e.g., bigeminy). Seizures can also occur in about 10% of patients; seizures can also occur with use of tramadol and meperidine.

27-58. **The answer is C** (Chapter 251). As detailed in Table 27-2, this patient has a class III hemorrhage. Although this is a somewhat arbitrary classification of hemorrhage, it helps differentiate the amount of blood loss

based on vital signs. Class III shock represents 30–40% blood loss and is manifested as hypotension and tachycardia.

27-59. **The answer is A** (Chapter 265). Although it is very difficult to place a concise time of incident to any bruise or contusion, wounds that are dark red or purple with well-defined margins have been inflicted within 48 hours of the exam. Bruises or contusions from injuries >48 hours old appear yellow or brown with margins that are fading. It is important to remember that bruising and contusions may have different appearances depending on the pigmentation of a patient's skin.

27-60. **The answer is C** (Chapter 11). This patient is presenting with pulseless electrical activity (PEA). PEA is defined by an organized rhythm without a pulse or signs of perfusion. More specifically, ventricular tachycardia (VT), ventricular fibrillation, and asystole are excluded from this definition. Patients with PEA rarely survive to hospital discharge. PEA can be caused by hypovolemia, hypoxia, cardiac tamponade, pulmonary embolism, tension, pneumothorax, massive myocardial infarction, or ingestion. Treatment of PEA should focus not only on following an algorithmic approach to treatment and appropriate pharmacologic intervention with epinephrine and atropine but also on identifying an underlying etiology. The physical finding of healing, self-inflicted wounds in conjunction with PEA should raise concern for a possible ingestion. Atropine is indicated in PEA only when a bradycardic rhythm is

TABLE 27-2. ESTIMATED FLUID AND BLOOD LOSSES BASED ON PATIENT'S INITIAL PRESENTATION

	Class I	Class II	Class III	Class IV
Blood loss (mL)*	Up to 750	750–1500	1500–2000	>2000
Blood loss (percent blood volume)	Up to 15	15–30	30–40	40
Pulse rate	<100	100–120	120–140	>140
Blood pressure	Normal	Normal	Decreased	Decreased
Pulse pressure (mmHg)	Normal or increased	Decreased	Decreased	Decreased

* Assumes a 70-kg patient with a preinjury circulating blood volume of 5 L.

present. Calcium would be indicated in the setting of calcium channel blocker toxicity, but the presence of tachycardia makes this ingestion unlikely. Amiodarone is indicated as a second-line agent for VT after epinephrine, but although these QRS complexes are wide, this rhythm is sinus in origin. This

patient ingested amitriptyline, a tricyclic antidepressant (TCA). A TCA should be suspected from the clinical presentation and the characteristic electrocardiogram findings. Sodium bicarbonate along with supportive care is the appropriate intervention.

Learning Objectives

After reviewing the above materials, individuals will be able to:

1. Determine their fund of knowledge with regard to acute and emergent care of system-based problems, including but not limited to cardiovascular emergencies, skin emergencies, gastrointestinal emergencies, and neurologic emergencies.

2. Determine their fund of knowledge with regard to non-system specific emergent care problems such as analgesia, anesthesia, and sedation; environmental emergencies; and toxicology.

3. Be able to assess their knowledge base of ABEM's 2004 and 2005 Continuous Certification Articles.

Directions

Please read before completing the answer sheet for *Emergency Medicine Examination & Board Review.*

1. Use a No. 2 pencil to complete the answer sheet. Erase all changes completely.
2. If you are an ACEP member, please record your 6-digit ACEP ID number (the 6 numbers that follow "A") in the area indicated on the answer sheet. Be sure to use "0" when appropriate. For example, if your member number is A98765, enter it as 098765. If you are not an ACEP member, you may leave this space blank.
3. Print your name and address and other contact information clearly in the area indicated on the answer sheet. ACEP will use this information to send you a report of your score and your CME certificate.
4. Complete the "Payment Information" section to indicate how you will pay the $20 CME processing fee. Please be sure to fill in all of the blanks; otherwise, ACEP will not be able to score your answer sheet. If you are paying by check, please make the check payable to ACEP (US funds only). If you are paying by credit or debit card, please be sure to provide all of the information requested and your signature.
5. Read each question and select one best answer. Indicate your answer by filling in the corresponding "bubble" on the answer sheet. Do not put marks outside the bubbles. Erase all changes completely.
6. Send your completed answer sheet to ACEP *unfolded* in a large, flat envelope, along with your payment or payment information.

Your completed answer sheet will be scored by ACEP. You will receive a report of your score and a CME certificate within 3 weeks after sending it to ACEP.

If you have questions about submitting your completed answer sheet, call ACEP Customer Service, 800-798-1822, touch 6, during business hours, or send an e-mail to customerservice@acep.org.

American College of Emergency Physicians®

▶ ACEP ID NUMBER

⓪	⓪	⓪	⓪	⓪	⓪
①	①	①	①	①	①
②	②	②	②	②	②
③	③	③	③	③	③
④	④	④	④	④	④
⑤	⑤	⑤	⑤	⑤	⑤
⑥	⑥	⑥	⑥	⑥	⑥
⑦	⑦	⑦	⑦	⑦	⑦
⑧	⑧	⑧	⑧	⑧	⑧
⑨	⑨	⑨	⑨	⑨	⑨

NAME_____

Mailing Address_____

City, State, Zip_____

Telephone Number_____

Payment Information

☐ My check for $20 is enclosed made payable to ACEP (US funds only).

☐ Please charge my: ☐ **VISA** ☐ **Master Card** ☐ **American Express**

Card #_____ Expiration Date_____

Name as it appears on card_____

Signature (required)_____

1 Ⓐ Ⓑ Ⓒ Ⓓ Ⓔ	16 Ⓐ Ⓑ Ⓒ Ⓓ Ⓔ	31 Ⓐ Ⓑ Ⓒ Ⓓ Ⓔ	46 Ⓐ Ⓑ Ⓒ Ⓓ Ⓔ
2 Ⓐ Ⓑ Ⓒ Ⓓ Ⓔ	17 Ⓐ Ⓑ Ⓒ Ⓓ Ⓔ	32 Ⓐ Ⓑ Ⓒ Ⓓ Ⓔ	47 Ⓐ Ⓑ Ⓒ Ⓓ Ⓔ
3 Ⓐ Ⓑ Ⓒ Ⓓ Ⓔ	18 Ⓐ Ⓑ Ⓒ Ⓓ Ⓔ	33 Ⓐ Ⓑ Ⓒ Ⓓ Ⓔ	48 Ⓐ Ⓑ Ⓒ Ⓓ Ⓔ
4 Ⓐ Ⓑ Ⓒ Ⓓ Ⓔ	19 Ⓐ Ⓑ Ⓒ Ⓓ Ⓔ	34 Ⓐ Ⓑ Ⓒ Ⓓ Ⓔ	49 Ⓐ Ⓑ Ⓒ Ⓓ Ⓔ
5 Ⓐ Ⓑ Ⓒ Ⓓ Ⓔ	20 Ⓐ Ⓑ Ⓒ Ⓓ Ⓔ	35 Ⓐ Ⓑ Ⓒ Ⓓ Ⓔ	50 Ⓐ Ⓑ Ⓒ Ⓓ Ⓔ
6 Ⓐ Ⓑ Ⓒ Ⓓ Ⓔ	21 Ⓐ Ⓑ Ⓒ Ⓓ Ⓔ	36 Ⓐ Ⓑ Ⓒ Ⓓ Ⓔ	51 Ⓐ Ⓑ Ⓒ Ⓓ Ⓔ
7 Ⓐ Ⓑ Ⓒ Ⓓ Ⓔ	22 Ⓐ Ⓑ Ⓒ Ⓓ Ⓔ	37 Ⓐ Ⓑ Ⓒ Ⓓ Ⓔ	52 Ⓐ Ⓑ Ⓒ Ⓓ Ⓔ
8 Ⓐ Ⓑ Ⓒ Ⓓ Ⓔ	23 Ⓐ Ⓑ Ⓒ Ⓓ Ⓔ	38 Ⓐ Ⓑ Ⓒ Ⓓ Ⓔ	53 Ⓐ Ⓑ Ⓒ Ⓓ Ⓔ
9 Ⓐ Ⓑ Ⓒ Ⓓ Ⓔ	24 Ⓐ Ⓑ Ⓒ Ⓓ Ⓔ	39 Ⓐ Ⓑ Ⓒ Ⓓ Ⓔ	54 Ⓐ Ⓑ Ⓒ Ⓓ Ⓔ
10 Ⓐ Ⓑ Ⓒ Ⓓ Ⓔ	25 Ⓐ Ⓑ Ⓒ Ⓓ Ⓔ	40 Ⓐ Ⓑ Ⓒ Ⓓ Ⓔ	55 Ⓐ Ⓑ Ⓒ Ⓓ Ⓔ
11 Ⓐ Ⓑ Ⓒ Ⓓ Ⓔ	26 Ⓐ Ⓑ Ⓒ Ⓓ Ⓔ	41 Ⓐ Ⓑ Ⓒ Ⓓ Ⓔ	56 Ⓐ Ⓑ Ⓒ Ⓓ Ⓔ
12 Ⓐ Ⓑ Ⓒ Ⓓ Ⓔ	27 Ⓐ Ⓑ Ⓒ Ⓓ Ⓔ	42 Ⓐ Ⓑ Ⓒ Ⓓ Ⓔ	57 Ⓐ Ⓑ Ⓒ Ⓓ Ⓔ
13 Ⓐ Ⓑ Ⓒ Ⓓ Ⓔ	28 Ⓐ Ⓑ Ⓒ Ⓓ Ⓔ	43 Ⓐ Ⓑ Ⓒ Ⓓ Ⓔ	58 Ⓐ Ⓑ Ⓒ Ⓓ Ⓔ
14 Ⓐ Ⓑ Ⓒ Ⓓ Ⓔ	29 Ⓐ Ⓑ Ⓒ Ⓓ Ⓔ	44 Ⓐ Ⓑ Ⓒ Ⓓ Ⓔ	59 Ⓐ Ⓑ Ⓒ Ⓓ Ⓔ
15 Ⓐ Ⓑ Ⓒ Ⓓ Ⓔ	30 Ⓐ Ⓑ Ⓒ Ⓓ Ⓔ	45 Ⓐ Ⓑ Ⓒ Ⓓ Ⓔ	60 Ⓐ Ⓑ Ⓒ Ⓓ Ⓔ

Please continue on the back. ➡

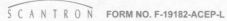

61. Please indicate your most important reason for completing the CME portion of *Emergency Medicine Examination & Board Review*.

- ☐ earn CME credit
- ☐ personal self-assessment, content review
- ☐ prepare for the emergency medicine board certification examination
- ☐ required by my group or residency program
- ☐ other

62. To what degree did *Emergency Medicine Examination & Board Review* meet that need?

- ☐ great degree
- ☐ moderate degree
- ☐ small degree
- ☐ not at all
- ☐ not sure

63. Are the stated learning objectives (page 307) met?

☐ yes   ☐ no   ☐ not sure

64. How helpful was the *Emergency Medicine Examination & Board Review* format?

- ☐ very helpful
- ☐ moderately helpful
- ☐ helpful
- ☐ not at all helpful
- ☐ not sure

65. Was the number of questions in the CME portion (60):

☐ just right   ☐ too many   ☐ too few

66. Was the level of content:

☐ just right   ☐ too advanced   ☐ too basic

67. To what degree will the CME portion of *Emergency Medicine Examination & Board Review* contribute to a change in your practice?

- ☐ great degree
- ☐ moderate degree
- ☐ small degree
- ☐ not at all
- ☐ not sure

68. Are you board certified in emergency medicine?

☐ yes   ☐ no

69. Do you plan to take the board certification examination in emergency medicine?

☐ yes   ☐ no

70. If yes to 69, when do you plan to take the certification examination?

- ☐ within 1 year
- ☐ within 2 years
- ☐ within 3 years
- ☐ within 4 years
- ☐ not sure

Place form in large envelope and mail to the address below. DO NOT FOLD.

CONFIDENTIAL
TEST MATERIALS ENCLOSED
Customer Service Department
American College of Emergency Physicians
PO BOX 619911
Dallas, TX 75261-9911